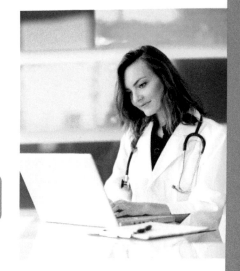

Biomarkers in Urologic Cancer

Editor

KEVIN R. LOUGHLIN

UROLOGIC CLINICS
OF NORTH AMERICA

www.urologic.theclinics.com

Consulting Editor
SAMIR S. TANEJA

February 2016 • Volume 43 • Number 1

ELSEVIER

1600 John F. Kennedy Boulevard • Suite 1800 • Philadelphia, Pennsylvania, 19103-2899

http://www.theclinics.com

UROLOGIC CLINICS OF NORTH AMERICA Volume 43, Number 1
February 2016 ISSN 0094-0143, ISBN-13: 978-0-323-41718-1

Editor: Kerry Holland
Developmental Editor: Alison Swety

Urologic Clinics of North America (ISSN 0094-0143) is published quarterly by Elsevier Inc., 360 Park Avenue South, New York, NY 10010-1710. Months of issue are February, May, August, and November. Business and Editorial Offices: 1600 John F. Kennedy Blvd., Suite 1800, Philadelphia, PA 19103-2899. Periodicals postage paid at New York, NY and additional mailing offices. Subscription prices are $360.00 per year (US individuals), $660.00 per year (US institutions), $415.00 per year (Canadian individuals), $825.00 per year (Canadian institutions), $515.00 per year (foreign individuals), and $825.00 per year (foreign institutions). Foreign air speed delivery is included in all *Clinics* subscription prices. All prices are subject to change without notice. **POSTMASTER:** Send address changes to *Urologic Clinics of North America*, Elsevier Health Sciences Division, Subscription Customer Service, 3251 Riverport Lane, Maryland Heights, MO 63043. **Customer Service: 1-800-654-2452 (US). From outside the United States, call 1-314-447-8871. Fax: 1-314-447-8029. E-mail: JournalsCustomerServiceusa@elsevier.com (for print support)** and **JournalsOnlineSupport-usa@elsevier.com (for online support)**.

Reprints. For copies of 100 or more, of articles in this publication, please contact the Commercial Reprints Department, Elsevier Inc., 360 Park Avenue South, New York, New York 10010-1710. Tel.: 212-633-3874; Fax: 212-633-3820; E-mail: reprints@elsevier.com.

Urologic Clinics of North America is covered in MEDLINE/PubMed (*Index Medicus*), *Excerpta Medica*, *Current Contents/Clinical Medicine*, *Science Citation Index*, and *ISI/BIOMED*.

PROGRAM OBJECTIVE
The goal of *Urologic Clinics of North America* is to keep practicing urologists and urology residents up to date with current clinical practice in urology by providing timely articles reviewing the state of the art in patient care.

TARGET AUDIENCE
Practicing urologists, urology residents and other health care professionals practicing in the discipline of urology.

LEARNING OBJECTIVES
Upon completion of this activity, participants will be able to:
1. Review the use of the Prostate Health Index and new genetic markers in diagnosing prostate cancer.
2. Discuss the current use of biomarkers for detection and targeted therapy of bladder cancer.
3. Recognize the diagnostic and prognostic roles of biomarkers in renal neoplasms and renal cell carcinomas.

ACCREDITATION
The Elsevier Office of Continuing Medical Education (EOCME) is accredited by the Accreditation Council for Continuing Medical Education (ACCME) to provide continuing medical education for physicians.

The EOCME designates this enduring material for a maximum of 15 *AMA PRA Category 1 Credit*(s)™. Physicians should claim only the credit commensurate with the extent of their participation in the activity.

All other health care professionals requesting continuing education credit for this enduring material will be issued a certificate of participation.

DISCLOSURE OF CONFLICTS OF INTEREST
The EOCME assesses conflict of interest with its instructors, faculty, planners, and other individuals who are in a position to control the content of CME activities. All relevant conflicts of interest that are identified are thoroughly vetted by EOCME for fair balance, scientific objectivity, and patient care recommendations. EOCME is committed to providing its learners with CME activities that promote improvements or quality in healthcare and not a specific proprietary business or a commercial interest.

The planning committee, staff, authors and editors listed below have identified no financial relationships or relationships to products or devices they or their spouse/life partner have with commercial interest related to the content of this CME activity:
Marc D. Bullock, MD, PhD; Kenneth M. Felsenstein, MS; Anjali Fortna; Mark L. Gonzalgo, MD, PhD; A. Ari Hakimi, MD; Kerry Holland; Robert T. Jones, BS; Li Yan Khor, MD; Julia Klap, MD; Laura-Maria Krabbe, MD; Lisa Krassnig, BSc; Indu Kumari; Michael S. Leapman, MD; Abbey Lepor; Hui Ling, MD, PhD; Yair Lotan, MD; Kevin R. Loughlin, MD, MBA; Ilaria Lucca, MD; Vitaly Margulis, MD; Romain Mathieu, MD; Aurélie Mbeutcha, MD; Michelle L. McDonald, MD; Maria C. Mir, MD, PhD; George J. Netto, MD; J. Kellogg Parsons, MD, MHS, FACS; Alan W. Partin, MD, PhD; Nicola Pavan, MD; Christian P. Pavlovich, MD; Martin Pichler, MD; Ashley E. Ross, MD, PhD; Shahrokh F. Shariat, MD; Lori J. Sokoll, PhD; Megan Suermann; Laura J. Tafe, MD; Puay Hoon Tan, MD, FRCPA; Dan Theodorescu, MD, PhD; Jeffrey J. Tosoian, MD, MPH; Camille Vuichoud, MD; Andrew G. Winer, MD.

The planning committee, staff, authors and editors listed below have identified financial relationships or relationships to products or devices they or their spouse/life partner have with commercial interest related to the content of this CME activity:
Peter R. Carroll, MD, MPH has research support from Genomic Health, Inc. and Myriad Genetics, Inc.
William J. Catalona, MD is on the speakers' bureau for Beckman Coulter, Inc. and Ohmx Corporation, is a consultant/advisor for, with research support from, Beckman Coulter, Inc.; deCODE Genetics; and Ohmx Corporation, and receives royalties/patents from Ohmx Corporation.
Stacy Loeb, MD, MSc is a consultant/advisor for Bayer AG.
Robert J. Motzer, MD is a consultant/advisor for Pfizer Inc. and Novartis AG, with research support from Pfizer Inc.; Novartis AG; Bristol-Myers Squibb Company; Genentech, Inc.; and GSK group of companies.
Samir S. Taneja, MD is a consultant/advisor for Bayer AG; Eigen Pharma LLC; GTx, Inc.; HealthTronics, Inc.; and Hitachi, Ltd.

UNAPPROVED/OFF-LABEL USE DISCLOSURE
The EOCME requires CME faculty to disclose to the participants:
1. When products or procedures being discussed are off-label, unlabelled, experimental, and/or investigational (not US Food and Drug Administration [FDA] approved); and
2. Any limitations on the information presented, such as data that are preliminary or that represent ongoing research, interim analyses, and/or unsupported opinions. Faculty may discuss information about pharmaceutical agents that is outside of FDA-approved labelling. This information is intended solely for CME and is not intended to promote off-label use of these medications. If you have any questions, contact the medical affairs department of the manufacturer for the most recent prescribing information.

TO ENROLL

To enroll in the *Urologic Clinics of North America* Continuing Medical Education program, call customer service at 1-800-654-2452 or sign up online at http://www.theclinics.com/home/cme. The CME program is available to subscribers for an additional annual fee of USD $270.

METHOD OF PARTICIPATION

In order to claim credit, participants must complete the following:
1. Complete enrolment as indicated above.
2. Read the activity.
3. Complete the CME Test and Evaluation. Participants must achieve a score of 70% on the test. All CME Tests and Evaluations must be completed online.

CME INQUIRIES/SPECIAL NEEDS

For all CME inquiries or special needs, please contact elsevierCME@elsevier.com.

Contributors

CONSULTING EDITOR

SAMIR S. TANEJA, MD
The James M. Neissa and Janet Riha Neissa
Professor of Urologic Oncology; Professor of
Urology and Radiology; Director, Division of
Urologic Oncology; Co-Director, Department
of Urology, Smilow Comprehensive Prostate
Cancer Center, NYU Langone Medical Center,
New York, New York

EDITOR

KEVIN R. LOUGHLIN, MD, MBA
Division of Urology, Brigham and Women's
Hospital, Harvard Medical School, Boston,
Massachusetts

AUTHORS

MARC D. BULLOCK, MD, PhD
Department of Experimental Therapeutics, The
University of Texas M.D. Anderson Cancer
Center, Houston, Texas

PETER R. CARROLL, MD, MPH
Professor and Chair, Department of Urology,
UCSF - Helen Diller Family Comprehensive
Cancer Center, University of California, San
Francisco, San Francisco, California

WILLIAM J. CATALONA, MD
Professor of Urology and Director of Clinical
Prostate Cancer Program, Department of
Urology, Northwestern Feinberg School of
Medicine, Chicago, Illinois

KENNETH M. FELSENSTEIN, MS
University of Colorado Cancer Center; Medical
Scientist Training Program, University of
Colorado School of Medicine, Aurora,
Colorado

MARK L. GONZALGO, MD, PhD
Department of Urology, Sylvester
Comprehensive Cancer Center, University of
Miami Miller School of Medicine, Miami, Florida

A. ARI HAKIMI, MD
Urology Service, Department of Surgery,
Memorial Sloan Kettering Cancer Center,
New York, New York

ROBERT T. JONES, BS
University of Colorado Cancer Center; Medical
Scientist Training Program, University of
Colorado School of Medicine, Aurora,
Colorado

LI YAN KHOR, MD
Department of Pathology, Singapore General
Hospital, Singapore, Singapore

JULIA KLAP, MD
Division of Urology, Brigham and Women's
Hospital, Harvard Medical School, Boston,
Massachusetts

LAURA-MARIA KRABBE, MD
Department of Urology, University of Texas
Southwestern Medical Center at Dallas, Dallas,
Texas; Resident, Department of Urology,
University of Muenster Medical Center,
Muenster, Germany

LISA KRASSNIG, BSc
Division of Oncology, Department of Internal Medicine, Medical University of Graz (MUG), Graz, Austria

MICHAEL S. LEAPMAN, MD
Clinical Fellow, Department of Urology, UCSF - Helen Diller Family Comprehensive Cancer Center, University of California, San Francisco, San Francisco, California

ABBEY LEPOR
Department of Urology, New York University, New York, New York

HUI LING, MD, PhD
Department of Experimental Therapeutics, The University of Texas M.D. Anderson Cancer Center, Houston, Texas

STACY LOEB, MD, MSc
Assistant Professor of Urology and Population Health, Department of Urology, New York University; Department of Population Health, Laura and Isaac Perlmutter Cancer Center, New York University, New York, New York

YAIR LOTAN, MD
Professor, Department of Urology, University of Texas Southwestern Medical Center, Dallas, Texas

KEVIN R. LOUGHLIN, MD, MBA
Division of Urology, Brigham and Women's Hospital, Harvard Medical School, Boston, Massachusetts

ILARIA LUCCA, MD
Department of Urology, Comprehensive Cancer Center, Vienna General Hospital, Medical University of Vienna, Vienna, Austria; Department of Urology, Centre Hospitalier Universitaire Vaudois, Lausanne, Switzerland

VITALY MARGULIS, MD
Associate Professor, Department of Urology, University of Texas Southwestern Medical Center at Dallas, Dallas, Texas

ROMAIN MATHIEU, MD
Department of Urology, Comprehensive Cancer Center, Vienna General Hospital, Medical University of Vienna, Vienna, Austria; Department of Urology, Rennes University Hospital, Rennes, France

AURÉLIE MBEUTCHA, MD
Department of Urology, Comprehensive Cancer Center, Vienna General Hospital, Medical University of Vienna, Vienna, Austria; Department of Urology, Hôpital Archet 2, Centre Hospitalier Universitaire de Nice, University of Nice Sophia-Antipolis, Nice, France

MICHELLE L. McDONALD, MD
Urology Resident Physician, Department of Urology, UC San Diego Health, San Diego, California

MARIA C. MIR, MD, PhD
Department of Urology, Sylvester Comprehensive Cancer Center, University of Miami Miller School of Medicine, Miami, Florida

ROBERT J. MOTZER, MD
Genitourinary Oncology Service, Division of Solid Tumor Oncology, Department of Medicine, Memorial Sloan Kettering Cancer Center, New York, New York

GEORGE J. NETTO, MD
Professor, Departments of Pathology, Oncology and Urology, The Johns Hopkins Medical Institutes, Baltimore, Maryland

J. KELLOGG PARSONS, MD, MHS, FACS
Associate Professor of Surgery, Department of Urology, UC San Diego Health, San Diego, California

ALAN W. PARTIN, MD, PhD
The James Buchanan Brady Urological Institute, Johns Hopkins Medical Institutions, Baltimore, Maryland

NICOLA PAVAN, MD
Department of Urology, Sylvester Comprehensive Cancer Center, University of Miami Miller School of Medicine, Miami, Florida; Department of Medical, Surgical and Health Science, Urology Clinic, University of Trieste, Trieste, Italy

CHRISTIAN P. PAVLOVICH, MD
The James Buchanan Brady Urological Institute, Johns Hopkins Medical Institutions, Baltimore, Maryland

MARTIN PICHLER, MD
Department of Experimental Therapeutics, The University of Texas M.D. Anderson Cancer Center, Houston, Texas; Division of Oncology, Department of Internal Medicine, Medical University of Graz (MUG), Graz, Austria

ASHLEY E. ROSS, MD, PhD
The James Buchanan Brady Urological Institute, Johns Hopkins Medical Institutions, Baltimore, Maryland

SHAHROKH F. SHARIAT, MD
Department of Urology, Comprehensive Cancer Center, Vienna General Hospital, Medical University of Vienna, Vienna, Austria; Adjunct Professor, Department of Urology, University of Texas Southwestern Medical Center, Dallas, Texas; Adjunct Professor of Urology and Medical Oncology, Department of Urology, Weill Cornell Medical College, Cornell University, New York, New York

LORI J. SOKOLL, PhD
Department of Pathology, Johns Hopkins Medical Institutions, Baltimore, Maryland

LAURA J. TAFE, MD
Assistant Professor, Department of Pathology, Dartmouth-Hitchcock Medical Center, Lebanon, New Hampshire; Geisel School of Medicine at Dartmouth, Hanover, New Hampshire

PUAY HOON TAN, MD, FRCPA
Department of Pathology, Singapore General Hospital; Departments of Anatomy and Pathology, Yong Loo Lin School of Medicine, National University of Singapore; Duke-NUS Graduate Medical School, Singapore, Singapore

DAN THEODORESCU, MD, PhD
Paul A Bunn Cancer Research Chair, Professor of Surgery and Pharmacology, Director, University of Colorado Cancer Center; Medical Scientist Training Program, University of Colorado School of Medicine, Aurora, Colorado

JEFFREY J. TOSOIAN, MD, MPH
The James Buchanan Brady Urological Institute, Johns Hopkins Medical Institutions, Baltimore, Maryland

CAMILLE VUICHOUD, MD
Division of Urology, Brigham and Women's Hospital, Harvard Medical School, Boston, Massachusetts

ANDREW G. WINER, MD
Urology Service, Department of Surgery, Memorial Sloan Kettering Cancer Center, New York, New York

Contents

cancer in appropriately counseled and selected men. Population-based screening with PSA decreases prostate cancer mortality; however, because of relatively poor specificity, PSA-based screening may also increase the detection of clinically insignificant cancers that would otherwise never require treatment. Use of newer biomarkers that increase the specificity for prostate cancer detection may aid in risk stratification and the appropriate identification of men for prostate biopsy. The authors review the 4-kallikrein panel and 4K probability score.

The standard of care for detection and surveillance of bladder cancer consists of cytology and cystoscopy, but both examinations suffer from many limitations, including issues related to accuracy, invasiveness, and cost. Several noninvasive methods for detection and surveillance of bladder cancer have been developed and urine-based biomarkers seem the most promising. This nonsystematic review critically analyzes the commercially available biomarkers and highlights some upcoming investigational biomarkers. To date, none of these biomarkers has sufficient validation to serve as a reliable alternative to cystoscopy.

Bladder cancer is a heterogeneous disease characterized by complex networks of molecular alterations and gene expression. This review summarizes some of the recent genomic studies that have further advanced the understanding of the pathways driving bladder cancer, highlighting several important biomarkers and potential targeted therapeutic strategies that are now in clinical trials. In addition, noninvasive techniques to evaluate biomarkers in patients' urine and serum for early detection and surveillance are discussed.

The clinical management of bladder cancer has seen little change over the last three decades and there is pressing need to identify more effective treatments for advanced disease. Low clinical use of neoadjuvant therapies stems from historical limitations in the ability to predict patients most likely to respond to combination chemotherapies. This article focuses on recent molecular and genetic studies, highlighting promising clinical trials and retrospective studies, and discusses emerging trials that use predictive biomarkers to match patients with therapies to which they are most likely to respond. The implementation of predictive genomic and molecular biomarkers will revolutionize urologic oncology and the clinical management of bladder cancer.

Incidental small renal masses identified on imaging are increasingly investigated via needle core or fine needle aspiration biopsies with limited material provided for rendering a diagnosis. Lesions with a prominent eosinophilic or oncocytic cell presence showing morphologic overlap between well-known eosinophilic neoplasms are challenging to diagnose. We review the range of known benign and malignant eosin-ophilic renal neoplasms and their immunoprofiles to elucidate a useful panel of stains that may assist the pathologist in making an accurate diagnosis.

Improved understanding of renal carcinoma disease biology has led to the discovery and approval of five novel therapies targeting specific molecules in the vascular endothelial growth factor (VEGF) biochemical pathway. Biomarker studies attempt-ing to predict response to VEGF-targeted therapies have largely focused on circu-lating proteins, tissue-based molecules, and germline polymorphisms. Thus far studies have yielded conflicting results that require prospective validation; therefore no definitive biomarker has yet been integrated into the clinician's armamentarium. However, early analyses featuring genomic biomarkers have generated promising findings. This article provides an overview of available biomarkers evaluated with respect to VEGF-targeted therapies in patients with advanced renal cell carcinoma.

The cell cycle is one of the most important regulatory mechanisms of cellular growth and proliferation. Dysregulation of this pathway is thought to be the first step in carci-nogenesis of renal cell carcinoma (RCC), important for tumor invasion and metasta-ses. Multiple different parts and regulators of the cell cycle are detectable via assays like immunohistochemistry and have been studied extensively. This review aims to provide an overview of current data regarding individual cell cycle and proliferative markers and their association with clinicopathologic parameters and their impact on prognosis for patients with RCC. Furthermore, the value of marker combinations is discussed.

Current use of testicular biomarkers for screening, diagnosis, and follow-up is re-viewed in the context of potential clinical utility of these tests. This information will be of value to clinicians to determine patient suitability for certain treatments and will also assist in reviewing current literature regarding potential biomarkers that may be used for testicular cancer.

Testicular cancer processes a unique and clear miRNA expression signature. This differentiates testicular cancer from most other cancer types, which are usually more ambiguous when assigning miRNA patterns. As such, testicular cancer may represent a unique cancer type in which miRNAs find their use as biomarkers for cancer diagnosis and prognosis, with a potential to surpass the current available markers usually with low sensitivity. In this review, we present literature findings on miRNAs associated with testicular cancer, and discuss their potential diagnostic and prognostic values, as well as their potential as indicators of drug response in patients with testicular cancer.

Camille Vuichoud, Julia Klap, and Kevin R. Loughlin

Penile cancer is a rare malignancy, which can be a source of devastating psychosexual distress because of its implication on sexual function and self-image. Current penile staging relies on invasive techniques and is often inaccurate. The authors review the promising biomarkers currently under investigation and their application to the staging and prognosis of penile cancer. Further development of such biomarkers provides the potential of improved clinical management of this disease.

UROLOGIC CLINICS OF NORTH AMERICA

THE CLINICS ARE AVAILABLE ONLINE!
Access your subscription at:
www.theclinics.com

Foreword
Biomarkers in Urologic Cancer

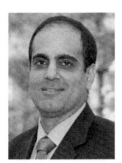

Samir S. Taneja, MD
Consulting Editor

This wonderful issue of *Urologic Clinics* explores the current and evolving role of biomarkers in urologic oncology. While we often consider biomarkers only in the clinical context of prostate cancer, the use of biomarkers extends beyond detection, and beyond the prostate in refining the art of cancer care.

Historically, the surgical treatment of urologic malignancies was limited by late detection. By the time tumors became symptomatic, it was too late for us to help the patient. In the case of prostate cancer, for which serum PSA has allowed early detection, and to a lesser extent kidney cancer, for which incidental detection on imaging has allowed earlier detection, survival following surgery has improved and the challenge of treatment has changed. We now must figure out if every tumor we find truly warrants therapy, and this question may be best answered through the use of alternate biomarkers capable of distinguishing indolent from aggressive disease. In the cases of bladder and testis, earlier detection has been achieved to some extent through patient education, but true screening tests do not exist. In these diseases, improvements in outcome have come solely through improvements in therapy. The application of aggressive therapy has resulted in improved outcomes for those destined to die of disease, but potentially leaves some overtreated (much as in the case of prostate cancer). As such, the role of biomarkers in these diseases may perhaps allow individualized treatment rather than avoidance of treatment. Biomarkers may allow us, in this case, to direct a treatment approach.

The use of biomarkers in clinical practice can range from screening, to refined detection in an at-risk population, to risk stratification following diagnosis, to prognostication following therapy. As such, an increasing knowledge of tumor biology and genetic heterogeneity will likely lead clinicians to adopt clinical paradigms that utilize sequences of biomarker assessments. It is critically important for urologists to remain at the forefront of the care of urologic malignancies, and knowledge of emerging biomarkers is an important component of this effort.

This issue, conceived and constructed by Dr Kevin R. Loughlin, provides a remarkably comprehensive overview of biomarkers in urologic oncology—not just for prostate cancer, but for all the cancers we treat. While the role of biomarkers may be more evident in some cancers than others (for now), their potential is truly pervasive. The authors have provided fantastic insight into individual biomarkers and the relationship of biomarkers to individual disease processes. I know the readers will be fascinated. We are deeply indebted to Dr Loughlin and all of the contributing authors for another truly outstanding issue of *Urologic Clinics*.

Samir S. Taneja, MD
Division of Urologic Oncology
Smilow Comprehensive Prostate Cancer Center
Department of Urology
NYU Langone Medical Center
150 East 32nd Street, Suite 200
New York, NY 10016, USA

E-mail address:
samir.taneja@nyumc.org

Urol Clin N Am 43 (2016) xv
http://dx.doi.org/10.1016/j.ucl.2015.10.002
0094-0143/16/$ – see front matter © 2016 Published by Elsevier Inc.

Preface
Biomarkers in Urologic Cancer

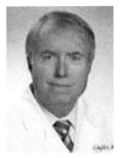

Kevin R. Loughlin, MD, MBA
Editor

This issue of *Urologic Clinics* is devoted to biomarkers. The writer Sean O'Casey said, "Nothing is so powerful as an idea whose time has come." That can be said of biomarkers today. As scientific research has continued to progress, we now have a better understanding of the molecular basis of the genesis and progression of many malignancies that can be applied to the clinical management of urologic cancers.

A Medline search of "biomarkers" by year demonstrates the inexorable increase of interest in the field. **Box 1** displays the number of biomarker citations by year. At the same time that the science has advanced, so too have the economic exigencies of health care delivery intensified. The continued development of biomarkers has the potential to enable us to deliver oncologic care more economically by perhaps decreasing the frequency of imaging and other diagnostic procedures.

Biomarkers have multiple potential clinical applications that include diagnosis, prognosis, selection of therapy, and surveillance. It is fair to say that the past decade and a half only represents the nascent stage of biomarker development. This issue of *Urologic Clinics* is intended to provide a state-of-the-art review of the current status of biomarker research in urologic oncology. I am delighted to have been able to assemble the work of these experts in a single volume and hope it is of value to the urologic community.

I dedicate this issue of *Urologic Clinics* to my three mentors—Ben Gittes, Scott McDougal, and Ed Mahoney.

Box 1
Medline citation-biomarker 2000–2014
2000-116
2001-189
2002-239
2003-298
2004-378
2005-562
2006-681
2007-932
2008-1103
2009-1385
2010-1753
2011-2017
2012-2555
2013-2634
2014-2988

Kevin R. Loughlin, MD, MBA
Division of Urology
Brigham and Women's Hospital
Harvard Medical School
75 Francis Street
Boston, MA 02115, USA

E-mail address:
kloughlin@partners.org

The Prostate Health Index
Its Utility in Prostate Cancer Detection

Abbey Lepor[a], William J. Catalona, MD[b],
Stacy Loeb, MD, MSc[a,c],*

KEYWORDS

- Prostate Health Index • Prostate cancer • Screening • Detection

KEY POINTS

- The Prostate Health Index (phi) is a mathematical formula that combines total, free, and proPSA.
- Phi is more specific for the detection of clinically significant prostate cancer than free and/or total PSA.
- Phi was approved by the US FDA in 2012 and is included in the National Comprehensive Cancer Network Guidelines for early prostate cancer detection.
- Increasing phi scores predict a greater risk of high-risk pathology and biochemical recurrence after radical prostatectomy.
- Phi performed at the initiation and during the course of active surveillance predicts subsequent biopsy reclassification.

INTRODUCTION

Prostate cancer is the second most common cause of cancer death in US men. In 2015, an estimated 220,800 men will be diagnosed with prostate cancer, and there will be 27,540 prostate cancer–related deaths. The prevalence of prostate cancer increases with age. Of all new prostate cancer cases, only 0.6% are diagnosed among men younger than 44 years of age, with most cases being diagnosed at ages 65 to 74.[1] Prostate cancer is generally asymptomatic until it has reached an advanced stage, a strong incentive to the widespread use of prostate-specific antigen (PSA)-based screening for early detection within the window of curability.

The goal of PSA screening is to test asymptomatic men and improve health outcomes by diagnosing the cancer at an early stage. A benefit of screening is a reduction in the proportion of advanced-stage cases at the time of diagnosis and a decrease in the prostate cancer–specific mortality rate. However, PSA screening has been controversial because of numerous limitations. Although higher PSA levels are a strong predictor of prostate cancer risk, the total PSA measurement is not specific for prostate cancer and is influenced by other factors, such as benign prostatic hyperplasia, prostatitis, and other benign conditions.[2] Consequently, many men undergo unnecessary biopsies leading to the overdetection of some indolent tumors.[3]

The Prostate Health Index (phi), approved by the US Food and Drug Administration (FDA) in June 2012, addresses many of the drawbacks associated with PSA screening. Its specificity is greater because phi is a combination of three different isoforms of PSA: total PSA, free PSA (fPSA), and [-2]

[a] Department of Urology, New York University, New York, NY, USA; [b] Department of Urology, Northwestern Feinberg School of Medicine, 675 North St. Clair Street, Galter Suite 20-150, Chicago, Illinois 60611, USA; [c] Department of Population Health, Laura and Isaac Perlmutter Cancer Center, New York University, New York, NY, USA
* Corresponding author. 550 1st Avenue VZ30, 6th Floor #612, New York, NY 10016.
E-mail address: stacyloeb@gmail.com

Urol Clin N Am 43 (2016) 1–6
http://dx.doi.org/10.1016/j.ucl.2015.08.001
0094-0143/16/$ – see front matter © 2016 Elsevier Inc. All rights reserved.

proPSA,[4] combined in the following mathematical formula: phi = ([-2]proPSA/fPSA) × $\sqrt{PSA}$. Phi is a simple blood test, but it outperforms any of its individual components for the identification of clinically significant prostate cancer.[5,6] This article reviews the major studies on phi in prostate cancer detection and risk stratification.

PHI AS A PREDICTOR OF BIOPSY OUTCOME

A large prospective multicenter study of phi was initiated in the United States from 2003 to 2009, and ultimately enrolled 892 men with total PSA levels of 2 to 10 ng/mL and findings that were not suspicious for cancer on digital rectal examination (DRE).[4] Participants underwent at least 10-core prostate biopsy, which was the initial biopsy in 79%, repeat biopsy in 18%, and unknown in 3%. The primary objective of the study was to compare the specificity of phi with percent free PSA (%fPSA) at 95% sensitivity for prostate cancer detection. The results showed that phi had significantly greater specificity at 95% sensitivity compared with %fPSA (16.0% vs 8.4%; P = .015). It was also more specific than total PSA. Similar patterns were observed at the 90%, 85%, and 80% sensitivity thresholds. On receiver operating characteristic analysis, phi outperformed both %fPSA (area under the curve [AUC], 0.703 vs 0.648; P = .004) and total PSA (AUC, 0.525). There was also a significant association between phi with the Gleason score on biopsy. Compared with the lowest phi category (scores of 0–24.9), men with the highest phi scores (>55) had a significantly higher risk of detecting any prostate cancer (relative risk, 4.7; 95% confidence interval [CI], 3.0–8.3), and Gleason score greater than or equal to seven disease on biopsy (relative risk, 1.61; 95% CI, 0.95–2.75).

A later study in this population examined the relationship of phi with clinically significant disease in greater detail.[6] Specifically, among 658 men from the prospective trial undergoing initial or repeat prostate biopsy for a PSA level of 4 to 10, phi was a more accurate predictor of clinically significant prostate cancer on biopsy using a variety of different criteria for significant disease. On receiver operating characteristic analysis, phi had a higher AUC for Gleason score greater than or equal to seven (0.707) and Epstein significant disease (0.698) compared with its components PSA (AUCs, 0.551 and 0.549), %fPSA (AUCs, 0.661 and 0.654), and p2PSA (AUCs, 0.661 and 0.654), respectively.

The specificity of phi for clinically significant prostate cancer also was evaluated in biopsy-naive men from the National Cancer Institute Early Detection Research Network Clinical Validation Center cohort.[5] Using Gleason score greater than or equal to seven disease on biopsy as the primary end point, de la Calle and colleagues[5] compared phi with its component parts. The first cohort included 561 men from Harvard with a mean PSA of 6.5 ng/mL and abnormal DRE in 23.7%. Of these men, 20.3% were found to have Gleason score greater than or equal to seven disease on biopsy, and phi had an AUC of 0.82 for high-grade disease. Using a cutoff of 24 as the criterion for biopsy would have avoided 41% of unnecessary biopsies among men without prostate cancer and 17% of overdiagnosed cases. These results were compared with a validation population including 395 men from two other US institutions (Weill Cornell Medical College and University of Michigan), with a mean PSA of 5.9 ng/mL and abnormal DRE in 10.6%. In this cohort, 30.9% had Gleason score greater than or equal to seven disease on biopsy, and the AUC for phi was 0.78. Using a phi cutoff of 24 as the criterion for biopsy would have avoided 36% of unnecessary biopsies among men without prostate cancer, and 24% of overdiagnosed indolent cancers in the validation population.

Phi also has been evaluated prospectively in several European populations. Guazzoni and colleagues[7] reported on 268 men with PSA levels of 2 to 10 ng/mL and negative DRE who were scheduled for extended prostate biopsy (18–22 cores) at a large academic center in Italy. The primary objective of the study was to compare phi with commonly used reference tests, including total PSA, %fPSA, and PSA density. Overall, 39.9% of the population was diagnosed with prostate cancer, and these men had a significantly higher phi (median, 44.3 vs 33.1; P<.001). At 90% specificity, phi had greater sensitivity (42.9%) than %fPSA (20.0%) or PSA density (26.5%). Predictive accuracy was higher for phi (AUC, 0.76) than for PSA density (61%), %fPSA (58%), and total PSA (53%). At 90% specificity, phi had greater sensitivity (42.9%) than %fPSA (20.0%) and PSA density (26.5%). The addition of phi to a multivariable model with age, prostate volume, and total and free PSA led to a significant gain in predictive accuracy (0.83 from 0.72; P<.001). Phi was also a significant independent predictor of high-grade disease.

Lazzeri and colleagues[8] subsequently reported on a large prospective evaluation of phi in 646 men age greater than 45 years from five European countries. All of the men in this study were undergoing initial prostate biopsy with at least 12 cores for a PSA level from 2 to 10 ng/mL with or without an abnormal DRE. The primary objective of the study was to compare the performance characteristics of phi with total and free PSA for prostate cancer detection; a secondary end point was to examine the relationship to Gleason score on biopsy. The 264 (40.1%) men diagnosed with prostate cancer had a significantly higher median phi compared with those with negative biopsy (48 vs 32; P<.001). On multivariable analysis including total, free, and %fPSA, the addition of phi led to a significant 6.4% and 7.5% gain in predictive accuracy for overall and Gleason score greater than or equal to seven prostate cancer on biopsy, respectively. At 90% sensitivity, use of phi would have avoided 100 unnecessary biopsies (15.5%) while missing only 1.1% of aggressive cancers (compared with 7.5% missed using %fPSA).

PHI AS A COMPONENT OF MULTIVARIABLE RISK STRATIFICATION

There has been a paradigm shift in prostate cancer decision-making from a one-size-fits-all approach using total PSA, as was done in the early 1990s, toward multivariable risk assessment taking into account individual patient characteristics. Such an approach is recommended by numerous contemporary clinical practice guidelines, such as the Melbourne Consensus statement.[9]

Given the substantial international evidence showing the superiority of phi over PSA, several tools have been created that combine phi with other clinical risk factors to aid in prostate biopsy decisions. Lughezzani and colleagues[10] reported a study including 729 men from a major tertiary referral center in Italy undergoing extended prostate biopsy (66.5% initial, 33.5% repeat). These men had total PSA levels ranging from 0.5 to 20 ng/mL, and 17.7% had a suspicious DRE. Similar to the previous studies, phi had superior predictive accuracy for biopsy outcome (AUC, 0.80) compared with %fPSA (AUC, 0.62) or total PSA (AUC, 0.51). The addition of phi to a multivariable model with age, prostate volume, DRE, and prostate biopsy history led to a statistically significant 7% gain in predictive accuracy. The authors created a nomogram combining these five variables, which had an AUC of 0.80. The nomogram was well calibrated for men at low to intermediate risk. Of note, using PSA or %fPSA in the nomogram instead of phi resulted in significantly inferior predictive accuracy (AUC, 0.73 and AUC, 0.75, respectively).

This nomogram was subsequently externally validated in an independent population of men undergoing initial or repeat greater than or equal to 12-core prostate biopsy at five European centers from the PRO-PSA Multicentric European Study Group described previously.[11] This study included 883 patients with total PSA levels of 0.5 to 20 ng/mL, of whom 17% had positive DRE. As in the previous study, phi on its own had a higher AUC (0.68) for prostate cancer detection than total or free PSA. The phi-based nomogram had an AUC of 0.75, was well-calibrated in men at low to intermediate risk, and showed the greatest net benefit on decision curve analysis.

Researchers from Ireland also created a multivariable phi-based nomogram to aid in prostate biopsy decisions.[12] From 2012 to 2014, 250 men aged greater than 40 years were referred to the Irish Rapid Access Clinic for prostate biopsy for an elevated age-specific PSA level or abnormal DRE. All of the men underwent at least 12-core prostate biopsy, and 112 (45%) had prostate cancer detected. Similar to other studies, phi as a stand-alone test had greater predictive accuracy for overall (AUC, 0.71) and particularly high-grade prostate cancer detection (AUC, 0.78) compared with total and free PSA. A multivariable model was then constructed including age, family history, DRE, previous negative biopsy, and either PSA or phi. The model using phi had an AUC of 0.77 for overall prostate cancer and 0.79 for high-grade disease, and significantly outperformed PSA-based model and the predictions of the online Prostate Cancer Prevention Trial risk calculator. In a subset of men undergoing repeat prostate biopsy, the phi-based multivariable model had an AUC of 0.85 for any prostate cancer, and 0.88 for Gleason score greater than or equal to seven disease. These studies confirm that phi is a useful addition to multivariable nomograms for initial or repeat biopsy to improve the accuracy of risk stratification. Phi has also been integrated into the Rotterdam Risk Calculator app, a multivariable prediction tool available on smartphones and tablets for easier use at the point of care.[13]

PHI AS A PREDICTOR OF TREATMENT OUTCOME

Numerous studies have demonstrated a significant relationship between phi and adverse tumor features at radical prostatectomy, including pathologic stage, grade, tumor volume, and composite outcome of clinically significant prostate cancer.[14-17] These studies include single-institution and prospective multicenter studies, and they corroborate the previously discussed evidence regarding the association of phi with more aggressive disease on biopsy among men with a full pathologic assessment.

More recently, Lughezzani and coworkers[18] took the next step by examining whether phi also predicts the risk of biochemical recurrence (BCR) in 313 men undergoing robotic-assisted radical prostatectomy from 2010 to 2011. The mean patient age was 64 years, and the median preoperative phi was 46. At a median follow-up of 28 months, 34 (10.9%) men had BCR. The 2-year BCR-free survival rate was 97.7% for men with a phi less than 82, versus 69.7% with phi levels greater than or equal to 82 (P<.001). Even among the 228 (72.8%) men with organ-confined disease, phi was able to significantly stratify the 2-year BCR-free survival (98.0% at phi <82 vs 83.3% at phi ≥82; P = .005). On multivariable analysis with age, prostate volume, clinical stage, and biopsy Gleason score, phi remained a significant independent predictor of BCR. Although the follow-up was relatively short, this study suggests that phi may be useful to help predict prognosis after radical prostatectomy.

Meanwhile, phi has been examined for a role in patient selection and monitoring during active surveillance, as was recently reviewed.[19] Hirama and colleagues[20] studied phi in a small group of men from a prospective active surveillance cohort in Japan. Inclusion criteria for the protocol were age 50 to 80, stage T1cN0M0, PSA less than or equal to 20 ng/mL, Gleason less than or equal to six in two or less cores with a maximum of 50% involvement. Among 67 men who underwent surveillance biopsy at 1 year, baseline phi was significantly higher among those who experienced reclassification (median, 60.3 vs 47.8; P = .01). On multivariable analysis with age, prostate volume, percentage of positive biopsy cores, and maximum core involvement, phi was the only significant independent predictor of biopsy reclassification (odds ratio, 3.7; 95% CI, 1.4–9.5; P = .008). Despite the limited sample size, this study suggests that the baseline phi score can help to further improve candidate selection for active surveillance.

Among US men in the Johns Hopkins active surveillance program, Tosoian and colleagues[21] examined baseline and longitudinal values of phi as a predictor of biopsy reclassification, defined as an increase in grade or volume of cancer on surveillance biopsy. In this program, men underwent PSA and DRE every 6 months with yearly surveillance biopsies. At a median follow-up of 4.3 years, 37.7% of men had biopsy reclassification, of which 16.7% were reclassified specifically by Gleason upgrading. In a multivariable Cox model adjusting for age, date, and PSA density, phi measurements at baseline predicted a significantly greater risk of biopsy reclassification. Similar results were reported in a separate model using longitudinal values of phi. Changes in phi over time were significantly greater among men with Gleason upgrading, and longitudinal measurements of phi had a concordance index of 0.82 for grade reclassification.

COMPARISON OF PHI WITH OTHER PROSTATE CANCER TESTS

Several other marker tests are commercially available for prostate biopsy decisions. One of these is the 4 kallikrein panel (4KScore), which is conceptually similar to phi by using a combination of PSA-based markers and has also been validated in US and European populations to improve specificity.[22] Both are presented as options in the 2015 National Comprehensive Cancer Network Guidelines.[23] Unlike phi, which is FDA approved, the 4KScore is a Clinical Laboratory Improvement Amendments–certified test and is currently more expensive in the United States. In a comparative study including 531 Swedish men, phi and the 4KScore had similar discrimination for overall prostate cancer detection (AUC, 0.704 vs 0.690) and high-grade disease (AUC, 0.711 vs 0.718).[24] Both markers provided significant incremental value compared with a model with PSA and age alone. A key difference between the tests in clinical practice is that the 4KScore uses a proprietary algorithm, which also incorporates the patient's age, DRE, and prior biopsy status along with the 4 kallikrein markers to estimate the number of men it is necessary to biopsy to find one high-grade prostate cancer. Although either test can be used for decisions about initial or repeat biopsy, the 4KScore does not yet have a validated algorithm for active surveillance.

The other major commercially available marker is urinary PCA3, which is FDA approved as an aid for repeat prostate biopsy decisions. Seisen and colleagues[25] recently evaluated 138 patients aged greater than 50 years undergoing initial prostate biopsy at an academic medical center in France for either a suspicious DRE and/or PSA level from 4 to 20 ng/mL. Overall, 44.9% of the cohort was found to have prostate cancer on biopsy. Men with prostate cancer had significantly higher median PCA3 and phi scores compared with those with negative biopsies and were significantly more likely to have a PCA3 greater than 35 (P = .01) and a phi greater than 40 (P = .01). On receiver operating characteristic analysis, PCA3 had better discrimination than phi for any prostate cancer (AUC, 0.71 vs 0.65; P = .03). However, the authors also compared the performance of these tests for identifying clinically significant prostate cancer (Gleason score ≥7, more than three positive cores, or >50% cancerous involvement of any core). They found that phi outperformed PCA3 for detection of clinically significant prostate cancer (AUC, 0.80 vs 0.55; P = .03). As a result, they concluded that phi should be used rather than PCA3 for decisions about initial biopsy to reduce overdiagnosis of insignificant disease.

Similarly, Cantiello and colleagues[15] compared the performance of phi and PCA3 to predict adverse pathologic features at radical prostatectomy. This study included 156 men undergoing radical prostatectomy at two institutions. In a multivariable model with age, body mass index, PSA, free PSA, prostate volume, biopsy Gleason score, percent of positive cores, and clinical stage, both phi and PCA3 led to a significant improvement in predictive accuracy for the end point of extracapsular tumor extension. However, only phi provided significant incremental predictive accuracy for the prediction of tumor volume greater than 0.5 mL, prostatectomy Gleason score greater than or equal to seven, seminal vesicle invasion, and a composite endpoint of clinically significant prostate cancer.

In a separate study, Cantiello and colleagues[16] specifically reported on 188 men who met the Prostate Cancer Research International Active Surveillance criteria and were given the option of active surveillance but chose radical prostatectomy instead, of which 96 men also met the more restrictive Epstein criteria for active surveillance. They found that although phi and PCA3 provided incremental predictive information regarding the presence of insignificant prostate cancer, phi was superior to PCA3.[16]

Finally, the use of MRI continues to increase for prostate cancer detection, treatment planning, and prognostication. Furthermore, recent studies have shown that MRI-ultrasound fusion biopsy can increase the detection of clinically significant prostate cancer.[26] Although high-quality multiparametric-based diagnostics are not yet universally available, within an imaging-based paradigm, phi can be used to guide the need for further assessment with MRI, because MRI is much more expensive and time-consuming than a simple blood test. It is likely that a combination of phi and MRI could further reduce the chances of finding low-grade insignificant tumors on biopsy. Together, these tests are promising noninvasive modalities that could be used in active surveillance protocols.

SUMMARY

Numerous large, prospective studies from geographically diverse regions have consistently demonstrated that phi is more specific for prostate cancer detection than existing standard reference tests of total and free PSA. It is a simple blood test that is approved by the US FDA and many other countries worldwide. Increasing phi scores predict a greater risk of clinically significant disease on biopsy and adverse prostatectomy outcomes. Phi outperforms PCA3 for identifying significant prostate cancer, and also predicts the risk of biopsy reclassification during active surveillance.

REFERENCES

1. Available at: www.seer.cancer.gov. Accessed August 1, 2015.
2. Nadler RB, Humphrey PA, Smith DS, et al. Effect of inflammation and benign prostatic hyperplasia on elevated serum prostate specific antigen levels. J Urol 1995;154(2 Pt 1):407–13.
3. Loeb S, Bjurlin MA, Nicholson J, et al. Overdiagnosis and overtreatment of prostate cancer. Eur Urol 2014; 65(6):1046–55.
4. Catalona WJ, Partin AW, Sanda MG, et al. A multicenter study of [-2] pro-prostate specific antigen combined with prostate specific antigen and free prostate specific antigen for prostate cancer detection in the 2.0 to 10.0 ng/ml prostate specific antigen range. J Urol 2011;185:1650–5.
5. de la Calle C, Patil D, Wei JT, et al. Multicenter evaluation of the Prostate Health Index (PHI) for detection of aggressive prostate cancer in biopsy-naive men. J Urol 2015;194(1):65–72.
6. Loeb S, Sanda MG, Broyles DL, et al. The Prostate Health Index selectively identifies clinically significant prostate cancer. J Urol 2015;193(4):1163–9.
7. Guazzoni G, Nava L, Lazzeri M, et al. Prostate-specific antigen (PSA) isoform p2PSA significantly improves the prediction of prostate cancer at initial extended prostate biopsies in patients with total PSA between 2.0 and 10 ng/ml: results of a prospective study in a clinical setting. Eur Urol 2011;60(2): 214–22.
8. Lazzeri M, Haese A, de la Taille A, et al. Serum isoform [-2]proPSA derivates (%p2PSA and phi) significantly improves the prediction of prostate cancer at initial biopsy in a tPSA range 2–10 ng/ml. A multicentric European Study. Eur Urol 2013;63(6):986–94.
9. Murphy DG, Ahlering T, Catalona WJ, et al. The Melbourne consensus statement on the early detection of prostate cancer. BJU Int 2014;113(2):186–8.
10. Lughezzani G, Lazzeri M, Larcher A, et al. Development and internal validation of a Prostate Health Index based nomogram for predicting prostate cancer at extended biopsy. J Urol 2012;188(4): 1144–50.
11. Lughezzani G, Lazzeri M, Haese A, et al. Multicenter European external validation of a prostate

health index-based nomogram for predicting prostate cancer at extended biopsy. Eur Urol 2014; 66(5):906–12.

12. Foley RW, Gorman L, Sharifi N, et al. Improving multivariable prostate cancer risk assessment using the Prostate Health Index. BJU Int 2015. [Epub ahead of print].

13. Roobol M, Salman J, Azevedo N. Abstract 857: the Rotterdam prostate cancer risk calculator: improved prediction with more relevant pre-biopsy information, now in the palm of your hand. Stockholm (Sweden): European Association of Urology; 2014.

14. Fossati N, Buffi NM, Haese A, et al. Preoperative prostate-specific antigen isoform p2PSA and its derivatives, %p2PSA and prostate health index, predict pathologic outcomes in patients undergoing radical prostatectomy for prostate cancer: results from a multicentric European prospective study. Eur Urol 2015;68(1):132–8.

15. Cantiello F, Russo GI, Ferro M, et al. Prognostic accuracy of Prostate Health Index and urinary prostate cancer antigen 3 in predicting pathologic features after radical prostatectomy. Urol Oncol 2015;33(4): 163.e15–23.

16. Cantiello F, Russo GI, Cicione A, et al. PHI and PCA3 improve the prognostic performance of PRIAS and Epstein criteria in predicting insignificant prostate cancer in men eligible for active surveillance. World J Urol 2015. [Epub ahead of print].

17. Guazzoni G, Lazzeri M, Nava L, et al. Preoperative prostate-specific antigen isoform p2PSA and its derivatives, %p2PSA and Prostate Health Index, predict pathologic outcomes in patients undergoing radical prostatectomy for prostate cancer. Eur Urol 2012;61(3):455–66.

18. Lughezzani G, Lazzeri M, Buffi NM, et al. Preoperative Prostate Health Index is an independent predictor of early biochemical recurrence after radical prostatectomy: results from a prospective single-center study. Urol Oncol 2015;33(8):337.e7–14.

19. Loeb S, Bruinsma SM, Nicholson J, et al. Active surveillance for prostate cancer: a systematic review of clinicopathologic variables and biomarkers for risk stratification. Eur Urol 2015;67(4):619–26.

20. Hirama H, Sugimoto M, Ito K, et al. The impact of baseline [-2]proPSA-related indices on the prediction of pathological reclassification at 1 year during active surveillance for low-risk prostate cancer: the Japanese multicenter study cohort. J Cancer Res Clin Oncol 2014;140(2):257–63.

21. Tosoian JJ, Loeb S, Feng Z, et al. Association of [-2] proPSA with biopsy reclassification during active surveillance for prostate cancer. J Urol 2012; 188(4):1131–6.

22. Parekh DJ, Punnen S, Sjoberg DD, et al. A multi-institutional prospective trial in the USA Confirms that the 4Kscore accurately identifies men with high-grade prostate cancer. Eur Urol 2015;68(3): 464–70.

23. NCCN clinical practice guidelines in oncology: prostate cancer early detection 2015. Available at: http://www.nccn.org/professionals/physician_gls/pdf/ prostate_detection.pdf. Accessed July 2, 2015.

24. Nordstrom T, Vickers A, Assel M, et al. Comparison between the four-kallikrein panel and prostate health index for predicting prostate cancer. Eur Urol 2015; 68(1):139–46.

25. Seisen T, Roupret M, Brault D, et al. Accuracy of the Prostate Health Index versus the urinary prostate cancer antigen 3 score to predict overall and significant prostate cancer at initial biopsy. Prostate 2015; 75(1):103–11.

26. Siddiqui MM, Rais-Bahrami S, Turkbey B, et al. Comparison of MR/ultrasound fusion-guided biopsy with ultrasound-guided biopsy for the diagnosis of prostate cancer. JAMA 2015;313(4):390–7.

New Genetic Markers for Prostate Cancer

Michael S. Leapman, MD, Peter R. Carroll, MD, MPH*

KEYWORDS

- Prostate cancer • Gene expression testing • Biomarker

KEY POINTS

- Novel gene-based tests have been developed to improve the prediction accuracy at various phases within the prostate cancer (PCa) disease course.
- Urine-based assays evaluating the expression levels of PCA3 and TMPRSS2:ERG aim to refine the selection for both initial and repeat prostate biopsy.
- Tissue-based gene expression tests have been developed to predict the occurrence of subsequent PCa events, including adverse characteristics, biochemical recurrence, metastatic progression, and PCa mortality.

INTRODUCTION

From a global perspective, prostate cancer (PCa) is a public health burden, detected in approximately 899,000 men per year and culminating in 258,000 deaths.[1] As a consequence of early detection resulting from population-based screening efforts, vigilant primary treatment, and the integration of advanced therapies in late-stage disease, declines in PCa mortality have been observed.[2] Yet as a highly prevalent malignancy with considerable variation in aggressiveness and an array of treatment options at numerous decision points within the disease, a need has emerged for increasingly reliable tools with which patients and clinicians alike may better predict the likelihood of downstream outcomes.[3] Such developments hold potential for informing accurate management decisions and may facilitate a reduction of both over and undertreatment. On this front, genomic characterization may provide prognostic insights not presently offered with other tools and may assist in the allocation of aggressive therapy for individuals at higher risk, while reducing the treatment burden for individuals less likely to derive benefit.

Conventional clinical stratification tools for PCa offer favorable delineation of downstream end points but will mistakenly categorize a proportion of patients as either higher or lower risk of experiencing a given disease-related event. Such information may be mobilized to assist in the selection of initial management strategy, increasingly rendered as initial definitive therapy or active surveillance.[4] Similarly, following primary treatment, prediction of the risk of failure is useful in determining the potential value of adjuvant or salvage therapy.[5,6] At initial diagnosis, instruments incorporating standard variables, including age, prostate-specific antigen (PSA), Gleason score, tumor volume, and clinical stage, estimate the risk of disease recurrence following treatment, including biochemical recurrence, metastases, and cancer-related mortality and overall mortality with accuracies in the range of 60% to 80%.[7–9] Uncertainty in these predictions may be a source of distress for patients and physicians and may also inform misdirected management decisions: intervention for biologically indolent tumors or, conversely, unwitting missed opportunities for intervention among those harboring insidious disease.[3,10]

Relevant disclosures: research funding support: Genomic Health Inc (Dr P.R. Carroll); none (Dr M.S. Leapman).
Department of Urology, UCSF - Helen Diller Family Comprehensive Cancer Center, University of California, San Francisco, San Francisco, CA, USA
* Corresponding author. 550 16th Street, Box 1695, San Francisco, CA 94143-1695.
E-mail address: peter.carroll@ucsf.edu

urologic.theclinics.com

On the heels of insights gained into PCa biology and technological advancements affording accessible, high throughput sequencing, assays have emerged that evaluate numerous junctures within the PCa disease process.[11] Spanning the prediagnostic, initial detection and posttreatment settings, this expanding battery of risk-stratification tools seek to offer improved assessment of outcome and gain widespread implementation in clinical practice. In light of the novelty of such developments, the authors aim to critically review the current body of tools that have appeared in recent years and the details of their supporting evidence and offer a contextualization of the pipeline of emerging tests under development.

PRINCIPLES OF DESIGN AND EVALUATION
Phases of Critical Evaluation

The evidence in support of an emerging prognostic genetic marker is established on several accounts addressing reproducibility and clinical performance. Although assays developed in a research setting may seem to offer reliability in measurement, it is essential that any gene-based test intended for widespread clinical utilization exhibit consistency when implemented in large-scale commercial laboratories.[12] Initial *analytical validation studies* address the ability of an assay to consistently measure a biological event within the context of a clinical laboratory. These studies yield valuable information relating to the variation that exists among clinical specimens.[13] Measures to ensure the quality and consistency of commercially available assays fall within the rubric of the Clinical Laboratory Improvement Amendment (CLIA) under the auspices of the Centers for Medicare and Medicaid Services. As the gene expression–based assays are increasingly used to inform clinical decision making, CLIA certification often serves as a valuable analytical standard.

Clinical validation studies address the relationship between the test and a prespecified clinical outcomes. In the setting of PCa, these end points may vary by tissue source and the proposed event of interest and often include adverse pathology, biochemical recurrence (BCR), progression to metastatic disease, or PCa-specific mortality (PCSM). Clinical validation studies often use archival, paraffin-embedded tissue of patients with extended follow. As a consequence, it is critical to note whether such retrospectively conceived studies adhere to blinded evaluation design, if specimens were collected in a standardized and prospective fashion, and whether the disease characteristics of the study populations remain valid today. Such measures act to minimize potential sources of bias in the selection of study subjects that may undermine the integrity and conclusions.[14]

TESTS BEFORE DIAGNOSIS

Most PCa detected worldwide are the result of biopsy undertaken in the setting of elevated PSA. Owing to the well-recognized deficiencies in specificity of PSA for the identification of clinically significant disease, a considerable number of individuals will undergo screening and biopsy to detect a single high-risk cancer.[15] The development of accurate markers to better select those at greatest risk for harboring significant and actionable disease would, therefore, be impactful for men who may be spared unneeded biopsy or detection of low-grade tumors in whom treatment may offer little benefit to longevity or quality of life. In this setting, new markers have emerged that seek to offer improvements in the selection for initial or repeat biopsy.

URINARY-BASED GENE EXPRESSION ASSAYS
Prostate Cancer Antigen 3

Urine-based PCa assays have been regarded as a promising means for the acquisition of markers highly specific to the prostate. Measurement of PCa antigen 3 (PCA3) mRNA expression within post–digital-rectal-examination (DRE) urine has been evaluated as a predictor for the detection of PCa on subsequent biopsy whereby higher expression levels have been associated with PCa discovery.[16] A urinary PCA3 assay (Progensa, Hologic Inc, Bedford, MA) is currently approved by the Food and Drug Administration in the setting of prior negative biopsy, where studies have examined the predictive value of using PCA3 thresholds for selecting men for repeat biopsy.[17] Among men with a minimum of one negative biopsy, the area under the receiver operating characteristic (AUROC) curve for PCa detection has ranged from 0.651 to 0.684; at a cutoff of 35, the sensitivity and specificity has ranged from 54% to 58% and 72% to 74%, respectively.[18–20] In the biopsy-naïve setting, PCA3 expression levels have been evaluated in several studies, including men with elevated PSA levels in the Rotterdam section of the European Randomized Study of Screening for Prostate Cancer (ERSPC) as well as in a prospective multicentered study of men using the Progensa PCA3 assay. At a PCA3 cutoff level of 35 or greater, the sensitivity and specificity for PCa detection ranged from 64% to 68% and 55.7% to 76.0%, respectively, and outperformed

PSA density, total PSA, and percentage of free PSA in predicting prostate biopsy outcomes.[21–23] With improvements in diagnostic sensitivity associated with lower PCA3 thresholds at the expense of diagnostic specificity, optimal PCA3 cutoff levels have yet to be established and may vary by clinical context.[24,25]

Transmembrane Protease Serine 2:ERG

Gene fusions of the transmembrane protease serine 2 (TMPRSS2) and the E26 transformation–specific ERG oncogene have been identified as a common event in human PCa development.[26] With high specificity for PCa, quantitative measurement of the TMPRSS2:ERG fusion in urine using quantitative nucleic acid amplification has been evaluated as a marker for disease in the prediagnosis setting. The addition of PCA3 to TMPRSS2:ERG measurement may to offer improved discrimination of disease on biopsy.[27,28] In a prospective multicentered study of men with clinical suspicion for PCa due to elevated PSA ($\geq$3 ng/mL), family history, or abnormal DRE, quantitative measurement of PCA3 and TMPRSS2:ERG was performed on first-catch urine before prostate biopsy. Using PCA3 thresholds of 25 and greater than 10 copies of TMPRSS2:ERG mRNA, investigators compared the prediction of biopsy outcome. Among 443 men, models composed of the ERSPC risk calculator with PCA3 and TMPRSS2:ERG demonstrated a predictive accuracy of 0.842, compared with 0.833 for the ERSPC calculator and PCA3 or 0.799 for the risk calculator alone. Of note, however, TMPRSS2:ERG but not PCA3 was associated with biopsy Gleason score and clinical tumor stage.[29] Emerging interest in evaluating the TMPRSS2:ERG and PCA3 markers with novel PSA isoforms to develop comprehensive panels with high predictive accuracy before diagnosis are currently under investigation.[30] From this perspective, efforts are warranted to identify parsimonious and cost-effective marker combinations likely to demonstrate clinical utility when implemented on a population level.

Urinary Exosomal Assays

Novel techniques have been developed to identify mRNA from urinary exosomes, nano-vesicles excreted from both malignant and benign cells.[31,32] The EXO106 score is derived from first-catch urine specimens to identify a gene signature with the intention of distinguishing high-grade (Gleason score 3 + 4 and greater) and low-grade disease. The emerging assay, which has not yet met clinical integration, examines expression levels of ERG and PCA3 mRNA using quantitative reverse transcription–polymerase chain reaction (RT-PCR) amplification techniques, normalized to the SPDEF gene and yields a score between 0 and 30, with higher scores reflecting a greater likelihood of high-grade PCa. The performance of the assay at a dichotomous threshold score of 10 was evaluated in 170 men with clinical suspicion of PCa undergoing prostate biopsy with PSA between 2 and 10 ng/mL in which the negative predictive value (NPV) and positive predictive value (PPV) for the detection of any PCa was 73.9% and 59.4%, respectively. For the detection of Gleason score 3 + 4 or greater disease, the NPV and PPV were 98.6% and 34.7%, respectively. When examined as a continuous (0–30) variable, the AUROC was 0.76 for distinguishing between Gleason 3 + 4 or greater versus Gleason 3 + 3 disease, which significantly outperformed the PCa prevention risk calculator (0.60).[33] A presumed advantage of the exosomal assay over other urinary markers is the lack of necessity for DRE before specimen acquisition. An important consideration that frames promising preliminary results, however, is the well-described limitation of conventional biopsy and a need for direct comparison with other biomarkers and imaging tools that aim to refine the performance of the initial biopsy.

TISSUE-BASED GENE EXPRESSION TESTS
ConfirmMDx (MDxHealth, Irvine, California)

Well-recognized poor NPV associated with standard template prostate biopsy for men with clinical suspicion of PCa results in a significant proportion of repeat biopsy among men with initially negative studies.[34] Investigational interest has emerged in identifying epigenetic signatures within histologically benign prostate tissue to select men at risk for harboring occult, undersampled PCa. Methylation of the GSTP1 has been extensively studied as a highly sensitive and specific diagnostic test for PCa, whereas other genes, including APC, RARbeta2, and RASSF1, may confer added diagnostic value in detecting epigenetic field effects within benign tissue.[35–37] The ConfirmMDx assay evaluates the status of methylation promoter genes GSTP1, APC, and RASSF1 in histologically negative prostate biopsy using multiplex methylation-specific PCR. The test has been studied for the ability to predict the subsequent detection of PCa at later biopsy and has demonstrated NPVs in the range of 88% to 90%.[38,39] As these validation studies regarded subsequent identification of PCa at any grade or volume, it is unclear whether similarly favorable performance characteristics will persist for the detection of high-grade disease. Moreover, the methylation assay has not been directly compared with other aforementioned tools that have similarly been evaluated in the setting of a prior negative biopsy. Furthermore, improvements in the performance of prostate biopsy including MRI guidance have culminated in improved detection yields for significant (high-grade) PCa; it is not known whether the NPV of the biopsy will be improved by such refined biopsy approaches.[40]

PROLARIS (MYRIAD GENETICS INC, SALT LAKE CITY, UTAH)

Cell cycle progression (CCP) genes serve to regulate the crucial functions relating to cellular replication. Therefore, aberrations in these genes are a key aspect of malignant transformation and the appearance of aggressive cancer phenotypes.[41] The Prolaris test calculates a 31-gene CCP score based on a list of genes refined from an initial group of 126 genes highly conserved among 96 commercially available formalin-fixed, paraffin-embedded (FFPE) prostate tumors. The signature includes the following: FOXM1, CDC20, CDKN3, CDC2, KIF11, KIAA0101, NUSAP1, CENPF, ASPM, BUB1B, RRM2, DLGAP5, BIRC5, KIF20A, PLK1, TOP2A, TK1, PBK, ASF1B, C18orf24, RAD54L, PTTG1, CDCA3, MCM10, PRC1, DTL, CEP55, RAD51, CENPM, CDCA8, and ORC6L. The selection of the final complement of genes was determined based on standardization of expression levels generating a reproducible profile of genes related to cellular proliferation.[42] The CCP score is calculated based on quantitative RT-PCR–based measurement of RNA expression, normalized to 15 housekeeping genes to account for sample quality and overall RNA yield. The result, reflecting aggregate CCP gene expression, is expressed as a positive (overexpression) or negative (underexpression) score normally distributed over a range of approximately −2 to +4.

At Initial Diagnosis: Prostate Biopsy Specimens

An appreciation of the outcome diversity of clinically localized PCa as well as the quality of life detriment associated with definitive PCa treatment via radical prostatectomy or radiation therapy has led to an interest in a strategy of active surveillance, a management strategy that involves the deferment of initial primary therapy and periodic monitoring to evaluate for disease progression.[43,44] Inadequacy of clinical models to definitively stratify patients by risk for adverse events during surveillance, including progression, disease reclassification, as well as distant occurrences, including BCR, is a source of early

diagnostic uncertainty.[3] From this vantage, tests derived from prostate biopsy specimens may improve the accuracy and experience at initial management planning.

The application of the Prolaris score to prostate biopsy specimens has been examined in the context of adverse clinical outcomes following treatment with both radiation therapy and radical prostatectomy. In a study of 141 men receiving external beam radiation therapy, alone or combined with androgen deprivation therapy between 1991 and 2006, the CCP score was evaluated for the ability to predict BCR by Phoenix criteria as well as PCSM.[45] On univariate analysis, CCP was significantly associated with BCR (hazard ratio [HR] 2.55, 95% confidence interval [CI] 1.43–4.55, $P = .002$). In a multivariate model incorporating PSA, Gleason score, hormonal therapy, and core positivity, the significance of CCP persisted (HR = 2.11, 95% CI 1.05–4.25, $P = .034$). In addition, the CCP score was also independently associated with PCSM ($P = .034$). The added value of the CCP score to a model composed of standard clinical variables and CCP yielded a concordance (c) index of 0.80 compared with 0.78 in a model consisting of clinical variables alone.

The CCP score derived from FFPE prostate biopsy specimens was also validated to predict adverse outcomes (BCR and metastasis) after radical prostatectomy (RP). Bishoff and colleagues[46] examined biopsy specimens from 3 biopsy cohorts: one simulated biopsy derived from formalin-fixed RP specimens and 2 actual diagnostic biopsy cohorts. Biopsy was performed by obtaining 0.6-mm tissue cores from 316 formalin-fixed RP specimens in patients with longitudinal follow-up at their institution, whereas diagnostic biopsies were used to identify 1 mm of tumor for RNA isolation in aggregate of 123 + 176 (299). This process yielded 582 evaluable patients with complete CCP scores and clinical data. Among the 299 patients who underwent diagnostic needle biopsies, increasing CCP score was a significant predictor of BCR and progression to metastatic disease in multivariate models incorporating Gleason score, though only 4 metastatic events occurred in this population. In the aggregate 582 patients, the CCP score was significantly predictive of BCR on multivariate analysis (HR = 1.47, 95% CI 1.23–1.76, $P.001$) as well as progression to metastatic disease (HR = 4.19, 95% CI 2.08–8.45, $P.001$).

Oncotype DX Genomic Prostate Score (Genomic Health, Redwood City, California)

The Oncotype DX Genomic Prostate Score (GPS) is a 17-gene RT-PCR assay derived from FFPE prostate biopsies. This gene signature assesses 12 cancer-related genes along 4 biological axes: (1) androgen response: AZGP1, KLK2, SRD5A2, and RAM13C; (2) cellular organization: FLNC, GSN, TPM2, and GSTM2; (3) proliferation: TPX2; (4) stromal response: BGN, COL1A1, and SFRP4. Five reference genes (ARF1, ATP5E, CLTC, GPS1, and PGK1), which exhibit little variability between patients and are used to normalize the cancer-related genes, adjust for differences that may affect expression levels, serving to control for analytical variability and RNA inputs.[47] Within these gene pathways, higher expression levels of stromal response and proliferation groups have been associated with an increased risk of clinical recurrence, whereas higher expression levels of androgen response and cellular organization were negatively associated with recurrence.

The assay involves tumor identification and microdissection by pathologists to exclude normal prostatic tissue and has demonstrated the ability to generate results with minimal tumor volumes. Expression levels are assessed by means of standard RNA extraction, fluorescence quantification, reverse transcription, and complementary DNA preamplification. A total of 1 mm of tumor was required for analysis, yielding evaluable scores in 96%; only 4% were excluded for insufficient RNA. At an RNA input of 10 ng, valid results were achieved in 99.5% of specimens. Quantitative PCR and genomic DNA detection occur for each gene assay; expression levels are calculated, and the GPS score is derived from an algorithm representing the 4 pathways.

Analysis of precision and reproducibility indicate the standard deviation for GPS is 1.86 units and reproducibility variation of 2.11 units. The commercial assay also provides a likelihood of favorable pathology derived from the GPS score and clinical risk as defined by high-grade (primary Gleason pattern 4) or non–organ-confined disease (pathologic stage at prostatectomy T3a or greater).[48]

Supporting Data: Prostate Biopsy Specimens

The 17-gene assay has recently been evaluated as a predictor for tumor aggressiveness in both a radical prostatectomy and prostate needle biopsy cohort. The initial discovery cohort consisted of 441 patients treated with radical prostatectomy at the Cleveland Clinic between 1987 and 2004 for clinically localized PCa: 110 patients with clinical recurrence matched 1:3 with recurrence-free controls. Of 727 genes evaluated in the prostatectomy group, 288 were identified, which were predictive of both primary and highest Gleason pattern in the RP specimen. Furthermore, in

multivariate analysis adjusting for clinical risk groups derived from PSA, Gleason score, and clinical stage, 198 genes (69%) remained significantly associated with clinical recurrence. A distinct biopsy cohort of FFPE tissue derived from 167 patients was performed involving quantitative RT-PCR analysis of 81 associated with adverse pathology at RP, of which 58 were identified that remained significantly associated with adverse pathology at surgery in the prostatectomy and biopsy studies. This number was further refined to 12 cancer-related genes that represented the most parsimonious gene sets from each representative pathway.

An independent clinical validation study was performed on a cohort of 395 patients with low to intermediate clinical risk (Cancer of the Prostate Risk Assessment score [CAPRA] <5 and biopsy Gleason pattern ≤3 + 4) who represented potential candidates for active surveillance who instead underwent immediate radical prostatectomy at the University of California, San Francisco between 1998 and 2011. The goal of the study was to determine whether or not analysis of the gene signature in the biopsy specimen could better predict those patients who were harboring high-risk disease (T3 or primary pattern 4 or 5 disease). Such a test may allow patients and physicians to consider active surveillance more confidently. Adjusting for biopsy Gleason score, the GPS score was a significant predictor of pathologic stage and grade ($P = .002$). The odds ratio (OR) for adverse pathology for each 20-point increase in GPS was 2.1 when adjusting for CAPRA score (95% CI 1.4–3.2) and 1.9 when adjusting for a de novo model incorporating age, PSA, clinical stage, and biopsy Gleason score (95% CI 1.2–2.8). Here, the area under the curve (AUC) for predicting favorable pathology was improved with GPS and CAPRA to 0.67 from CAPRA alone (0.63). Decision-curve analysis modeling indicated an improved net benefit for the CAPRA and GPS scores together compared with the CAPRA score alone.[48]

Further downstream clinical end points including biochemical or distant failure have also recently been evaluated in historical cohorts treated with radical prostatectomy. The GPS score was shown to predict BCR in a racially diverse cohort of 402 men treated surgically at 2 US military medical centers. In a model including limited adjustment for the National Comprehensive Cancer Network risk group, the HR per 20-unit GPS score was 2.73 (95% CI 1.84–3.96, P.01) and remained a predictor of time to recurrence within subgroups of race and other clinical and pathologic factors. In the same study, GPS per 20 units was also predictive of metastasis (OR 3.83, 95% CI 1.13–12.60, $P = .032$).[49] In a multivariate model adjusting for prostatectomy grade and stage, GPS was independently associated with clinical recurrence (HR 1.69, 95% CI 1.08–2.66, $P = .022$).

DECIPHER (GENOMEDX, VANCOUVER, BRITISH COLUMBIA)

The Decipher assay is a 22-gene genomic classifier (GC) evaluated as a prediction tool for adverse events following definitive treatment.[50] The marker set was developed using a nested case-control design from a cohort of patients treated with RP at the Mayo Clinic between 1987 and 2001 and stratified by outcomes (no evidence of disease, PSA recurrence without metastasis within 5 years, or clinical metastasis following BCR). A methodological distinction in the development of the Decipher assay is that genes included in the sequence high-density, transcriptosome-wide arrays evaluating coding and noncoding sequences reflecting approximately 1.4 million features. Further statistical refinement was used to identify robust features, and a random forest machine learning algorithm was used to integrate selected features into a classifier. Training and validation sets were derived from 545 samples, and the eventual GC was derived from 1.1 million RNA features on the microarray. The resulting markers include LASP1, IQGAP3, NFIB, S1PR4, THBS2, ANO7, PCDH7, MYBPC1, EPPK1, TSBP, PBX1, NUS AP1, ZWILCH, UBE2C, CAMK2N1, RABGAP1, PCAT-32, GLYATL1P4/PCAT-80, and TNFRSF19. In addition, clinical and pathologic variables were evaluated in logistic regression models to generate an integrated classifier model. The resulting score is generated on a 0 to 1 scale, with scores greater than 0.5 classified as high risk.

Following Definitive Treatment

The performance of the Decipher GC in the prediction of metastatic progression following RP was examined in a validation study of 256 men treated at the Mayo Clinic with adverse clinical and pathologic features. In this setting, the Decipher GC alone predicted metastasis after RP with an AUC of 0.79. Adjusting for clinical pathologic factors and adjuvant treatment, 10% increases in GC were independently associated with metastatic progression (HR 1.51, 95% CI 1.29–1.76, $P.001$).[51] The addition of the Decipher GC to the postsurgical Cancer of the Prostate Risk Assessment score (CAPRA-S) score has also been evaluated in the Mayo Clinic cohort to predict PCSM. Among 185 patients culled from the high-risk cohort, of which 28 patients

experienced death due to PCa, both CAPRA-S (c-index 0.75, 95% CI 0.55–0.84) and the GC (c-index 0.78, 95% CI 0.68–0.87) performed well; however, the addition of these tools together did not significantly improve the predictive ability.[52] In a multivariate model adjusting for GC, CAPRA-S, and adjuvant therapy, 0.1-unit incremental increases in the GC score were associated with a significant increase in PCSM (HR 1.81, 95% CI 1.48–2.25, $P.001$). When further stratified by GC category (≥ 0.6), the HR for PCSM was 11.26 (95% CI 4.69–30.37, $P<.001$); for CAPRA-S greater than 5, the HR was 2.36 (95% CI 1.06–5.68, $P = .04$).

The Decipher test was also evaluated in a cohort of 143 men who received either adjuvant or salvage post-RP radiotherapy in the setting of advanced-stage (pT3) or margin-positive PCa. Among 139 evaluable patients, the GC predicted freedom from BCR and metastasis, AUC 0.75 (95% CI 0.67–0.84) and 0.78 (95% CI 0.64–0.91) for BCR and distant metastasis (DM), respectively. When added to clinical models, the GC improved the AUC for the Stephenson nomogram from 0.70 to 0.78 (95% CI 0.69–0.86) for BCR and from 0.70 to 0.80 (95% CI 0.68–0.93) for DM, with a similar effect for CAPRA-S.[53] In addition, the Decipher test has also received evaluation as a prognostic tool for individuals experiencing BCR in which higher GC scores were significantly associated with progression to metastatic disease, independent of clinical or pathologic factors.[54–56]

SUMMARY

The development of new clinical tools to improve the accuracy and experience of PCa decision making holds considerable promise. From the prediagnostic setting, noninvasive assays may stem the burden of PSA-guided biopsy, whereas tissue-based tests may foster greater certainty in initial management or following primary treatment failure. Enthusiasm for technological innovation must be framed by the strength of supporting clinical evidence and an as-yet unevaluated phase of clinical and cost-effectiveness studies.

Future areas of investigation that have not yet met clinical application include the acquisition and analysis of circulating genomic information that may facilitate noninvasive testing. Because of their abundance in serum, small single-stranded miR-NAs that function in posttranscriptional regulation have been studied as independently predictive, readily accessible PCa biomarkers.[57] If validated, such markers may potentially facilitate liquid biopsy and obviate or reduce the necessity of repeated prostate biopsy during active surveillance.[58,59] Moreover, in light of the pace of biomarker discovery and validation studies within similar clinical domains, the authors anticipate the performance of larger cross-sectional validation studies that will better address the clinical utility of these emerging advancements.

REFERENCES

1. Center MM, Jemal A, Lortet-Tieulent J, et al. International variation in prostate cancer incidence and mortality rates. Eur Urol 2012;61(6):1079–92.

2. Schröder FH, Hugosson J, Roobol MJ, et al. Screening and prostate cancer mortality: results of the European Randomised Study of Screening for Prostate Cancer (ERSPC) at 13 years of follow-up. Lancet 2014;384(9959):2027–35.

3. Wang SY, Cowan JE, Cary KC, et al. Limited ability of existing nomograms to predict outcomes in men undergoing active surveillance for prostate cancer. BJU Int 2014;114(6b):E18–24.

4. Womble PR, Montie JE, Ye Z, et al. Contemporary use of initial active surveillance among men in Michigan with low-risk prostate cancer. Eur Urol 2015; 67(1):44–50.

5. Briganti A, Karnes RJ, Joniau S, et al. Prediction of outcome following early salvage radiotherapy among patients with biochemical recurrence after radical prostatectomy. Eur Urol 2014;66(3): 479–86.

6. Brockman JA, Alanee S, Vickers AJ, et al. Nomogram predicting prostate cancer-specific mortality for men with biochemical recurrence after radical prostatectomy. Eur Urol 2015;67(6):1160–7.

7. Cooperberg MR, Pasta DJ, Elkin EP, et al. The University of California, San Francisco Cancer of the Prostate Risk Assessment score: a straightforward and reliable preoperative predictor of disease recurrence after radical prostatectomy. J Urol 2005; 173(6):1938–42.

8. Korets R, Motamedinia P, Yeshchina O, et al. Accuracy of the Kattan nomogram across prostate cancer risk-groups. BJU Int 2011;108(1):56–60.

9. Greene KL, Meng MV, Elkin EP, et al. Validation of the Kattan preoperative nomogram for prostate cancer recurrence using a community based cohort: results from cancer of the prostate strategic urological research endeavor (capsure). J Urol 2004;171(6 Pt 1):2255–9.

10. Parker PA, Davis JW, Latini DM, et al. Relationship between illness uncertainty, anxiety, fear of progression and quality of life in men with favourable-risk prostate cancer undergoing active surveillance. BJU Int 2015. [Epub ahead of print].

11. Boutros PC, Fraser M, Harding NJ, et al. Spatial genomic heterogeneity within localized, multifocal prostate cancer. Nat Genet 2015;47(7):736–45.

12. McShane LM, Altman DG, Sauerbrei W, et al. Reporting recommendations for tumor marker prognostic studies. J Clin Oncol 2005;23(36):9067–72.

13. Simon R. Clinical trial designs for evaluating the medical utility of prognostic and predictive biomarkers in oncology. Per Med 2010;7(1):33–47.

14. Pepe MS, Feng Z, Janes H, et al. Pivotal evaluation of the accuracy of a biomarker used for classification or prediction: standards for study design. J Natl Cancer Inst 2008;100(20):1432–8.

15. Loeb S, Vonesh EF, Metter EJ, et al. What is the true number needed to screen and treat to save a life with prostate-specific antigen testing? J Clin Oncol 2011;29(4):464–7.

16. Fradet Y, Saad F, Aprikian A, et al. uPM3, a new molecular urine test for the detection of prostate cancer. Urology 2004;64(2):311–5 [discussion: 315–6].

17. Wei JT, Feng Z, Partin AW, et al. Can urinary PCA3 supplement PSA in the early detection of prostate cancer? J Clin Oncol 2014;32(36):4066–72.

18. Deras IL, Aubin SM, Blase A, et al. PCA3: a molecular urine assay for predicting prostate biopsy outcome. J Urol 2008;179(4):1587–92.

19. Marks LS, Fradet Y, Deras IL, et al. PCA3 molecular urine assay for prostate cancer in men undergoing repeat biopsy. Urology 2007;69(3):532–5.

20. Haese A, de la Taille A, van Poppel H, et al. Clinical utility of the PCA3 urine assay in European men scheduled for repeat biopsy. Eur Urol 2008;54(5): 1081–8.

21. de la Taille A, Irani J, Graefen M, et al. Clinical evaluation of the PCA3 assay in guiding initial biopsy decisions. J Urol 2011;185(6):2119–25.

22. Roobol MJ, Schroder FH, van Leeuwen P, et al. Performance of the prostate cancer antigen 3 (PCA3) gene and prostate-specific antigen in prescreened men: exploring the value of PCA3 for a first-line diagnostic test. Eur Urol 2010;58(4):475–81.

23. Auprich M, Chun FK, Ward JF, et al. Critical assessment of preoperative urinary prostate cancer antigen 3 on the accuracy of prostate cancer staging. Eur Urol 2011;59(1):96–105.

24. Nakanishi H, Groskopf J, Fritsche HA, et al. PCA3 molecular urine assay correlates with prostate cancer tumor volume: implication in selecting candidates for active surveillance. J Urol 2008;179(5): 1804–9 [discussion: 1809–10].

25. Ploussard G, Durand X, Xylinas E, et al. Prostate cancer antigen 3 score accurately predicts tumour volume and might help in selecting prostate cancer patients for active surveillance. Eur Urol 2011;59(3):422–9.

26. Tomlins SA, Rhodes DR, Perner S, et al. Recurrent fusion of TMPRSS2 and ETS transcription factor

genes in prostate cancer. Science 2005;310(5748): 644–8.

27. Salami SS, Schmidt F, Laxman B, et al. Combining urinary detection of TMPRSS2:ERG and PCA3 with serum PSA to predict diagnosis of prostate cancer. Urol Oncol 2013;31(5):566–71.

28. Hessels D, Smit FP, Verhaegh GW, et al. Detection of TMPRSS2-ERG fusion transcripts and prostate cancer antigen 3 in urinary sediments may improve diagnosis of prostate cancer. Clin Cancer Res 2007;13(17):5103–8.

29. Leyten GH, Hessels D, Jannink SA, et al. Prospective multicentre evaluation of PCA3 and TMPRSS2-ERG gene fusions as diagnostic and prognostic urinary biomarkers for prostate cancer. Eur Urol 2014;65(3):534–42.

30. Tallon L, Luangphakdy D, Ruffion A, et al. Comparative evaluation of urinary PCA3 and TMPRSS2: ERG scores and serum PHI in predicting prostate cancer aggressiveness. Int J Mol Sci 2014;15(8): 13299–316.

31. Duijvesz D, Luider T, Bangma CH, et al. Exosomes as biomarker treasure chests for prostate cancer. Eur Urol 2011;59(5):823–31.

32. Nilsson J, Skog J, Nordstrand A, et al. Prostate cancer-derived urine exosomes: a novel approach to biomarkers for prostate cancer. Br J Cancer 2009;100(10):1603–7.

33. Donovan MJ, Noerholm M, Bentink S, et al. A first catch, non-DRE urine exosome gene signature to predict Gleason 7 prostate cancer on an initial prostate needle biopsy. Abstract #45/Poster#C12 2015 Genitourinary Cancers Symposium. Orlando, FL, 2015.

34. Lughezzani G, Budaus L, Isbarn H, et al. Head-to-head comparison of the three most commonly used preoperative models for prediction of biochemical recurrence after radical prostatectomy. Eur Urol 2010;57(4):562–8.

35. Van Neste L, Herman JG, Otto G, et al. The epigenetic promise for prostate cancer diagnosis. Prostate 2012;72(11):1248–61.

36. Mehrotra J, Varde S, Wang H, et al. Quantitative, spatial resolution of the epigenetic field effect in prostate cancer. Prostate 2008;68(2):152–60.

37. Trock BJ, Brotzman MJ, Mangold LA, et al. Evaluation of GSTP1 and APC methylation as indicators for repeat biopsy in a high-risk cohort of men with negative initial prostate biopsies. BJU Int 2012; 110(1):56–62.

38. Stewart GD, Van Neste L, Delvenne P, et al. Clinical utility of an epigenetic assay to detect occult prostate cancer in histopathologically negative biopsies: results of the MATLOC study. J Urol 2013;189(3): 1110–6.

39. Partin AW, Van Neste L, Klein EA, et al. Clinical validation of an epigenetic assay to predict negative histopathological results in repeat prostate biopsies. J Urol 2014;192(4):1081–7.

40. Siddiqui MM, Rais-Bahrami S, Turkbey B, et al. Comparison of MR/ultrasound fusion-guided biopsy with ultrasound-guided biopsy for the diagnosis of prostate cancer. JAMA 2015;313(4):390–7.

41. Whitfield ML, Sherlock G, Saldanha AJ, et al. Identification of genes periodically expressed in the human cell cycle and their expression in tumors. Mol Biol Cell 2002;13(6):1977–2000.

42. Cuzick J, Swanson GP, Fisher G, et al. Prognostic value of an RNA expression signature derived from cell cycle proliferation genes in patients with prostate cancer: a retrospective study. Lancet Oncol 2011;12(3):245–55.

43. Cooperberg MR, Carroll PR, Klotz L. Active surveillance for prostate cancer: progress and promise. J Clin Oncol 2011;29(27):3669–76.

44. Dall'era MA, Cooperberg MR, Chan JM, et al. Active surveillance for early-stage prostate cancer: review of the current literature. Cancer 2008;112(8): 1650–9.

45. Freedland SJ, Gerber L, Reid J, et al. Prognostic utility of cell cycle progression score in men with prostate cancer after primary external beam radiation therapy. Int J Radiat Oncol Biol Phys 2013;86(5): 848–53.

46. Bishoff JT, Freedland SJ, Gerber L, et al. Prognostic utility of the cell cycle progression score generated from biopsy in men treated with prostatectomy. J Urol 2014;192(2):409–14.

47. Knezevic D, Goddard AD, Natraj N, et al. Analytical validation of the oncotype DX prostate cancer assay - a clinical RT-PCR assay optimized for prostate needle biopsies. BMC Genomics 2013;14:690.

48. Klein EA, Cooperberg MR, Magi-Galluzzi C, et al. A 17-gene assay to predict prostate cancer aggressiveness in the context of Gleason grade heterogeneity, tumor multifocality, and biopsy undersampling. Eur Urol 2014;66(3):550–60.

49. Cullen J, Rosner IL, Brand TC, et al. A biopsy-based 17-gene genomic prostate score predicts recurrence after radical prostatectomy and adverse surgical pathology in a racially diverse population of men with clinically low- and intermediate-risk prostate cancer. Eur Urol 2015;68(1):123–31.

50. Nakagawa T, Kollmeyer TM, Morlan BW, et al. A tissue biomarker panel predicting systemic progression after PSA recurrence post-definitive prostate cancer therapy. PLoS One 2008;3(5): e2318.

51. Karnes RJ, Bergstralh EJ, Davicioni E, et al. Validation of a genomic classifier that predicts metastasis following radical prostatectomy in an at risk patient population. J Urol 2013;190(6):2047–53.

52. Cooperberg MR, Davicioni E, Crisan A, et al. Combined value of validated clinical and genomic risk

stratification tools for predicting prostate cancer mortality in a high-risk prostatectomy cohort. Eur Urol 2015;67(2):326–33.

53. Den RB, Feng FY, Showalter TN, et al. Genomic prostate cancer classifier predicts biochemical failure and metastases in patients after postoperative radiation therapy. Int J Radiat Oncol Biol Phys 2014;89(5):1038–46.

54. Antonarakis ES, Feng Z, Trock BJ, et al. The natural history of metastatic progression in men with prostate-specific antigen recurrence after radical prostatectomy: long-term follow-up. BJU Int 2012; 109(1):32–9.

55. Simmons MN, Stephenson AJ, Klein EA. Natural history of biochemical recurrence after radical prostatectomy: risk assessment for secondary therapy. Eur Urol 2007;51(5):1175–84.

56. Ross AE, Feng FY, Ghadessi M, et al. A genomic classifier predicting metastatic disease progression in men with biochemical recurrence after prostatectomy. Prostate Cancer Prostatic Dis 2014;17(1):64–9.

57. Brett SI, Kim Y, Biggs CN, et al. Extracellular vesicles such as prostate cancer cell fragments as a fluid biopsy for prostate cancer. Prostate Cancer Prostatic Dis 2015;18(3):213–20.

58. Zheng Q, Peskoe SB, Ribas J, et al. Investigation of miR-21, miR-141, and miR-221 expression levels in prostate adenocarcinoma for associated risk of recurrence after radical prostatectomy. Prostate 2014;74(16):1655–62.

59. Wang SY, Shiboski S, Belair CD, et al. miR-19, miR-345, miR-519c-5p serum levels predict adverse pathology in prostate cancer patients eligible for active surveillance. PLoS One 2014;9(6):e98597.

Urinary Biomarkers for Prostate Cancer

Jeffrey J. Tosoian, MD, MPH[a],*, Ashley E. Ross, MD, PhD[a], Lori J. Sokoll, PhD[b],
Alan W. Partin, MD, PhD[a], Christian P. Pavlovich, MD[a]

KEYWORDS

- Prostate cancer • Biomarkers • Urine • PCA3 • TMPRSS2:ERG • GSTP1 • Metabolomics
- Microbiota

KEY POINTS

- Prostate cancer antigen 3 scores less than 20 seem to reliably rule out the presence of prostate cancer and particularly higher-risk prostate cancer on repeat biopsy; complementary RNA-based markers, such as TMPRSS2:ERG, and DNA-based markers, such as GSTP1, may improve its predictive ability and require additional study.
- In addition to traditional RNA, DNA, and protein-based biomarkers, emerging areas of study include urinary microRNA, long noncoding RNA, metabolomics, exosomes, and microbiota.
- Optimal diagnostic ability is generally obtained when novel biomarkers are added to multivariable models, including clinical factors, such as age, prostate-specific antigen, digital rectal examination, and prostate volume.
- Studies comparing urinary biomarkers with other promising diagnostic tools, such as the Prostate Health Index and multi-parametric MRI, are limited but will be necessary to optimize accurate and efficient disease detection.
- Future biomarker studies should consistently report the rate of biopsy avoidance with marker use, rate of undiagnosed cancers if biopsy omitted, performance associated with specific threshold values, marker utility in multivariable models, and marker utility in diagnosing high-grade cancers.

INTRODUCTION

Significant technological advances in analytical methods and a greater understanding of molecular carcinogenesis has paved the way toward a new era of disease detection.[1–3] Potential biomarkers of human disease range from whole-cell analysis to characterization of cell-free components, such as proteins and nucleic acids.[4] In addition to traditional serum or plasma, urine has been proposed as an easily obtained substrate for prostatic biomarkers.[5] To date, several urinary biomarkers have been identified and considered for use in prostate cancer (PCa), each with varying levels of evidence. In the subsequent review, the authors' primary aim is to assess the evidence basis and potential applications of urinary biomarkers for PCa.

Urine as a Substrate

Before considering the multitude of molecular isolation and quantification techniques, successful urine-based screening largely depends on the (1) the shedding of PCa cells or their components into urine and (2) successful acquisition, processing, and preservation of urine.[6] The technical aspects of such methodologies have been previously reviewed in significant detail.[4,5] Initial questions considering the type (single void vs 24 hour)

The authors report no relevant disclosures or conflicts of interest.
[a] The James Buchanan Brady Urological Institute, Department of Urology, Johns Hopkins Medical Institutions, 600 North Wolfe Street, Baltimore, MD 21287, USA; [b] Department of Pathology, Johns Hopkins Medical Institutions, 600 North Wolfe Street, Baltimore, MD 21287, USA
* Corresponding author. Department of Urology, Johns Hopkins Hospital, Marburg 144, 600 North Wolfe Street, Baltimore, MD 21287.
E-mail address: jt@jhmi.edu

Urol Clin N Am 43 (2016) 17–38
http://dx.doi.org/10.1016/j.ucl.2015.08.003
0094-0143/16/$ – see front matter © 2016 Elsevier Inc. All rights reserved.

and timing (first catch vs midstream) of specimen collection have come out largely in favor of single-void, first-catch sampling.[4–6] From a clinical perspective, evidence supports collection of urine after prostatic manipulation (eg, digital rectal examination [DRE]) to optimize assay yield, and collection after transrectal ultrasonography (TRUS)–guided biopsy has proven feasible as well.[7,8] The authors have herein considered potential urinary markers of PCa with attention to clinically relevant factors impacting their use.

RNA-BASED MARKERS
Prostate Cancer Antigen 3

From bench to bedside
In 1999, Bussemakers and colleagues[9] first described *Differential Display Code 3* as a potential urinary biomarker for PCa. Based on differential display analysis, the investigators described a messenger RNA that was highly overexpressed in 95% of PCa tissue and absent from benign prostate tissue and other tumor types. Subsequently identified as PCa antigen 3 (PCA3), it was further characterized as a noncoding RNA that was indeed highly specific for PCa.[10,11] Early quantification with quantitative real-time–polymerase chain reaction (qRT-PCR) demonstrated a 34-fold increased expression in malignant prostate tissue and high discriminative value as demonstrated by an area under the receiver operating characteristic curve (AUC) of 0.98 (**Table 1** includes key definitions in the assessment of diagnostic tests).[10] These findings were subsequently replicated by other investigators, and the introduction of a novel urinary assay to detect PCA3 helped lead its transition to the clinical setting.[11,12]

In 2006, a functional platform for clinical use was introduced as the Progensa PCA3 assay.[12] Urine specimens were obtained after attentive DRE (3 strokes to each prostate lobe), and PCA3 was quantified based on transcription-mediated

Table 1
Measures of diagnostic performance

	Meaning	Equation	Practical Use	Threshold[a]
Sn	Ability of a test to correctly identify those who have the disease	$\dfrac{TP}{TP + FN}$	Emphasize sensitivity when penalty for missing a case is high (eg, disease spreads easily and is fatal but can be successfully treated)	Decrease threshold = test is more sensitive, less specific
Sp	Ability of a test to correctly identify those who do not have the disease	$\dfrac{TN}{TN + FP}$	Emphasize specificity when consequence (eg, treatment, additional testing) of positive test is significant (eg, invasive, toxic)	Increase threshold = test is more specific, less sensitive
PPV[b]	The proportion of patients who truly *do* have the disease out of all who test positive	$\dfrac{TP}{TP + FP}$	If a person tests positive, what is the probability that he or she *does* have the disease?	—
NPV[b]	The proportion of patients who truly *do not* have the disease out of all who test negative	$\dfrac{TN}{TN + FN}$	If a person tests negative, what is the probability that he or she *does not* have the disease?	—
AUC[a]	The probability the test score of a randomly selected diseased subject will be greater than that of a randomly selected nondiseased subject	—	Quantifies the diagnostic performance of a test in terms of sensitivity and specificity independent of a specific threshold value	

Abbreviations: FN, false negatives; FP, false positives; NPV, negative predictive value; PPV, positive predictive value; Sn, sensitivity; Sp, specificity; TN, true negatives; TP, true positives.
  [a] Assuming higher/increased values are positive test results.
  [b] Predictive values (ie, positive predictive value, negative predictive value) are *not* fixed characteristics of a test; they depend on the disease prevalence in the tested population.
  Data from Refs.[209–212]

amplification and hybridization. Using prostate-specific antigen (PSA) transcripts to control for RNA quality and confirm the presence of nuclear material, PCA3 scores were generated as a simple PCA3 to PSA ratio. Promising data emerged suggesting that PCA3 may be superior to PSA in the diagnostic setting.[13,14] Deras and colleagues[13] demonstrated univariable AUC of 0.69 for PCA3 as compared with 0.55 for PSA. In a multivariable model with other clinical factors, PCA3 conferred an AUC up to 0.75. Furthermore, PCA3 was shown to be independent of age, prostate volume, and PSA.[14] Follow-up studies also suggested a role for PCA3 in men with previous negative biopsies.[15,16] In this population, Marks and colleagues[15] reported an AUC of 0.68 for PCA3 as compared with 0.52 for PSA. Importantly, reports of PCA3 have consistently yielded informative rates ranging from 94% to 99%.[7,12,15]

Repeat biopsy: diagnosis

Based on these findings and others, PCA3 was approved by the Food and Drug Administration in 2012 for use in men with a previous negative biopsy.[15–18] Although multiple studies demonstrated improved diagnostic accuracy compared with PSA, the optimal threshold for clinical use was the focus of further investigation. Eleven studies of moderate to high quality were included in a 2014 meta-analysis from Luo and colleagues.[19] The investigators examined performance characteristics using PCA3 threshold values of 20 and 35. Based on a threshold score of 20, sensitivity and specificity measured up to 93% and 64%, respectively. High sensitivity and negative predictive values (NPVs) approaching 90% across multiple populations (ie, predictive values are not inherent to diagnostic tests but also vary with disease prevalence in the study population; see **Table 1**) suggested potential use for excluding PCa in men who tested negative. The performance characteristics of PCA3 across multiple studies using threshold scores of 20 and 35 are listed in **Table 2**.[19]

Based on their findings, Luo and colleagues concluded that a cutoff score of 20 was superior to 35 in the repeat biopsy setting. As others had observed,[20] the investigators reported that use of PCA3 could reduce unnecessary repeat biopsies by more than 50% in some settings. Similar results were replicated in prospective multicenter cohorts of Italian and American men.[21,22] In the repeat biopsy cohort of the National Cancer Institute Early Detection Research Network validation trial, Wei and colleagues[22] confirmed that PCA3 scores below a threshold of 20 were associated with a very low rate of high-grade cancers; this finding was not observed, however, in men undergoing initial biopsy. In addition to corroborating previous findings in the repeat biopsy population, the study by Wei and colleagues[22] added to the growing literature aiming to clarify the prognostic role of PCA3.

The contemporary era

Studies of PCA3 since 2012 generally varied from the previous era in 3 ways.[23] First, PCA3 was more frequently assessed in the setting of initial biopsy.

Table 2
Performance characteristics of PCA3 with threshold scores 20 and 35 in men who underwent repeat biopsy

Study, Year	N	Threshold PCA3 = 20				Threshold PCA3 = 35			
		Sn (%)	Sp (%)	PPV (%)	NPV (%)	Sn (%)	Sp (%)	PPV (%)	NPV (%)
Wei et al,[22] 2014	297	76	52	32	88	54	73	36	84
Pepe & Aragona,[178] 2013	100	93	17	30	86	79	24	29	74
Goode et al,[179] 2013	167	—	—	—	—	42	71	16	91
Wu et al,[180] 2012	103	67	64	52	78	38	77	50	66
Pepe et al,[20] 2012	118	91	28	32	89	72	42	32	80
Bollito et al,[181] 2012	509	88	44	41	90	75	70	52	87
Barbera et al,[182] 2012	177	92	26	32	90	73	42	35	81
Auprich et al,[183] 2012	127	85	25	38	78	75	58	49	81
Pepe & Aragona,[184] 2011	74	93	21	43	89	70	44	42	72
Aubin et al,[185] 2010	1072	71	57	26	90	48	79	33	88
Haese et al,[16] 2008	463	73	51	36	83	47	72	39	78
Composite range		67–93	17–64	26–52	78–90	38–79	24–79	16–52	66–91

Abbreviations: PPV, positive predictive value; Sn, sensitivity; Sp, specificity.
Data from Ref.[19]

At the same time, many contemporary reports considered the presence of high-grade PCa (HGPCa, defined herein as Gleason sum ≥ 7) in addition to PCa. Finally, additional studies examined PCA3 in the setting of multiple biomarkers as part of a multivariable model or nomogram. In addition to total PSA, other PSA isoforms and permutations have been frequently considered, including percent free PSA (%fPSA = fPSA/total PSA), percent (−2)proenzyme PSA (%percent pro PSA = [(percent pro PSA pg/mL/10)/fPSA ng/mL]), and the Prostate Health Index (PHI = [(percent pro PSA pg/mL/fPSA ng/mL) × (total PSA ng/mL)$^{1/2}$]).

Initial biopsy: diagnosis and prognosis

In 2013, Scattoni and colleagues[24] found that PCA3 did not improve the predictive accuracy of a baseline multivariable model (BMM) including PSA, %fPSA, and prostate volume (PV) in men presenting for initial biopsy (AUC 0.79 vs 0.80, P = .69). PHI, on the other hand, improved the model by 5%, although statistical significance was not reached (0.79 vs 0.84, P = .144). Ferro and colleagues[25] further explored these markers in men with PSA 2 to 10 ng/mL, reporting AUC values of 0.77, 0.76, and 0.73 for PHI, %p2PSA, and PCA3, respectively. Although PHI did not significantly outperform PCA3 on a pairwise comparison (P = .247), PHI did outperform PCA3 on decision curve analysis when the threshold probability (ie, the probability of cancer at which the benefit of biopsy and no biopsy are considered equal) exceeded 25%. For example, using a threshold probability of 30%, the use of PHI conferred 21% fewer biopsies without increasing PCa underdetection as compared with only 11% when using PCA3.

Several reports have considered the role of PCA3 in PCa diagnosis and in prognosis through assessment of HGPCa. Hansen and colleagues[26] explored various PCA3 thresholds and noted improvements ranging from 5.0% to 7.1% (all P<.001) compared with the BMM. Similarly, prediction of HGPCa improved by 3.6% to 5.4% (all P<.001). For both outcomes, the PCA3 threshold score of 21 optimized predictive accuracy. Ruffion and colleagues[27] examined PCA3 in conjunction with established nomograms in a large French cohort. The projected rates of biopsies avoided and HGPCa underdiagnosed were as follows: 43% and 6% for the Hansen nomogram, 48% and 6% for the Chun nomogram, and 22% and 3% for the Prostate Cancer Prevention Trial (PCPT) risk calculator (PCPTrc).[28] In the largest such study to date, Chevli and colleagues[29] demonstrated that PCA3 significantly improved the baseline model for both PCa (AUC 0.70 vs

0.75, P<.001) and HGPCa (AUC 0.80 vs 0.81, P = .015). Notable studies of PCA3 in initial biopsy populations are summarized in **Table 3**.

Most recently, Seisen and colleagues[30] directly compared PCA3 and PHI in an initial biopsy cohort of 138 men. Although PCA3 significantly outperformed PHI in predicting overall PCa (AUC 0.71 vs 0.65, P = .03), PHI was a superior predictor of significant PCa defined using Epstein criteria (AUC 0.80 vs 0.55, P = .03) and was the lone independent predictor of significant PCa on multivariable analysis. Recognizing the limitations of prostate biopsy, Cantiello and colleagues[31] compared these markers in a radical prostatectomy (RP) cohort. The investigators found that PHI significantly and substantially improved the baseline model ability to predict tumor volume less than 0.5 mL and seminal vesicle invasion compared with PCA3. In men with a biopsy Gleason score of 6 or less, the use of PHI was associated with a 7.6% increase in the ability to predict significant PCa (defined by non–organ-confined cancer, volume ≥ 0.5 mL, or Gleason pattern ≥ 4) as compared with the baseline model (97.3% vs 89.7%, P<.05), whereas PCA3 did not improve the model. These findings were corroborated in a recent cohort of 78 men who underwent RP, as PHI was again superior to PCA3 in predicting tumor volume greater than 0.5 mL, Gleason score of 7 or greater, and pathologic T3 disease.[32]

Unique applications

In addition to use in traditional settings, others have tested various adaptations of the PCA3 score. Like PSA density,[33] Siegrist and colleagues[34] investigated the ratio of PCA3 score to PV (ie, PCA3 density [PCA3D]). In 288 men undergoing initial (63.5%) or repeat (36.5%) diagnostic biopsy, they observed AUC of 0.72 for PCA3D as compared with 0.49 for PSA, 0.59 for PSA density (PSAD), and 0.69 for PCA3. In a follow-up study, PCA3D of 1 or greater was associated with a 70% risk of positive biopsy as compared with 29% if PCA3D was 1 or less. Notably, PSAD was superior to PCA3D in predicting HGPCa.[35] Elsewhere, De Luca and colleagues[36] investigated trends in PCA3 over time; over a median period of 16 months, intraindividual PCA3 scores were stable relative to threshold values (eg, 20, 35, and 50) in 80% of men. In a subsequent study of 108 men in which repeat PCA3 either upgraded (ie, increased from below a threshold to above it) or downgraded (ie, decreased from above a threshold to below it), they observed upgrading in 83% of men found to have PCa.[37] As in other settings, however, the ease of clinical use was limited by the absence of a robust threshold value. Finally, among men with

Table 3
Assessment of PCA3 as diagnostic test for PCa and HGPCa on initial biopsy

	N	BMM Variables	BMM	BMM + PCA3	Bx Avoided (%)	Sn (%)	Sp[a] (%)	NPV (%)	Optimal Threshold
Scattoni et al,[24] 2013	116	PSA, %fPSA, PV	0.79	0.80	—	—	—	—	—
Ferro et al,[25] 2013	300	Age, PSA, fPSA, DRE, PV	0.72	0.77	—	—	—	—	—
Hansen et al,[26] 2013	692	Age, PSA, DRE, PV	0.74	0.81	23	94	36	87	21
HGPCa		Age, PSA, DRE, PV	0.78	0.83	23	98.5	36	99	21
Ruffion et al,[27] 2013	594	Age, PSA, DRE, PV	0.71	0.78	13	97	22	92	21
HGPCa		Age, PSA, DRE, PV	0.77	0.80	13	99	22	98	21
Chevli et al,[29] 2014	3073	Age, PSA, fPSA, DRE, PV, FH, BMI	0.70	0.75	—	—	—	—	—
HGPCa		Age, PSA, fPSA, DRE, PV, FH, BMI	0.80	0.81	—	—	—	—	—

Abbreviations: BMI, body mass index; Bx, biopsy; FH, family history; PV, prostate volume; Sn, sensitivity; Sp, specificity.
[a] Specificity is equivalent to the proportion of biopsies avoided among the population that did not have PCa/HGPCa.

high-grade prostatic intraepithelial neoplasia, PCA3 had limited application individually but demonstrated increased utility in multiplex models considering additional markers.[38]

Others have studied the impact of multiparametric MRI (mpMRI) on PCA3 and other biomarkers. In 2013, Leyten and colleagues[39] studied 290 men who underwent PCA3 testing and biopsy, including 115 men who also underwent mpMRI. The investigators reported that PCA3 predicted biopsy outcome based on the detection of PCa in 55% of men with a PCA3 of 35 or greater compared with 23% of men with a PCA3 less than 35 (P<.001). Assessment of the 115 men exposed to all 3 tests, however, suggests that mpMRI was vastly superior to PCA3 (**Table 4**). Porpiglia and colleagues[40] examined PCA3, PHI, and MRI in 170 men with a history of negative biopsy. They found that PCA3 and PHI were independent predictors of PCa only when mpMRI was not considered. In the multivariable model including all 3 tests, mpMRI was the only significant predictor of PCa (odds ratio 98.1, P<.001). This study used binary (ie, suspicious vs nonsuspicious) MRI reporting from a single expert radiologist as opposed to a standardized reporting system, such as the Prostate Imaging and Data System (PI-RADS) or PI-RADS2.[41–43] Therefore, additional study will be necessary to determine the reproducibility of their findings.

Active surveillance

There are limited data exploring emerging biomarkers in active surveillance (AS) populations.[44] One preliminary study measured PCA3 in 294 men with very-low-risk disease.[45] In this cohort, PCA3 was obtained at a median of 2.5 years after diagnosis and subjects were followed for a median of 3.7 years from diagnosis and underwent yearly biopsy. PCA3 showed a nonsignificant trend toward being increased in the 38 (13%) men who were reclassified during follow-up (mean 50.8 in nonreclassified vs 60.0 in reclassified, P = .131).

Table 4
Performance characteristics of PCA3 and mpMRI in 115 men

	Sn (%)	Sp (%)	PPV (%)	NPV (%)
PCA3	69	46	74	39
mpMRI	95	49	81	81

Abbreviations: PPV, positive predictive value; Sn, sensitivity; Sp, specificity.
Data from Leyten GH, Wierenga EA, Sedelaar JP, et al. Value of PCA3 to predict biopsy outcome and its potential role in selecting patients for multiparametric MRI. Int J Mol Sci 2013;14(6):11347–55.

In a limited number of subjects, it is notable that the PCA3 scores were higher in men who underwent grade reclassification (ie, Gleason score upgrading) as compared with those who underwent volume reclassification (mean 72.0 vs 51.2, respectively; P = .174) or no reclassification (mean 72.0 vs 50.8; P = .304) during follow-up. The relationship of PCA3 with tumor multifocality has obvious applications to the AS setting as well.[46] The limited data available underscore the need for additional research.

Prostate cancer antigen 3: summary

Although PCA3 has demonstrated incremental superiority to PSA in many settings, in-depth analyses have concluded there is insufficient evidence of improved health outcomes associated with its use.[47,48] Other limitations include the need for DRE before collection and the observation that, although based on very limited data, PCA3 may be less informative than other tests, such as PHI and mpMRI. Regardless, the marker is making a strong case for selective use in specific clinical settings; but what are those settings, and what is the risk of its use?

The strength of PCA3 lies in the rarity of false-negative tests when a low threshold value, such as 20, is used. At this threshold, as evident in **Table 2**, the test is highly sensitive and carries a high negative predictive value in most populations. To patients and providers, this means that if a PCA3 score is less than 20, the possibility that a cancer exists is low, ranging from 10% to just more than 20% in the repeat biopsy population. In the setting of multivariable models with clinical factors, these risks become even smaller. Perhaps most importantly, the risk of missing high-grade cancer seems to be even lower. Which values are low enough to avoid or delay biopsy is of course a shared decision to be made in the context of each patient's overall health and personal preferences. The accumulation of data from additional populations will help to characterize these risks and further clarify the potential uses of PCA3.

TMPRSS2:ERG

From bench to bedside

Previously described in hematologic malignancies, Tomlins and Colleagues first reported the presence of gene fusions in PCa in 2005.[49] Their landmark report described fusions of the androgen-regulated transmembrane protease, serine 2 (TMPRSS2) gene and members of the E26 transformation specific (ETS) oncogene family, which were strongly associated with marked overexpression of the latter. Of the ETS transcription factors, ERG (v-ets avian erythroblastosis virus E26 oncogene homolog) is regarded as a key PCa oncogene and is located in tandem to TMPRSS2 on chromosome 21.[50,51] Throughout the literature, TMPRSS2:ERG has been identified in 50% of tumor foci and 75% to 80% of PCa cases,[52–54] with greater than 99% histologic specificity for PCa.[54] In 2006, a urinary assay for TMPRSS2:ERG fusion transcripts was developed based on the transcription-mediated amplification platform used for PCA3 testing.[55,56] An initial study of this assay demonstrated 37% sensitivity, 93% specificity, and 94% positive predictive value (PPV) for PCa.[57] As there exists heterogeneity of TMPRSS2:ERG status among intraprostatic tumor foci, Young and colleagues[58] importantly demonstrated that TMPRSS2:ERG scores were strongly correlated to total ERG-positive cancer tissue.

The contemporary era

Given early findings reflecting its high specificity, it was proposed that TMPRSS2:ERG could be most useful in combination with a more sensitive marker, such as PCA3. A baseline assessment can be gained from the work of Salami and colleagues.[59] In 45 men scheduled for biopsy, they found PCA3 was the most sensitive marker (sensitivity = 93%, specificity = 37%), whereas TMPRSS2:ERG (sensitivity = 67%, specificity = 87%) and PSA (using threshold 10.0 ng/mL; sensitivity = 40%, specificity = 93%) were substantially more specific. Ultimately, TMPRSS2:ERG had the highest discriminatory value for diagnosis as compared with PCA3 and PSA (AUC of 0.77, 0.65, and 0.67, respectively). A multivariable model including all 3 markers conferred an AUC of 0.88 (95% confidence interval: 0.75–0.98). In a similar setting, however, Stephan and colleagues[60] fixed sensitivity at 90% and found that PCA3 yielded greater specificity, particularly in the repeat biopsy cohort

(PCA3 36%, PHI 19%, TMPRSS2:ERG 4%). The performance characteristics obtained from these studies are listed in **Table 5**.

Building on their novel discovery, Tomlins and colleagues[56] showed that TMPRSS2:ERG significantly increased AUC for PCa detection compared with PSA in their academic biopsy cohort (AUC 0.71 vs 0.61). Furthermore, the addition of PCA3 led to further improvement of the TMPRSS2:ERG model (AUC = 0.77). In multivariable models considering the PCPTrc,[61] optimal discriminative ability was obtained in the model including both PCA3 and TMPRSS2:ERG (AUC = 0.79). Several other studies have explored the impact of these markers on multivariable models; these findings are listed in **Table 6**. Cornu and colleagues[62] found that PSAD, PCA3, and TMPRSS2:ERG each contributed to the BMM, yielding an AUC of 0.73. In the HGPCa model, the combined model AUC was 0.80. Tallon and colleagues[63] subsequently found that PCA3, TMPRSS2:ERG, and PHI independently predicted a tumor volume of 0.5 mL or greater in men who underwent RP; but PHI was the only test predictive of a Gleason score of 7 or greater.

In conjunction with the European Randomized Study of Screening for Prostate Cancer risk calculator variables (PSA, DRE, TRUS, and PV), Leyten and colleagues[64] considered TMPRSS2:ERG as a dichotomous variable; they demonstrated very high discriminative ability for both PCa (AUC = 0.84) and HGPCa (AUC = 0.84; PCA3 did not independently contribute to this model). Most recently, Tomlins and colleagues[65] validated multivariable models, which include TMPRSS2:ERG and PCA3 scores along with serum PSA (deriving the Mi-Prostate Score [MiPS]) or the PCPTrc (MiPS-PCPT). Their findings were robust across multiple cohorts within the study population, and the clinical benefits were

Table 5
Diagnostic performance of urinary TMPRSS2:ERG

Study, N (Prevalence)	Setting	Variables	AUC PCa	Sn (%)	Sp (%)	PPV	NPV
Salami et al,[59]	IBx (53%)	PSA	0.67	40	93	—	—
2011, 45 (33%)	RBx (47%)	PCA3	0.65	93	37	42	92
		TMPRSS2:ERG	0.77	67	87	71	84
		PSA + PCA3 + T2E	0.88	80	90	80	90
Stephan et al,[60]	IBx (55%)	PCA3	0.70	90	32	—	—
2013, 246 (45%)		PHI	0.68	90	29		
		TMPRSS2:ERG	0.68	90	21		
	RBx (45%)	PCA3	0.77	90	36	—	—
		PHI	0.69	90	19		
		TMPRSS2:ERG	0.53	90	4		

Abbreviations: IBx, initial biopsy; Prevalence, PCa prevalence in the study population; RBx, repeat biopsy; Sn, sensitivity; Sp, specificity; T2E, TMPRSS2:ERG.

Table 6
Discriminative ability of TMPRSS2:ERG and other candidate biomarkers

Study	N (Prevalence)	Setting	Variables	AUC PCa	AUC HGPCa
Tomlins et al,[56] 2011	606 (44%)	Bx (70% IBx)	PSA	0.61	—
			TMPRSS2:ERG	0.71	
			PCA3 + T2E	0.77	
			PCPTrs	0.64	
			PCPTrs + PCA3 + T2E	0.79	
Cornu et al,[62] 2013	291 (59%)	Bx (63% IBx)	PSAD	0.57	—
			PCA3	0.66	—
			TMPRSS2:ERG	0.67	—
			BMM[a] + greater	0.73	0.80
Tallon et al,[63] 2014	154 (100%)	Pre-RP	PCA3	—	—
			PHI		0.66
			TMPRSS2:ERG		—
			BMM[b]		0.81
			BMM + PHI		0.86
Leyten et al,[64] 2014	497 (44%)	Bx (79% IBx)	PCA3	0.72	0.53
			TMPRSS2:ERG	0.59	0.64
			ERSPCrc	0.80	0.80
			ERSPCrc + PCA3	0.83	—
			ERSPCrc + T2E	0.84	0.84
Tomlins et al,[65] 2015[c]	1225 (42%)	Bx (80% IBx)	PSA	0.59	0.65
			PSA + T2E	0.69	0.73
			PSA + PCA3	0.73	0.75
			PSA + T2E + PCA3	0.75	0.77
			PCPTrc	0.64	0.71
			PCPTrc + T2E	0.72	0.75
			PCPTrc + PCA3	0.74	0.75
			PCPTrc + T2E + PCA3	0.76	0.78

Abbreviations: Bx, biopsy; ERSPCrc, European Randomized Study of Screening for Prostate Cancer risk calculator; GS, Gleason score; IBx, initial biopsy; Prevalence, PCa prevalence in the study population.
  [a] BMM including age, family history, and bioavailable testosterone.
  [b] BMM including age, PSA, DRE, biopsy GS.
  [c] Separate analyses performed in a single validation cohort.

well described at various risk thresholds. For example, at a risk threshold of 40%, the MiPS-PCPT model provided avoidance of 47.0% of biopsies and delayed the diagnosis in only 2.3% of high-grade cancers. At more conservative thresholds, the model avoided 35% of biopsies and delayed the diagnosis of only 1% of HGPCa. Certainly, biomarker panels combining TMPRSS2:ERG and PCA3 seem to hold great promise.

Active surveillance

In 2013, Lin and colleagues[66] studied PCA3 and TMPRSS2:ERG in 387 men enrolled in the Canary Prostate Active Surveillance Study. The investigators observed an increase in the median baseline PCA3 scores based on follow-up biopsy results: 27 for a negative biopsy, 31 for a Gleason score of 6 or less, and 48 for a Gleason score of 7 ($P = .02$). The corresponding median TMPRSS2:ERG values were 5, 14, and 29,

respectively ($P = .001$). The AUC for a Gleason score of 7 was 0.68 for PSA versus 0.70 for PCA3 and TMPRSS2:ERG scores ($P = .08$), demonstrating a trend toward significance. Although this study, like most in active surveillance (AS) populations, was limited by sample size and follow-up, there seems to be an association with follow-up biopsy results such that PCA3 and TMPRSS2:ERG could play a role in AS populations moving forward.

TMPRSS2:ERG summary

With a remarkably high specificity for PCa, TMPRSS2:ERG has been largely explored in combination with the more sensitive PCA3 assay. Combining these markers with baseline predictive models like the PCPTrc have produced AUC values approximating 0.80 and upward, providing an opportunity to spare 50% of men from unnecessary biopsies with minimal delays in diagnosing clinically significant cancers. Although these data are encouraging, studies of TMPRSS2:ERG and

PCA3 in the context of other promising diagnostic aids, such as PHI and mpMRI, remain limited. Further investigation is necessary to compare these tools and identify how to combine them for maximal clinical benefit.

Other RNA-Based Markers

Although PCA3 and TMPRSS2:ERG are the most thoroughly studied RNA biomarkers, other RNA-based markers have also been studied in urine, often in combination. In 2008, Tomlins and colleagues[67] described outlier expression of serine peptidase inhibitor Kazal type 1 (SPINK1) indicating an aggressive subtype of PCa not secondary to ETS fusion events. The investigators subsequently demonstrated urinary measurement of SPINK1 and its association with biochemical recurrence after RP. Alpha-methylacyl-CoA racemase (AMACR) is a mitochondrial enzyme preferentially overexpressed in PCa tissue.[68] Its use as a biomarker was derived by Zielie and colleagues[69] using RNA transcripts in prostatic secretions, and an assay for use in urine was subsequently developed.[70] Ouyang and colleagues[71] later investigated AMACR in 43 men with PCa and 49 controls. The investigators established a threshold of 10.7 for diagnosis, at which AMACR had 70% sensitivity and 71% specificity for PCa. In combination with PCA3, these measures increased to 81% and 84%. Pertinent studies exploring these and other biomarkers detected in urine are listed in **Table 7**. Most recently, Leyten and colleagues[72] identified a 3-gene panel for prediction of a Gleason score of 7 or greater disease. The panel included HOXC6, TDRD1, and DLX1 and outperformed PCA3 (AUC 0.77 vs 0.68) and PSA (AUC 0.77 vs 0.72). In combination with PSA, these markers conferred an AUC of 0.81 for HGPCa and hold great promise moving forward.

MicroRNA

MicroRNAs (miRNAs) are small, noncoding RNAs that regulate gene expression in various biological processes.[73,74] To this end, miRNAs seem to have important roles during key stages of carcinogenesis, including proliferation, avoidance of apoptosis, epithelial-to-mesenchymal transition, and castration resistance.[74,75] Differential expression of serum miRNA has been previously described in men with PCa.[76,77] In 2012, Bryant and colleagues[78] found that miR-107 and miR-574-3p were overexpressed in urine of men with PCa as compared with controls. Srivastava and colleagues[79] found that miR-205 and miR-214 were downregulated in 36 men with PCa versus healthy controls and yielded combined sensitivity of 89% and specificity of 80%. More recently,

however, Stephan and colleagues[80] aimed to validate observations in tissue that miR-183 and miR-205 were differentially expressed in men with PCa. In a randomly selected cohort of men with and without PCa, these urinary miRNAs offered no predictive ability. These findings, in addition to other studies of urinary miRNAs, are listed in **Table 8**.

Long noncoding RNA

In contrast to miRNAs, long noncoding RNAs (lncRNAs) contain greater than 200 nucleotides.[81] PCA3 is one well-studied example of lncRNA, but others have been similarly implicated in the biology of cancer. These molecules are thought to impact carcinogenesis at the interface of proliferation and apoptosis, through either transcriptional or post-transcriptional effects.[82] One promising marker, metastasis associated lung adenocarcinoma transcript 1 (MALAT1), was recently studied in a validation cohort and demonstrated an AUC of 0.83 in a base model with age, PSA, DRE, PV, and %fPSA.[83] The investigators demonstrated that use of the MALAT1-based model would result in avoidance of 30% of unnecessary biopsies without failing to diagnose a single cancer.[83–85] Another lncRNA, second chromosome locus associated with prostate-1, is the first lncRNA demonstrated to impair a major epigenetic complex with an established tumor suppressor function.[86,87] This finding has been associated with aggressive PCa in tissue.[88] The use of these lncRNAs in an effective urinary assay holds great potential.

DNA-BASED MARKERS

The presence of cell-free DNA (cfDNA) in human plasma has been well established in both healthy individuals and in various cancer types.[89,90] Cancer detection using DNA-based markers is centered on the identification of (1) cfDNA content or (2) tumor-specific alterations.[91–93] As compared with RNA, DNA is relatively stable in urine and requires less intensive methods of preservation.[94] Although glutathione S-transferase pi 1 (GSTP1) has been extensively studied in the setting of PCa, other potential DNA markers have only recently come under investigation. As in related disciplines, advancing technologies will continue to play a prominent role in use of DNA-based platforms.[95]

Cell-free DNA

Although less than 10% of cfDNA is derived from tumor cells,[96–99] there is substantial evidence of higher circulating cfDNA levels in patients with

Table 7
Studies of RNA-based urinary biomarkers

Study, N (PCa Prevalence)	Candidates	AUC	Sn (%)	Sp (%)	PPV (%)	NPV (%)
Laxman et al,[55] 2008, 234 (59%)	PSA	0.51	—	—	—	—
	AMACR	—	—	—	—	—
	ERG	—	—	—	—	—
	GOLPH2	0.66	—	—	—	—
	PCA3	0.66	75	56	71	61
	SPINK1	0.64	—	—	—	—
	TFF3	—	—	—	—	—
	TMPRSS2:ERG	—	—	—	—	—
	MPM	0.76	66	76	80	61
Talesa et al,[186] 2009, 90 (49%)	PSA[a]	0.67	—	—	—	—
	PCA3	0.68				
	PSMA	0.64				
	HEPSIN	0.48				
	GalNAC-T3	0.64				
	PSMA + PSA	0.82				
	PSMA + PCA3	0.80				
Rigau et al,[187] 2010, 215 (34%)	PSA	0.60	—	—	—	—
	PSGR	0.68	59	73	—	—
	PCA3	0.66	69	59	—	—
	PSGR, PCA3	0.73	77	60	50	83
Rigau et al,[188] 2011, 154 (37%)	PSMA	0.62	81	41	—	—
	PSGR	0.65	63	64		
	PCA3	0.60	86	35		
	PSMA, PSGR, PCA3	0.74	89	45		
	Above + PSA	0.77	—	—		
Jamaspishvili et al,[189] 2011, 104 (60%)	PCA3	0.57	—	—	—	—
	AMACR[b]	0.63	63	65	68	53
	TRPM8, MSMB	0.67	68	62	72	54
	TRPM8, MSMB, AMACR	0.73	77	62	75	63
	TRPM8, MSMB, AMACR, PCA3	0.74	72	71	79	60
	Above + SPINK1, EZH2, GOLM1	0.74	81	62	77	68
Ouyang et al,[71] 2009, 92 (47%)	PSA	0.59	77	45	55	66
	AMACR	0.65	70	71	68	73
	PCA3	0.67	72	59	61	71
	AMACR, PCA3	—	81	84	—	—
Dimitriades et al,[190] 2013, 66 (21%)	DRE	0.70	—	—	—	—
	PSA	0.54				
	PCA3	0.73				
	TMPRSS2:ERG	0.75				
	DRE, PSA, PCA3, T2E	0.89				

Multiplex model: GOLPH2, PCA3, SPINK1, TMPRSS2:ERG.
Abbreviations: MPM, multiplex model; Prevalence, PCa prevalence in the study population.
[a] All models include age.
[b] Only significant marker on univariable analysis.

cancer, including men with PCa.[100–104] Altimari and colleagues[105] observed that circulating cfDNA concentration was predictive of PCa diagnosis with 80% sensitivity and 82% specificity; others have similarly correlated cfDNA with the Gleason score, extraprostatic extension, and pathologic stage.[106] Casadio and colleagues[107,108] were the first to explore this relationship in urine. In their 2013 study, the investigators successfully quantified urinary cfDNA from all 54 subjects tested, and they demonstrated an AUC of 0.63. Notably, there was no significant difference in overall cfDNA concentration based on PCa status, although others have pointed out this study was not adjusted for creatinine and differential effects of diuresis.[4,108]

Table 8
Studies of urinary microRNA markers

Study	Candidates	Sn (%)	Sp (%)	AUC
Bryant et al,[78] 2012	miR-107	—	—	0.74
	miR-574-3p	—	—	0.66
Srivastava et al,[79] 2013	miR-205[a]	—	—	0.71
	miR-214[a]	—	—	0.74
	Combined	89	80	—
Haj-Ahmad et al,[75] 2014	miR-1825	60	69	—
	miR-484	80	19	—
	Combined	45	75	—
	Combined + PSA	40	81	—
Stephan et al,[80] 2015	miR-183	90	3	0.58
	miR-205[a]	90	3	0.56

Abbreviations: Sn, sensitivity; Sp, specificity.
[a] Underexpression.

In addition to the impact of total cfDNA concentration alone, qRT-PCR has allowed for assessment of DNA fragmentation patterns based on evidence that necrotic (eg, cancer) cells release DNA with a higher index of integrity, whereas apoptotic (eg, healthy) cells undergo DNA processing and release shorter ($\sim$180 base pairs) fragments.[97,109–111] Again, Casadio and colleagues[108] pioneered this study of urinary cfDNA by calculating the integrity index of men with and without PCa. Although their study was limited to 29 patients and 25 controls, they demonstrated a significantly higher integrity index in men with PCa, yielding diagnostic sensitivity of 79%, specificity of 84%, and AUC of 0.80. Ultimately, aside from this one report, urinary cfDNA remains largely unstudied in PCa. Previous findings in plasma, as well as the findings of Casadio and colleagues,[108] are encouraging.

Tumor-Specific Alterations

Genetic alterations

Although elevated cfDNA levels are a near-universal feature of cancer, cancer-specific DNA changes have been considered for improving diagnostic specificity. Tumor-specific alterations include genetic and epigenetic modifications.[5] Genetic alterations, such as gene amplification or loss of heterozygosity (LOH), were well described in the context of PCa tissue but scarcely described in urine.[112,113] In 2001, however, Cussenot and colleagues[114] assessed post-DRE urinary specimens for LOH at the 7q, 8p, 13q, and 16q loci as compared with %fPSA in 32 men undergoing biopsy. Considering one LOH as a positive test, they observed sensitivity of 72% and specificity of 67%, as compared with 45% and 52% for %fPSA. Thuret and colleagues[92] aimed to build on

these findings by adding the 12p and 18q regions in their study. Although 18 (18%) men lacked sufficient cells for analysis, in the remaining 81 men they observed 87% sensitivity and 44% specificity for PCa detection, as compared with 55% and 74% using %fPSA. Perhaps most interesting, the investigators harvested noncancerous epithelial cells from near the tumor in 19 men who underwent RP. They found that more than 50% of allelic deletions observed in the tumor were also present in neighboring benign cells, implying a potential field defect. Nonetheless, pursuit of these and other genetic alterations in urine has been limited.

Epigenetic alterations

Epigenetic modifications are heritable and reversible biochemical changes that alter gene expression without affecting the primary DNA sequence.[115] Methylation of clusters of CpG dinucleotides (termed *CpG islands* or *CGIs*) near the promoter region of genes is the most thoroughly studied epigenetic alteration.[116] In normal cells, unmethylated CGIs are permissive but not sufficient for gene expression. Hypermethylation of these regions is widely observed in prostatic carcinogenesis and thought to function in long-term silencing of genes associated with tumor suppression and cell cycle regulation.[117,118] Therefore, aberrant methylation of DNA has been extensively studied in tissue and urine, a practice facilitated by the stability of DNA in body fluids. GSTP1 functions in the detoxification of electrophiles, and its promoter region is hypermethylated in up to 90% of PCa cells,[93,119] making it an ideal marker of disease.

Like in its RNA counterparts, diagnostic yield seems to be highest when urine is obtained after prostatic massage.[120] In 2005, Hoque and colleagues[121] tested urinary sediment of 9 promoter regions and detected hypermethylation of at least one of the study genes in men with PCa; at the same time, 4 of the genes demonstrated no methylation from all 91 controls, although 27% of the control population was female. In 2011, a comprehensive review of 22 studies considering GSTP1 methylation in serum, plasma, and urine demonstrated a pooled specificity of 89% with consistently high specificity across multiple populations.[119] Given an associated sensitivity of 52%, GSTP1 has been recommended for further evaluation in combination with other biomarkers. Most recently, Jatkoe and colleagues[122] assessed the ability of a clinical model to predict a Gleason score of 7 or greater cancer. The addition of GSTP1 and APC (the adenomatous polyposis coli gene promoter) to a predictive model using conventional clinical factors increased the AUC from 0.69 to 0.82. Previous studies have suggested that urinary detection of methylated DNA may prove useful in prognosis, a possibility that merits further examination.[123,124]

Table 9 lists pertinent diagnostic reports. On the whole, these preliminary studies indicate GSTP1 to be a highly specific biomarker. Although they have provided point estimates for further exploration moving forward, the quality of these studies was not sufficient for consideration of clinical use without further validation.

PROTEIN-BASED MARKERS

Protein-based biomarkers tend to require fewer preanalytical considerations than nucleic acid-based markers, and the standard use of reliable immunologic assays such as ELISA makes protein-based markers an inexpensive and desirable clinical entity.[4,6] Moreover, the development of multiple new proteomic technologies have revolutionized the search for candidate markers. Namely, the ability to investigate thousands of proteins using a nonhypothesis driven approach is critical as deeper understanding of molecular pathways in PCa only procures additional candidate biomarkers.[125,126] In one recent study, Jedinak and colleagues[127] analyzed 173 urine samples in men with PCa (n = 90) or benign prostatic hyperplasia (BPH) (n = 83) using the isobaric tags for relative and absolute concentration (iTRAQ) approach to quantitative mass spectrometry.[128] The investigators identified 25 differentially expressed proteins, ranging in function across categories, including cell assembly and

Table 9
Studies of DNA-based urinary biomarkers

	N (Prev)	Variables	AUC	Sn (%)	Sp (%)
Roupret et al,[191] 2007	133 (71%)	GSTP1, APC, RASSF1, RARB2	—	87	89
Woodson et al,[192] 2008	100 (24%)	GSTP1	—	75	98
Vener et al,[193] 2008	121 (45%)	GSTP1	0.65	33	95
		RARB	0.59	40	84
		APC	0.59	36	91
		GSTP1, APC	0.68	51	89
		GSTP1, APC, RARB	0.69	55	80
Vener et al,[193] 2008	113 (50%)	GSTP1	0.64	36	91
		RARB	0.64	29	91
		APC	0.62	51	83
		GSTP1, APC	0.67	53	80
		GSTP1, APC, RARB	0.65	53	76
Payne et al,[194] 2009	—	GSTP1	0.69	45	80
		RASSF2	0.66	28	80
		HIST1H4K	0.64	43	80
		TFAP2E	0.65	47	80
Baden et al,[123] 2009	337 (53%)	GSTP1	0.66	—	—
		APC	0.59	—	—
		RARB2	0.71	—	—
		GSTP1, RARB2, APC	0.72	60	81
Baden et al,[195] 2011	515 (45.1%)	GSTP1	0.68	—	—
		RARB2	0.64	—	—
		APC	0.63	—	—
		GSTP1, RARB2, APC, B-actin	0.73	—	—

Abbreviations: Prev, prevalence; Sn, sensitivity; Sp, specificity.

organization, signaling, morphology, metabolism, growth and proliferation, replication, and others. Ultimately, 3 proteins were identified that increased the AUC from 0.73 in a baseline model using PSA categories to 0.81 (P value for improvement = .004). There is great promise for the future in proteomics, largely rooted in the dynamic advances in technology witnessed over the last decade. Although emerging methods for peptide discovery and validation are beyond the scope of this review, clinically relevant urinary proteomic studies are listed in **Table 10**.

OTHER URINARY MARKERS
Metabolomics

Metabolomics can be defined as the comprehensive assessment of all metabolites in a biological system or physiologic state.[129,130] Thus, in the setting of cancer, metabolomics provides an attractive approach for distinguishing malignant cells from normal cells based on observed differences in physiology and biochemical activity.[131] In 2009, Sreekumar and colleagues[132] profiled more than 1126 metabolites from 262 clinical samples (including 110 urine specimens). Based on these profiles, the investigators were able to distinguish benign prostate from localized and metastatic PCa. In this landmark study, the glycine derivative sarcosine was markedly elevated in invasive and metastatic PCa. Furthermore, sarcosine was differentially expressed in urine, conferring significant predictive value for invasive and metastatic cancer cell lines. Although these findings were not reproduced in a separate independent cohort,[133] the work of Sreekumar and

Table 10
Studies of protein-based urinary biomarkers

Author	Proteins	Approach	Findings
Rogers et al,[196] 2004	AMACR	Western blot	Sn 100%, Sp 58%
M'Koma et al,[197] 2007	Uromodulin, semenogelin	MALDI-TOF	Sn 71%, Sp 67%
Roy et al,[198] 2008	MMP-9, multiple dimers	Gelatin zymography	Sn 74%, Sp 82%
Theodorescu et al,[199] 2008	12 protein panel	CE-MS	Sn 91%, Sp 69% in multivariable model
Fujita et al,[200] 2008	HGF, IL18Bpa	ELISA	Association with tumor volume
Schostak et al,[201] 2009	Annexin A3	Western blot	AUC = 0.82 (annexin A3 + PSA)
Fujita et al,[202] 2009	Endoglin (CD105)	ELISA	AUC = 0.72 (endoglin + PSA)
Morgan et al,[203] 2011	Engrailed-2	ELISA	Sn 66%, Sp 88%
Pandha et al,[204] 2012	Engrailed-2	ELISA	Association with tumor volume and stage
Katafigiotis et al,[205] 2012	ZAG	Western blot + IHC	AUC = 0.75 (ZAG + PSA)
Mhatre et al,[206] 2014	sPSP94/sPSA	ELISA	AUC = 0.86, Sn 91%, Sp 70%
Haj-Ahmad et al,[75] 2014	Fibronectin	LC-MS/MS, qRT-PCR	Sn 75%, Sp 50%
Davalieva et al,[207] 2015	HP, AMBP	2-D DIGE, MS, bioinformatics	AUC = 0.85 (HP + AMBP)
Vermassen et al,[208] 2015	UGM	N-glycosylation profiling	AUC = 0.84 (UGM + PSA)
Jedinak et al,[127] 2015	B2M, PGA3, MUC3	iTRAQ, MS	AUC = 0.81 (3 proteins + PSA)

Abbreviations: 2-D DIGE, 2-dimensional difference in gel polyacrylamide gel electrophoresis; AMBP, alpha-1-microglobulin/bikunin; B2M, β-2-microglobulin; CE-MS, capillary electrophoresis coupled to mass spectrometry; ELISA, enzyme-linked immunosorbent assay; HGF, hepatocyte growth factor; HP, haptoglobin; IL18Bpa, interleukin 18 binding protein a; LC-MS/MS, 2-dimensional liquid chromatography-tandem mass spectrometry; MALDI-TOF, matrix-assisted laser desorption-mass spectrometry time of flight; MMP-9, matrix metalloprotease 9; MUC3, intestinal mucin 3; PGA3, pepsinogen 3 group 1; sPSA, serum PSA; sPSP94, serum prostate secretory protein of 94 amino acids; UGM, urinary glycoprofile marker; ZAG, zinc alpha-2-glycoprotein.

colleagues[134] was most significant in its proof of concept for the use of metabolomic profiling to identify potential biomarkers, rather than in sarcosine itself.[135,136] Other investigators have subsequently reported significant alterations in tissue-based metabolomic profiles from PCa and benign subjects,[137,138] confirming a potential role for this approach moving forward. Although metabolomic profiles have not been explored at the same depth as genetic and proteomic profiles, technological standardization and innovation will continue to close this gap as additional efforts are directed toward this emerging field.[139]

Exosomes

As described by Nilsson and colleagues[140] and Jansen and others,[141] prostatic fluids contain 2 types of microvesicles: (1) prostasomes, which are secreted by ductal epithelial cells and are a normal component of semen, and (2) exosomes, which are specialized 30 to 100 nm nanovesicles secreted by normal and cancerous cells.[142,143] Exosomes containing mRNA, miRNA, and proteins are secreted by tumor cells and subsequently taken up and translated by recipient cells.[144] Therefore, exosomes expressed in urine may serve as a noninvasive source of densely concentrated tumor-specific data with potential diagnostic utility.[145–147]

To this point, most of the efforts have been focused on establishing sound methods for successfully exploring exosomal data.[148] Dijkstra and colleagues[149] demonstrated exosomes to be a stable substrate for analysis that, similar to other markers, are made more sensitive by prevoid DRE. Other groups have begun to describe and characterize exosomal proteins.[150,151] Bijnsdorp and colleagues[151] revealed 2 proteins, ITGA3 and ITGB1, which were more abundant in the exosomes of men with metastatic PCa. In PCa cell lines, others have similarly demonstrated a differential pattern of peptide expression in benign prostasomes and malignant cell-derived vesicles.[152] In an early clinical study, Donovan and colleagues[153] described the use of a 3-gene signature including ERG, PCA3, and SPDEF (for normalization) to predict biopsy results in 170 men with PSA between 2 and 10 ng/mL. The overall AUC was 0.73 for PCa and 0.76 for HGPCa, as compared with 0.54 and 0.60 using the PCPTrc. Most notably, for HGPCa, the investigators reported a sensitivity of 97.2% (specificity 50.7%) and NPV of 98.6% (PPV 34.7%), suggesting the potential for use as a reliable test to rule out high-grade disease. Certainly, with further standardization and advancement of analytical technologies, the study of exosomes

and exosomal material will continue to evolve and improve.[154–157]

The Microbiome

With the establishment of the human microbiome project came the acknowledgment that humans are in fact supraorganisms living in symbiosis with the microbes that live inside and on us (the microbiota).[158] In this light, our collective genetic profile is the summation of our human genome and the genome of our microbial symbionts (the microbiome).[159] There are extensive data supporting the importance of this symbiotic relationship in maintaining host health.[160–162] Although urine has historically been considered sterile,[163] the development of advanced molecular techniques, such as 16S ribosomal RNA sequencing, has revealed extensive bacterial sequences in the urine of healthy individuals.[164–166] Therefore, investigators have sought to understand the impact of our urinary microbiome, both positive and negative, on urologic health.[167] Although more commonly studied in the context of urothelial cancers and benign conditions,[167,168] Yu and colleagues[169] sought to characterize the microbiota in men with PCa as compared with those with BPH. The investigators identified and quantified bacteria in urine, prostatic secretions, and seminal fluid obtained from 13 men with PCa and 21 men with BPH. They identified significant differences in the quantities of specific bacterial strains in men with PCa as compared with BPH (**Table 11**). These findings, like those of others, may suggest a role for inflammation or infection in prostate carcinogenesis. Certainly the varying presence of unique bacterial strains in this study does not prove causation, and it remains equally possible that the presence of PCa drives the establishment of particular microbiota. Regardless, additional studies are needed to better understand the potential clinical implications of these findings.

Table 11
Relative urinary presence of microbial species in PCa and BPH

Species Increased in PCa	Species Decreased in PCa
Bacteroidetes bacteria	Eubacterium
Alphaproteobacteria	Defluviicoccus
Firmicutes bacteria	Escherichia coli
Lachnospiraceae	—
Propionicimonas	—
Sphingomonas	—
Ochrobactrum	—

SUMMARY

Once heralded as the most meaningful tumor marker in cancer biology, the shortcomings of PSA have been well documented and highly scrutinized.[170–173] To date, science has yet to uncover a magic bullet biomarker for PCa[174]; but significant progress has been made nonetheless.[127,175–177] Although preliminary studies of emerging concepts, such as metabolomics, exosomes, and microbiota, are encouraging, other biomarkers, such as PCA3 and TMPRSS2:ERG, are better understood at present. Still, questions are prevalent, particularly surrounding when exactly to use these markers and the risks associated with doing so.

Based on studies to date, men with PCA3 scores less than 20 could be spared repeat biopsy, with less than 20% of them ultimately found to harbor cancer and far fewer found to have HGPCa. Although such estimates have been reproduced with some consistency in the repeat biopsy population, similar studies of men considering initial biopsy are both less promising and less prevalent, making it particularly difficult to identify guidelines for use without additional research. At the same time, although comparative studies have been rare, initial data seem to indicate that serum-based PHI and mpMRI may be superior to PCA3, which requires clinical examination (ie, DRE) as well. One goal moving forward should be to better characterize these diagnostic tools in a comparative or combined approach.

Although an abundance of time and resources has been devoted to biomarker research, existing data reveal that our efforts have lacked a unified approach. More specifically, greater emphasis must be placed on sharing study results in a consistent, clinically meaningful way. The presentation of odds ratios, though capable of demonstrating the relative significance of particular biomarkers, provides little value to the patients and clinicians faced with a difficult decision. Much like recent reports from Hansen and colleagues[26] and Ruffion and colleagues,[27] emerging studies should aim to illustrate the most pertinent applications of new data in context of the most useful existing data. For detection of PCa, the rate of biopsy avoidance and the corresponding rate of missed diagnoses are most essential. Given that these measures vary based on threshold values, multiple cutoffs should be considered and optimal cutoffs identified. When possible, these values should reflect incorporation with multivariable models, such as risk calculators or nomograms. Finally, in light of the heterogeneous nature of PCa, high-grade cancers should invariably be considered as a study outcome, if not the primary outcome. A unified approach such as this will allow that future studies more seamlessly build on existing data and will greatly enhance our ability to produce useful, clinically relevant research in an efficient manner.

REFERENCES

1. DeMarzo AM, Nelson WG, Isaacs WB, et al. Pathological and molecular aspects of prostate cancer. Lancet 2003;361(9361):955–64.
2. Tomlins SA, Mehra R, Rhodes DR, et al. Integrative molecular concept modeling of prostate cancer progression. Nat Genet 2007;39(1):41–51.
3. Logothetis CJ, Gallick GE, Maity SN, et al. Molecular classification of prostate cancer progression: foundation for marker-driven treatment of prostate cancer. Cancer Discov 2013;3(8):849–61.
4. Ralla B, Stephan C, Meller S, et al. Nucleic acid-based biomarkers in body fluids of patients with urologic malignancies. Crit Rev Clin Lab Sci 2014; 51(4):200–31.
5. Müller H, Brenner H. Urine markers as possible tools for prostate cancer screening: review of performance characteristics and practically. Clin Chem 2006;52(4):562–73.
6. Truong M, Yang B, Jarrard DF. Toward the detection of prostate cancer in urine: a critical analysis. J Urol 2013;189(2):422–9.
7. Sokoll LJ, Ellis W, Lange P, et al. A multicenter evaluation of the PCA3 molecular urine test: pre-analytical effects, analytical performance, and diagnostic accuracy. Clin Chim Acta 2008;389(1–2):1–6.
8. Gonzalgo ML, Pavlovich CP, Lee SM, et al. Prostate cancer detection by GSTP1 methylation analysis of postbiopsy urine specimens prostate cancer detection by gstp1 methylation analysis of postbiopsy urine specimens 1. Clin Cancer Res 2003; 9(7):2673–7.
9. Bussemakers MJG, Van Bokhoven A, Verhaegh GW, et al. DD3: a new prostate-specific gene, highly overexpressed in prostate cancer. Cancer Res 1999; 59(23):5975–9.
10. De Kok JB, Verhaegh GW, Roelofs RW, et al. DD3(PCA3), a very sensitive and specific marker to detect prostate tumors. Cancer Res 2002; 62(9):2695–8.
11. Hessels D, Klein Gunnewiek JMT, Van Oort I, et al. DD3PCA3-based molecular urine analysis for the diagnosis of prostate cancer. Eur Urol 2003;44(1): 8–16.
12. Groskopf J, Aubin SMJ, Deras IL, et al. APTIMA PCA3 molecular urine test: development of a method to aid in the diagnosis of prostate cancer. Clin Chem 2006;52(6):1089–95.

13. Deras IL, Aubin SMJ, Blase A, et al. PCA3: a molecular urine assay for predicting prostate biopsy outcome. J Urol 2008;179(4):1587–92.

14. Chun FK, de la Taille A, van Poppel H, et al. Prostate cancer gene 3 (PCA3): development and internal validation of a novel biopsy nomogram. Eur Urol 2009;56(4):659–68.

15. Marks LS, Fradet Y, Lim Deras I, et al. PCA3 molecular urine assay for prostate cancer in men undergoing repeat biopsy. Urology 2007;69(3):532–5.

16. Haese A, de la Taille A, van Poppel H, et al. Clinical utility of the PCA3 urine assay in European men scheduled for repeat biopsy. Eur Urol 2008;54(5):1081–8.

17. Auprich M, Haese A, Walz J, et al. External validation of urinary PCA3-based nomograms to individually predict prostate biopsy outcome. Eur Urol 2010;58(5):727–32.

18. Hessels D, Schalken JA. The use of PCA3 in the diagnosis of prostate cancer. Nat Rev Urol 2009;6(5):255–61.

19. Luo Y, Gou X, Huang P, et al. The PCA3 test for guiding repeat biopsy of prostate cancer and its cut-off score: a systematic review and meta-analysis. Asian J Androl 2014;16(3):487–92.

20. Pepe P, Fraggetta F, Galia A, et al. PCA3 score and prostate cancer diagnosis at repeated saturation biopsy. Which cut-off? 20 or 35? Int Braz J Urol 2012;38(4):489–95.

21. Capoluongo E, Zambon CF, Basso D, et al. PCA3 score of 20 could improve prostate cancer detection: results obtained on 734 Italian individuals. Clin Chim Acta 2014;429:46–50.

22. Wei JT, Feng Z, Partin AW, et al. Can urinary PCA3 supplement PSA in the early detection of prostate cancer? J Clin Oncol 2014;32(36):4066–72.

23. Dijkstra S, Mulders PFA, Schalken JA. Clinical use of novel urine and blood based prostate cancer biomarkers: a review. Clin Biochem 2014;47(10–11):889–96.

24. Scattoni V, Lazzeri M, Lughezzani G, et al. Head-to-head comparison of prostate health index and urinary PCA3 for predicting cancer at initial or repeat biopsy. J Urol 2013;190(2):496–501.

25. Ferro M, Bruzzese D, Perdonà S, et al. Prostate health index (Phi) and prostate cancer antigen 3 (PCA3) significantly improve prostate cancer detection at initial biopsy in a total PSA range of 2-10 ng/ml. PLoS One 2013;8(7):e67687.

26. Hansen J, Auprich M, Ahyai SA, et al. Initial prostate biopsy: development and internal validation of a biopsy-specific nomogram based on the prostate cancer antigen 3 assay. Eur Urol 2013;63(2):201–9.

27. Ruffion A, Devonec M, Champetier D, et al. PCA3 and PCA3-based nomograms improve diagnostic accuracy in patients undergoing first prostate biopsy. Int J Mol Sci 2013;14(9):17767–80.

28. Ankerst DP, Groskopf J, Day JR, et al. Predicting prostate cancer risk through incorporation of prostate cancer gene 3. J Urol 2008;180:1303–8 [discussion: 1308]; [Erratum appears in J Urol 2009; 181(3):1507].

29. Chevli KK, Duff M, Walter P, et al. Urinary PCA3 as a predictor of prostate cancer in a cohort of 3,073 men undergoing initial prostate biopsy. J Urol 2014;191(6):1743–8.

30. Seisen T, Rouprêt M, Brault D, et al. Accuracy of the prostate health index versus the urinary prostate cancer antigen 3 score to predict overall and significant prostate cancer at initial biopsy. Prostate 2015;75(1):103–11.

31. Cantiello F, Russo GI, Ferro M, et al. Prognostic accuracy of prostate health index and urinary prostate cancer antigen 3 in predicting pathologic features after radical prostatectomy. Urol Oncol 2015;33(4):163.e15–23.

32. Ferro M, Lucarelli G, Bruzzese D, et al. Improving the prediction of pathologic outcomes in patients undergoing radical prostatectomy: the value of prostate cancer antigen 3 (PCA3), prostate health index (Phi) and sarcosine. Anticancer Res 2015; 1024(2):1017–23.

33. Jones TD, Koch MO, Bunde PJ, et al. Is prostate-specific antigen (PSA) density better than the preoperative PSA level in predicting early biochemical recurrence of prostate cancer after radical prostatectomy? BJU Int 2006;97(3):480–4.

34. Siegrist TC, Panagopoulos G, Armenakas NA. PCA3 permutation increases the prostate biopsy yield. Commun Oncol 2012;9(8):243–6.

35. Ruffion a, Perrin P, Devonec M, et al. Additional value of PCA3 density to predict initial prostate biopsy outcome. World J Urol 2014;32(4):917–23.

36. De Luca S, Passera R, Cappia S, et al. Fluctuation in prostate cancer gene 3 (PCA3) score in men undergoing first or repeat prostate biopsies. BJU Int 2014;114(6b):E56–61.

37. De Luca SDE, Passera R, Cappia S, et al. Pathological patterns of prostate biopsy in men with fluctuations of prostate cancer gene 3 score: a preliminary report. Anticancer Res 2015;2422:2417–22.

38. Sequeiros T, Bastarós JM, Sánchez M, et al. Urinary biomarkers for the detection of prostate cancer in patients with high-grade prostatic intraepithelial neoplasia. Prostate 2015;75(10):1102–13.

39. Leyten GH, Wierenga EA, Sedelaar JPM, et al. Value of PCA3 to predict biopsy outcome and its potential role in selecting patients for multiparametric MRI. Int J Mol Sci 2013;14(6):11347–55.

40. Porpiglia F, Russo F, Manfredi M, et al. The roles of multiparametric magnetic resonance imaging, PCA3 and prostate health index-which is the best predictor of prostate cancer after a negative biopsy? J Urol 2014;192(1):60–6.

41. Rosenkrantz AB, Kim S, Lim RP, et al. Prostate cancer localization using multiparametric MR imaging: comparison of prostate imaging reporting and data system (PI-RADS) and Likert scales. Radiology 2013;269(2):482–92.

42. Roethke MC, Kuru TH, Schultze S, et al. Evaluation of the ESUR PI-RADS scoring system for multiparametric MRI of the prostate with targeted MR/TRUS fusion-guided biopsy at 3.0 Tesla. Eur Radiol 2014; 24(2):344–52.

43. Hamoen EHJ, de Rooij M, Witjes JA, et al. Use of the prostate imaging reporting and data system (PI-RADS) for prostate cancer detection with multiparametric magnetic resonance imaging: a diagnostic meta-analysis. Eur Urol 2014;67(6):1112–21.

44. Loeb S, Bruinsma SM, Nicholson J, et al. Active surveillance for prostate cancer: a systematic review of clinicopathologic variables and biomarkers for risk stratification. Eur Urol 2015; 67(4):619–26.

45. Tosoian JJ, Loeb S, Kettermann A, et al. Accuracy of PCA3 measurement in predicting short-term biopsy progression in an active surveillance program. J Urol 2010;183(2):534–8.

46. Vlaeminck-Guillem V, Devonec M, Colombel M, et al. Urinary PCA3 score predicts prostate cancer multifocality. J Urol 2011;185(4):1234–9.

47. Bradley LA, Palomaki GE, Gutman S, et al. Comparative effectiveness review: prostate cancer antigen 3 testing for the diagnosis and management of prostate cancer. J Urol 2013;190(2):389–98.

48. Calonge N. Recommendations from the EGAPP Working Group: does PCA3 testing for the diagnosis and management of prostate cancer improve patient health outcomes? Genet Med 2014;16(4): 338–46.

49. Tomlins SA, Rhodes DR, Perner S, et al. Recurrent fusion of TMPRSS2 and ETS transcription factor genes in prostate cancer. Science 2005; 310(5748):644–8.

50. Iljin K, Wolf M, Edgren H, et al. TMPRSS2 fusions with oncogenic ETS factors in prostate cancer involve unbalanced genomic rearrangements and are associated with HDAC1 and epigenetic reprogramming. Cancer Res 2006;66(21):10242–6.

51. Mehra R, Tomlins SA, Shen R, et al. Comprehensive assessment of TMPRSS2 and ETS family gene aberrations in clinically localized prostate cancer. Mod Pathol 2007;20(5):538–44.

52. Mosquera J-M, Mehra R, Regan MM, et al. Prevalence of TMPRSS2-ERG fusion prostate cancer among men undergoing prostate biopsy in the United States. Clin Cancer Res 2009;15(14): 4706–11.

53. Magi-Galluzzi C, Tsusuki T, Elson P, et al. TMPRSS2-ERG gene fusion prevalence and class are significantly different in prostate cancer of Caucasian, African-American and Japanese patients. Prostate 2011;71(5):489–97.

54. Pettersson A, Graff RE, Bauer SR, et al. The TMPRSS2:ERG rearrangement, ERG expression, and prostate cancer outcomes: a cohort study and meta-analysis. Cancer Epidemiol Biomarkers Prev 2012;21(9):1497–509.

55. Laxman B, Morris DS, Yu J, et al. A first-generation multiplex biomarker analysis of urine for the early detection of prostate cancer. Cancer Res 2008; 68(3):645–9.

56. Tomlins SA, Aubin SMJ, Siddiqui J, et al. Urine TMPRSS2:ERG fusion transcript stratifies prostate cancer risk in men with elevated serum PSA. Sci Transl Med 2011;3(94):94ra72.

57. Hessels D, Smit FP, Verhaegh GW, et al. Detection of TMPRSS2-ERG fusion transcripts and prostate cancer antigen 3 in urinary sediments may improve diagnosis of prostate cancer. Clin Cancer Res 2007;13(17):5103–8.

58. Young A, Palanisamy N, Siddiqui J, et al. Correlation of urine TMPRSS2:ERG and PCA3 to ERG+ and total prostate cancer burden. Am J Clin Pathol 2012;138(5):685–96.

59. Salami SS, Schmidt F, Laxman B, et al. Combining urinary detection of TMPRSS2:ERG and PCA3 with serum PSA to predict diagnosis of prostate cancer. Urol Oncol 2013;31(5):566–71.

60. Stephan C, Jung K, Semjonow A, et al. The TMPRSS2:ERG rearrangement, ERG expression, and prostate cancer outcomes: a cohort study and meta-analysis. Urol Oncol Semin Orig Investig 2013;9(5):566–71.

61. Individualized risk assessment of prostate cancer PCPTRC 1.0. Available at: http://deb.uthscsa.edu/URORiskCalc/Pages/calcs.jsp. Accessed September 20, 2015.

62. Cornu JN, Cancel-Tassin G, Egrot C, et al. Urine TMPRSS2: ERG fusion transcript integrated with PCA3 score, genotyping, and biological features are correlated to the results of prostatic biopsies in men at risk of prostate cancer. Prostate 2013;73(3):242–9.

63. Tallon L, Luangphakdy D, Ruffion A, et al. Comparative evaluation of urinary PCA3 and TMPRSS2: ERG scores and serum PHI in predicting prostate cancer aggressiveness. Int J Mol Sci 2014;15(8):13299–316.

64. Leyten GH, Hessels D, Jannink SA, et al. Prospective multicentre evaluation of PCA3 and TMPRSS2-ERG gene fusions as diagnostic and prognostic urinary biomarkers for prostate cancer. Eur Urol 2014;65(3):534–42.

65. Tomlins SA, Day JR, Lonigro RJ, et al. Urine TMPRSS2:ERG plus PCA3 for individualized prostate cancer risk assessment. Eur Urol 2015;1–9. [Epub ahead of print].

66. Lin DW, Newcomb LF, Brown EC, et al. Urinary TMPRSS2:ERG and PCA3 in an active surveillance

cohort: results from a baseline analysis in the canary prostate active surveillance study. Clin Cancer Res 2013;19(9):2442–50.

67. Tomlins SA, Rhodes DR, Yu J, et al. The role of SPINK1 in ETS rearrangement-negative prostate cancers. Cancer Cell 2008;13(6):519–28.

68. Jiang N, Zhu S, Chen J, et al. A-methylacyl-CoA racemase (AMACR) and prostate-cancer risk: a meta-analysis of 4,385 participants. PLoS One 2013;8(10):e74386.

69. Zielie PJ, Mobley JA, Ebb RG, et al. A novel diagnostic test for prostate cancer emerges from the determination of alpha-methylacyl-coenzyme a racemase in prostatic secretions. J Urol 2004; 172(3):1130–3.

70. Zehentner BK, Secrist H, Zhang X, et al. Detection of alpha-methylacyl-coenzyme-A racemase transcripts in blood and urine samples of prostate cancer patients. Mol Diagn Ther 2006;10(6):397–403.

71. Ouyang B, Bracken B, Burke B, et al. A duplex quantitative polymerase chain reaction assay based on quantification of alpha-methylacyl-CoA racemase transcripts and prostate cancer antigen 3 in urine sediments improved diagnostic accuracy for prostate cancer. J Urol 2009;181(6):2508–13 [discussion: 2513–4].

72. Leyten GH, Hessels D, Smit FP, et al. Identification of a candidate gene panel for the early diagnosis of prostate cancer. Clin Cancer Res 2015;3(13): 3061–71.

73. Ilic D, Neuberger MM, Djulbegovic M, et al. Screening for prostate cancer. Cochrane Database Syst Rev 2013;(1):CD004720.

74. Sapre N, Selth L. Circulating MicroRNAs as biomarkers of prostate cancer: the state of play. Prostate Cancer 2013;2013:539680.

75. Haj-Ahmad TA, Abdalla MA, Haj-Ahmad Y. Potential urinary protein biomarker candidates for the accurate detection of prostate cancer among benign prostatic hyperplasia patients. J Cancer 2014;5(3): 182–91.

76. Mitchell PS, Parkin RK, Kroh EM, et al. Circulating microRNAs as stable blood-based markers for cancer detection. Proc Natl Acad Sci U S A 2008; 105(30):10513–8.

77. Brase JC, Johannes M, Schlomm T, et al. Circulating miRNAs are correlated with tumor progression in prostate cancer. Int J Cancer 2011;128(3): 608–16.

78. Bryant RJ, Pawlowski T, Catto JWF, et al. Changes in circulating microRNA levels associated with prostate cancer. Br J Cancer 2012; 106(4):768–74.

79. Srivastava A, Goldberger H, Dimtchev A, et al. MicroRNA profiling in prostate cancer–the diagnostic potential of urinary miR-205 and miR-214. PLoS One 2013;8(10):e76994.

80. Stephan C, Jung M, Rabenhorst S, et al. Urinary miR-183 and miR-205 do not surpass PCA3 in urine as predictive markers for prostate biopsy outcome despite their highly dysregulated expression in prostate cancer tissue. Clin Chem Lab Med 2015;53(7):1109–18.

81. Zhang W, Ren S-C, Shi X-L, et al. A novel urinary long non-coding RNA transcript improves diagnostic accuracy in patients undergoing prostate biopsy. Prostate 2015;75(6):653–61.

82. Yang X, Gao L, Guo X, et al. A network based method for analysis of lncRNA-disease associations and prediction of lncRNAs implicated in diseases. PLoS One 2014;9(1):e87797.

83. Wang F, Ren S, Chen R, et al. Development and prospective multicenter evaluation of the long non-coding RNA MALAT-1 as a diagnostic urinary biomarker for prostate cancer. Oncotarget 2014; 5(22):11091–102.

84. Ren S, Liu Y, Xu W, et al. Long noncoding RNA MALAT-1 is a new potential therapeutic target for castration resistant prostate cancer. J Urol 2013; 190(6):2278–87.

85. Su Y-J, Yu J, Huang Y-Q, et al. Circulating long noncoding RNA as a potential target for prostate cancer. Int J Mol Sci 2015;16(6):13322–38.

86. Prensner JR, Iyer MK, Sahu A, et al. The long noncoding RNA SChLAP1 promotes aggressive prostate cancer and antagonizes the SWI/SNF complex. Nat Genet 2013;45(11):1392–8.

87. Atala A. Re: the long noncoding RNA SChLAP1 promotes aggressive prostate cancer and antagonizes the SWI/SNF complex. J Urol 2014;192(2):613.

88. Mehra R, Shi Y, Udager AM, et al. A novel RNA in situ hybridization assay for the long noncoding RNA SChLAP1 predicts poor clinical outcome after radical prostatectomy in clinically localized prostate cancer. Neoplasia 2014;16(12):1121–7.

89. Leon SA, Shapiro B, Sklaroff DM, et al. Free DNA in the serum of cancer patients and the effect of therapy. Cancer Res 1977;37(3):646–50.

90. Shapiro B, Shapiro B, Chakrabarty M, et al. Determination of circulating DNA levels in patients with benign or malignant gastrointestinal disease. Cancer 1983;51(11):2116–20.

91. Ellinger J, Müller SC, Stadler TC, et al. The role of cell-free circulating DNA in the diagnosis and prognosis of prostate cancer. Urol Oncol 2011;29(2): 124–9.

92. Thuret R, Chantrel-Groussard K, Azzouzi A-R, et al. Clinical relevance of genetic instability in prostatic cells obtained by prostatic massage in early prostate cancer. Br J Cancer 2005;92(2):236–40.

93. Meiers I, Shanks JH, Bostwick DG. Glutathione S-transferase pi (GSTP1) hypermethylation in prostate cancer: review 2007. Pathology 2007;39(3): 299–304.

94. Cannas A, Kalunga G, Green C, et al. Implications of storing urinary DNA from different populations for molecular analyses. PLoS One 2009;4(9):e6985.

95. Wee EJH, Ngo TH, Trau M. Colorimetric detection of both total genomic and loci-specific DNA methylation from limited DNA inputs. Clin Epigenetics 2015;7(1):65.

96. Stroun M, Anker P, Maurice P, et al. Neoplastic characteristics of the DNA found in the plasma of cancer patients. Oncology 1989;46(5):318–22.

97. Jahr S, Hentze H, Englisch S, et al. DNA fragments in the blood plasma of cancer patients: quantitations and evidence for their origin from apoptotic and necrotic cells. Cancer Res 2001;61(4):1659–65.

98. Ellinger J, Bastian PJ, Haan KI, et al. Noncancerous PTGS2 DNA fragments of apoptotic origin in sera of prostate cancer patients qualify as diagnostic and prognostic indicators. Int J Cancer 2008;122(1):138–43.

99. Ellinger J, Haan K, Heukamp LC, et al. CpG island hypermethylation in cell-free serum DNA identifies patients with localized prostate cancer. Prostate 2008;68(1):42–9.

100. Huang ZH, Li LH, Hua D. Quantitative analysis of plasma circulating DNA at diagnosis and during follow-up of breast cancer patients. Cancer Lett 2006;243(1):64–70.

101. Ellinger J, Albers P, Müller SC, et al. Circulating mitochondrial DNA in the serum of patients with testicular germ cell cancer as a novel noninvasive diagnostic biomarker. BJU Int 2009;104(1):48–52.

102. Ellinger J, Bastian PJ, Ellinger N, et al. Apoptotic DNA fragments in serum of patients with muscle invasive bladder cancer: a prognostic entity. Cancer Lett 2008;264(2):274–80.

103. Jung K, Stephan C, Lewandowski M, et al. Increased cell-free DNA in plasma of patients with metastatic spread in prostate cancer. Cancer Lett 2004;205(2):173–80.

104. Gordian E, Ramachandran K, Reis IM, et al. Serum free circulating DNA is a useful biomarker to distinguish benign versus malignant prostate disease. Cancer Epidemiol Biomarkers Prev 2010;19(8):1984–91.

105. Altimari A, Grigioni AD, Benedettini E, et al. Diagnostic role of circulating free plasma DNA detection in patients with localized prostate cancer. Am J Clin Pathol 2008;129(5):756–62.

106. Bastian PJ, Palapattu GS, Yegnasubramanian S, et al. CpG island hypermethylation profile in the serum of men with clinically localized and hormone refractory metastatic prostate cancer. J Urol 2008;179(2):529–34.

107. Casadio V, Calistri D, Salvi S, et al. Urine cell-free DNA integrity as a marker for early prostate cancer diagnosis: a pilot study. Biomed Res Int 2013;2013:270457.

108. Casadio V, Calistri D, Tebaldi M, et al. Urine cell-free DNA integrity as a marker for early bladder cancer diagnosis: preliminary data. Urol Oncol 2013;31(8):1744–50.

109. Chang H-W, Lee SM, Goodman SN, et al. Assessment of plasma DNA levels, allelic imbalance, and CA 125 as diagnostic tests for cancer. J Natl Cancer Inst 2002;94(22):1697–703.

110. Boynton KA, Summerhayes IC, Ahlquist DA, et al. DNA integrity as a potential marker for stool-based detection of colorectal cancer. Clin Chem 2003;49(7):1058–65.

111. Hanley R, Rieger-Christ KM, Canes D, et al. DNA integrity assay: a plasma-based screening tool for the detection of prostate cancer. Clin Cancer Res 2006;12(15):4569–74.

112. Barbieri CE, Bangma CH, Bjartell A, et al. The mutational landscape of prostate cancer. Eur Urol 2013;64(4):567–76.

113. Gonzalgo ML, Isaacs WB. Molecular pathways to prostate cancer. J Urol 2003;170(6 Pt 1):2444–52.

114. Cussenot O, Teillac P, Berthon P, et al. Noninvasive detection of genetic instability in cells from prostatic secretion as a marker of prostate cancer. Eur J Intern Med 2001;12(1):17–9.

115. Wolffe AP, Matzke MA. Epigenetics: regulation through repression. Science 1999;286(5439):481–6.

116. Jones PA. Functions of DNA methylation: islands, start sites, gene bodies and beyond. Nat Rev Genet 2012;13(7):484–92.

117. Strand SH, Orntoft TF, Sorensen KD. Prognostic DNA methylation markers for prostate cancer. Int J Mol Sci 2014;15(9):16544–76.

118. Haldrup C, Mundbjerg K, Vestergaard EM, et al. DNA methylation signatures for prediction of biochemical recurrence after radical prostatectomy of clinically localized prostate cancer. J Clin Oncol 2013;31(26):3250–8.

119. Wu T, Giovannucci E, Welge J, et al. Measurement of GSTP1 promoter methylation in body fluids may complement PSA screening: a meta-analysis. Br J Cancer 2011;105(1):65–73.

120. Goessl C, Müller M, Heicappell R, et al. DNA-based detection of prostate cancer in urine after prostatic massage. Urology 2001;58(3):335–8.

121. Hoque MO, Topaloglu O, Begum S, et al. Quantitative methylation-specific polymerase chain reaction gene patterns in urine sediment distinguish prostate cancer patients from control subjects. J Clin Oncol 2005;23(27):6569–75.

122. Jatkoe TA, Karnes RJ, Freedland SJ, et al. A urine-based methylation signature for risk stratification within low-risk prostate cancer. Br J Cancer 2015;112(5):802–8.

123. Baden J, Green G, Painter J, et al. Multicenter evaluation of an investigational prostate cancer methylation assay. J Urol 2009;182(3):1186–93.

124. Daniūnaitė K, Berezniakovas A, Jankevičius F, et al. Frequent methylation of RASSF1 and RARB in urine sediments from patients with early stage prostate cancer. Medicina (Kaunas) 2011;47(3):147–53.

125. Geisler C, Gaisa NT, Pfister D, et al. Identification and validation of potential new biomarkers for prostate cancer diagnosis and prognosis using 2D-DIGE and MS. Biomed Res Int 2015;2015:454256.

126. Li C, Zang T, Wrobel K, et al. Quantitative urinary proteomics using stable isotope labelling by peptide dimethylation in patients with prostate cancer. Anal Bioanal Chem 2015;407(12):3393–404.

127. Jedinak A, Curatolo A, Zurakowski D, et al. Novel non-invasive biomarkers that distinguish between benign prostate hyperplasia and prostate cancer. BMC Cancer 2015;15(1):259.

128. Afkarian M, Bhasin M, Dillon ST, et al. Optimizing a proteomics platform for urine biomarker discovery. Mol Cell Proteomics 2010;9(10):2195–204.

129. Monteiro MS, Carvalho M, Bastos ML, et al. Metabolomics analysis for biomarker discovery: advances and challenges. Curr Med Chem 2013;20(2):257–71.

130. Griffiths WJ, Koal T, Wang Y, et al. Targeted metabolomics for biomarker discovery. Angew Chem Int Ed Engl 2010;49(32):5426–45.

131. Spratlin JL, Serkova NJ, Eckhardt SG. Clinical applications of metabolomics in oncology: a review. Clin Cancer Res 2009;15(2):431–40.

132. Sreekumar A, Poisson LM, Rajendiran TM, et al. Metabolomic profiles delineate potential role for sarcosine in prostate cancer progression. Nature 2009;457(7231):910–4.

133. Jentzmik F, Stephan C, Miller K, et al. Sarcosine in urine after digital rectal examination fails as a marker in prostate cancer detection and identification of aggressive tumours. Eur Urol 2010;58(1):12–8 [discussion: 20–1].

134. Sreekumar A, Poisson LM, Rajendiran TM, et al. Re: Florian Jentzmik, Carsten Stephan, Kurt Miller, et al. Sarcosine in urine after digital rectal examination fails as a marker in prostate cancer detection and identification of aggressive tumours. Eur Urol 2010;58:12–8. Eur Urol 2010;58(3):e29–30 [author reply: e31–2].

135. Trock BJ. Application of metabolomics to prostate cancer. Urol Oncol 2011;29(5):572–81.

136. Cernei N, Heger Z, Gumulec J, et al. Sarcosine as a potential prostate cancer biomarker-a review. Int J Mol Sci 2013;14(7):13893–908.

137. McDunn JE, Li Z, Adam K-P, et al. Metabolomic signatures of aggressive prostate cancer. Prostate 2013;73(14):1547–60.

138. Thapar R, Titus MA. Recent advances in metabolic profiling and imaging of prostate cancer. Curr Metabolomics 2014;2(1):53–69.

139. Emwas A-H, Luchinat C, Turano P, et al. Standardizing the experimental conditions for using urine in NMR-based metabolomic studies with a particular focus on diagnostic studies: a review. Metabolomics 2014;11(4):872–94.

140. Nilsson J, Skog J, Nordstrand A, et al. Prostate cancer-derived urine exosomes: a novel approach to biomarkers for prostate cancer. Br J Cancer 2009;100(10):1603–7.

141. Jansen FH, Krijgsveld J, van Rijswijk A, et al. Exosomal secretion of cytoplasmic prostate cancer xenograft-derived proteins. Mol Cell Proteomics 2009;8(6):1192–205.

142. Burden HP, Holmes CH, Persad R, et al. Prostasomes–their effects on human male reproduction and fertility. Hum Reprod Update 2006;12(3):283–92.

143. Mitchell PJ, Welton J, Staffurth J, et al. Can urinary exosomes act as treatment response markers in prostate cancer? J Transl Med 2009;7:4.

144. Skog J, Würdinger T, van Rijn S, et al. Glioblastoma microvesicles transport RNA and proteins that promote tumour growth and provide diagnostic biomarkers. Nat Cell Biol 2008;10(12):1470–6.

145. Taylor DD, Gercel-Taylor C. MicroRNA signatures of tumor-derived exosomes as diagnostic biomarkers of ovarian cancer. Gynecol Oncol 2008;110(1):13–21.

146. Tompkins AJ, Chatterjee D, Maddox M, et al. The emergence of extracellular vesicles in urology: fertility, cancer, biomarkers and targeted pharmacotherapy. J Extracell Vesicles 2015;4:23815.

147. Øverbye A, Skotland T, Koehler CJ, et al. Identification of prostate cancer biomarkers in urinary exosomes. Oncotarget 2015. [Epub ahead of print].

148. Duijvesz D, Luider T, Bangma CH, et al. Exosomes as biomarker treasure chests for prostate cancer. Eur Urol 2011;59(5):823–31.

149. Dijkstra S, Birker IL, Smit FP, et al. Prostate cancer biomarker profiles in urinary sediments and exosomes. J Urol 2014;191(4):1132–8.

150. Principe S, Jones EE, Kim Y, et al. In-depth proteomic analyses of exosomes isolated from expressed prostatic secretions in urine. Proteomics 2013;13(10–11):1667–71.

151. Bijnsdorp IV, Geldof AA, Lavaei M, et al. Exosomal ITGA3 interferes with non-cancerous prostate cell functions and is increased in urine exosomes of metastatic prostate cancer patients. J Extracell Vesicles 2013;2.

152. Dubois L, Stridsberg M, Kharaziha P, et al. Malignant cell-derived extracellular vesicles express different chromogranin epitopes compared to prostasomes. Prostate 2015;75(10):1063–73.

153. Donovan MJ, Noerholm M, Bentink S, et al. A first-catch, non-DRE urine exosome gene signature to predict Gleason 7 prostate cancer on an initial prostate biopsy. Genitourinary Cancers Symposium taking place. Orlando, February 26–28, 2015.

154. Drake RR, Kislinger T. The proteomics of prostate cancer exosomes. Expert Rev Proteomics 2014; 11(2):167–77.

155. György B, Hung ME, Breakefield XO, et al. Therapeutic applications of extracellular vesicles: clinical promise and open questions. Annu Rev Pharmacol Toxicol 2015;55(1):439–64.

156. An T, Qin S, Xu Y, et al. Exosomes serve as tumour markers for personalized diagnostics owing to their important role in cancer metastasis. J Extracell Vesicles 2015;4:27522.

157. Brett SI, Kim Y, Biggs CN, et al. Extracellular vesicles such as prostate cancer cell fragments as a fluid biopsy for prostate cancer. Prostate Cancer Prostatic Dis 2015;18(3):213–20.

158. Turnbaugh PJ, Ley RE, Hamady M, et al. The human microbiome project. Nature 2007;449(7164):804–10.

159. Gill SR, Pop M, Deboy RT, et al. Metagenomic analysis of the human distal gut microbiome. Science 2006;312(5778):1355–9.

160. Guarner F, Malagelada JR. Gut flora in health and disease. Lancet 2003;361(9356):512–9.

161. Marrazzo JM. Interpreting the epidemiology and natural history of bacterial vaginosis: are we still confused? Anaerobe 2011;17(4):186–90.

162. Proctor LM. The human microbiome project in 2011 and beyond. Cell Host Microbe 2011;10(4):287–91.

163. Fouts DE, Pieper R, Szpakowski S, et al. Integrated next-generation sequencing of 16S rDNA and metaproteomics differentiate the healthy urine microbiome from asymptomatic bacteriuria in neuropathic bladder associated with spinal cord injury. J Transl Med 2012;10(1):174.

164. Lewis DA, Brown R, Williams J, et al. The human urinary microbiome; bacterial DNA in voided urine of asymptomatic adults. Front Cell Infect Microbiol 2013;3:41.

165. Nelson DE, van der Pol B, Dong Q, et al. Characteristic male urine microbiomes associate with asymptomatic sexually transmitted infection. PLoS One 2010;5(11):e14116.

166. Siddiqui H, Nederbragt AJ, Lagesen K, et al. Assessing diversity of the female urine microbiota by high throughput sequencing of 16S rDNA amplicons. BMC Microbiol 2011;11(1):244.

167. Whiteside SA, Razvi H, Dave S, et al. The microbiome of the urinary tract–a role beyond infection. Nat Rev Urol 2015;12(2):81–90.

168. Xu W, Yang L, Lee P, et al. Mini-review: perspective of the microbiome in the pathogenesis of urothelial carcinoma. Am J Clin Exp Urol 2014;2(1):57–61.

169. Yu H, Meng H, Zhou F, et al. Urinary microbiota in patients with prostate cancer and benign prostatic hyperplasia. Arch Med Sci 2015;11(2): 385–94.

170. Stamey TA, Kabalin JN. Prostate specific antigen in the diagnosis and treatment of adenocarcinoma of the prostate. I. Untreated patients. J Urol 1989; 141(5):1070–5.

171. Oesterling JE. Prostate specific antigen: a critical assessment of the most useful tumor marker for adenocarcinoma of the prostate. J Urol 1991; 145(5):907–23.

172. el-Shirbiny AM. Prostatic specific antigen. Adv Clin Chem 1994;31:99–133.

173. Stamey T, Caldwell M, Mcneal J, et al. The prostate specific antigen era in the United States is over for prostate cancer: what happened in the last 20 years? J Urol 2004;172(4):1297–301.

174. Strebhardt K, Ullrich A. Paul Ehrlich's magic bullet concept: 100 years of progress. Nat Rev Cancer 2008;8(6):473–80.

175. Tosoian J, Loeb S. PSA and beyond: the past, present, and future of investigative biomarkers for prostate cancer. ScientificWorldJournal 2010;10: 1919–31.

176. Wei JT. Urinary biomarkers for prostate cancer. Curr Opin Urol 2015;25(1):77–82.

177. Stephan C, Ralla B, Jung K. Prostate-specific antigen and other serum and urine markers in prostate cancer. Biochim Biophys Acta 2014;1846(1):99–112.

178. Pepe P, Aragona F. Prostate cancer detection rate at repeat saturation biopsy: PCPT risk calculator versus PCA3 score versus case-finding protocol. Can J Urol 2013;20(1):6620–4.

179. Goode RR, Marshall SJ, Duff M, et al. Use of PCA3 in detecting prostate cancer in initial and repeat prostate biopsy patients. Prostate 2013;73(1):48–53.

180. Wu AK, Reese AC, Cooperberg MR, et al. Utility of PCA3 in patients undergoing repeat biopsy for prostate cancer. Prostate Cancer Prostatic Dis 2012;15(1):100–5.

181. Bollito E, De Luca S, Cicilano M, et al. Prostate cancer gene 3 urine assay cutoff in diagnosis of prostate cancer: a validation study on an Italian patient population undergoing first and repeat biopsy. Anal Quant Cytol Histol 2012;34(2):96–104.

182. Barbera M, Pepe P, Paola Q, et al. PCA3 score accuracy in diagnosing prostate cancer at repeat biopsy: our experience in 177 patients. Arch Ital Urol Androl 2012;84(4):227–9.

183. Auprich M, Augustin H, Budäus L, et al. A comparative performance analysis of total prostate-specific antigen, percentage free prostate-specific antigen, prostate-specific antigen velocity and urinary prostate cancer gene 3 in the first, second and third repeat prostate biopsy. BJU Int 2012; 109(11):1627–35.

184. Pepe P, Aragona F. PCA3 score vs PSA free/total accuracy in prostate cancer diagnosis at repeat saturation biopsy. Anticancer Res 2011;31(12): 4445–9.

185. Aubin SMJ, Reid J, Sarno MJ, et al. PCA3 molecular urine test for predicting repeat prostate biopsy

outcome in populations at risk: validation in the placebo arm of the dutasteride REDUCE trial. J Urol 2010;184(5):1947–52.

186. Talesa VN, Antognelli C, Del Buono C, et al. Diagnostic potential in prostate cancer of a panel of urinary molecular tumor markers. Cancer Biomark 2009;5(6):241–51.

187. Rigau M, Morote J, Mir MC, et al. PSGR and PCA3 as biomarkers for the detection of prostate cancer in urine. Prostate 2010;70(16):1760–7.

188. Rigau M, Ortega I, Mir MC, et al. A three-gene panel on urine increases PSA specificity in the detection of prostate cancer. Prostate 2011; 71(16):1736–45.

189. Jamaspishvili T, Kral M, Khomeriki I, et al. Quadriplex model enhances urine-based detection of prostate cancer. Prostate Cancer Prostatic Dis 2011;14(4):354–60.

190. Dimitriadis E, Kalogeropoulos T, Velaeti S, et al. Study of genetic and epigenetic alterations in urine samples as diagnostic markers for prostate cancer. Anticancer Res 2013;33(1):191–7.

191. Rouprêt M, Hupertan V, Yates DR, et al. Molecular detection of localized prostate cancer using quantitative methylation-specific PCR on urinary cells obtained following prostate massage. Clin Cancer Res 2007;13(6):1720–5.

192. Woodson K, O'Reilly KJ, Hanson JC, et al. The usefulness of the detection of GSTP1 methylation in urine as a biomarker in the diagnosis of prostate cancer. J Urol 2008;179(2):508–11 [discussion: 511–2].

193. Vener T, Derecho C, Baden J, et al. Development of a multiplexed urine assay for prostate cancer diagnosis. Clin Chem 2008;54(5):874–82.

194. Payne SR, Serth J, Schostak M, et al. DNA methylation biomarkers of prostate cancer: confirmation of candidates and evidence urine is the most sensitive body fluid for non-invasive detection. Prostate 2009;69(12):1257–69.

195. Baden J, Adams S, Astacio T, et al. Predicting prostate biopsy result in men with prostate specific antigen 2.0 to 10.0 ng/mL using an investigational prostate cancer methylation assay. J Urol 2011; 186(5):2101–6.

196. Rogers CG, Yan G, Zha S, et al. Prostate cancer detection on urinalysis for alpha methylacyl coenzyme a racemase protein. J Urol 2004;172(4 Pt 1):1501–3.

197. M'Koma AE, Blum DL, Norris JL, et al. Detection of pre-neoplastic and neoplastic prostate disease by MALDI profiling of urine. Biochem Biophys Res Commun 2007;353(3):829–34.

198. Roy R, Louis G, Loughlin KR, et al. Tumor-specific urinary matrix metalloproteinase fingerprinting: identification of high molecular weight urinary matrix metalloproteinase species. Clin Cancer Res 2008;14(20):6610–7.

199. Theodorescu D, Schiffer E, Bauer HW, et al. Discovery and validation of urinary biomarkers for prostate cancer. Proteomics Clin Appl 2008;2(4):556–70.

200. Fujita K, Ewing CM, Sokoll LJ, et al. Cytokine profiling of prostatic fluid from cancerous prostate glands identifies cytokines associated with extent of tumor and inflammation. Prostate 2008;68(8):872–82.

201. Schostak M, Schwall GP, Poznanović S, et al. Annexin A3 in urine: a highly specific noninvasive marker for prostate cancer early detection. J Urol 2009;181(1):343–53.

202. Fujita K, Ewing CM, Chan DYS, et al. Endoglin (CD105) as a urinary and serum marker of prostate cancer. Int J Cancer 2009;124(3):664–9.

203. Morgan R, Boxall A, Bhatt A, et al. Engrailed-2 (EN2): a tumor specific urinary biomarker for the early diagnosis of prostate cancer. Clin Cancer Res 2011;17(5):1090–8.

204. Pandha H, Sorensen KD, Orntoft TF, et al. Urinary engrailed-2 (EN2) levels predict tumour volume in men undergoing radical prostatectomy for prostate cancer. BJU Int 2012;110(6 Pt B):E287–92.

205. Katafigiotis I, Tyritzis SI, Stravodimos KG, et al. Zinc α2-glycoprotein as a potential novel urine biomarker for the early diagnosis of prostate cancer. BJU Int 2012;110(11 Pt B):E688–93.

206. Mhatre DR, Mahale SD, Khatkhatay MI, et al. Development of an ELISA for sPSP94 and utility of the sPSP94/sPSA ratio as a diagnostic indicator to differentiate between benign prostatic hyperplasia and prostate cancer. Clin Chim Acta 2014;436: 256–62.

207. Davalieva K, Kiprijanovska S, Komina S, et al. Proteomics analysis of urine reveals acute phase response proteins as candidate diagnostic biomarkers for prostate cancer. Proteome Sci 2015; 13(1):2.

208. Vermassen T, Van Praet C, Lumen N, et al. Urinary prostate protein glycosylation profiling as a diagnostic biomarker for prostate cancer. Prostate 2015;75(3):314–22.

209. Hanley JA, McNeil BJ. The meaning and use of the area under a receiver operating characteristic (ROC) curve. Radiology 1982;143(1):29–36.

210. Eng J. Receiver operating characteristic analysis: a primer. Acad Radiol 2005;12(7):909–16.

211. Parikh R, Mathai A, Parikh S, et al. Understanding and using sensitivity, specificity and predictive values. Indian J Ophthalmol 2008;56(1):45–50.

212. Kanchanaraksa S. Evaluation of Diagnostic and Screening Tests: Validity and Reliability. Baltimore: Johns Hopkins University; 2012. Available at: http:// ocw.jhsph.edu/courses/fundepi/PDFs/Lecture11.pdf.

4-Kallikrein Test and Kallikrein Markers in Prostate Cancer Screening

Michelle L. McDonald, MD, J. Kellogg Parsons, MD, MHS*

KEYWORDS

- Prostate cancer • Biomarker • Kallikrein panel (4K panel) • Kallikrein score (4Kscore) • Screening
- Detection

KEY POINTS

- Overdetection of prostate cancer is in part attributable to the relatively low specificity and positive predictive value of prostate-specific antigen (PSA)-based screening.
- Biomarkers that enhance the performance characteristics of PSA and differentiate between indolent and lethal prostate cancers are needed.
- Tests with increased specificity for clinically significant cancer may decrease the number of men undergoing prostate biopsy and diminish the detection of indolent, clinically insignificant disease.
- As observed in multiple studies, the serum 4-kallikrein (4K) panel accurately predicts the risk of biopsy-detectable high-grade cancer (Gleason score ≥7) in men who have never undergone prostate biopsy or in those with a prior negative biopsy.
- The 4Kscore provides a probability score for the risk of biopsy-detectable cancer and may inform care in men who have never undergone prostate biopsy and in those with a prior negative biopsy.

INTRODUCTION

Since the early 1990s,[1] prostate cancer mortality has decreased 45%, a trend largely attributed to early detection through widespread use of prostate-specific antigen (PSA)–based prostate cancer screening.[2–4] Screen-detected prostate cancers constitute a spectrum of disease ranging from the indolent to the highly aggressive.[5] The goal of screening is to maximize the early diagnosis of potentially aggressive but curable disease while minimizing both the detection of indolent disease and the number of invasive confirmatory tests.[6,7] However, the relatively poor specificity of PSA has contributed to the overdetection of indolent disease. Efforts have, therefore, focused on identifying new robust tools, such as novel biomarkers, that increase specificity for prostate cancer detection. A newer biomarker, the serum 4-kallikrein (4K) panel, may inform initial screening in men who have never undergone biopsy as well as in those with a prior negative biopsy. The authors review the 4K panel and its potential ability to improve prostate cancer screening.

Disclosure statement: The authors have nothing to disclose.
Department of Urology, UC San Diego Health, 200 West Arbor Drive #8897, San Diego, CA 92103-8897, USA
* Corresponding author. Department of Urology, UC San Diego Moores Cancer Center, UC San Diego Health, 3855 Health Sciences Drive #0987, La Jolla, CA 92093-0987.
E-mail address: jkparsons@ucsd.edu

Urol Clin N Am 43 (2016) 39–46
http://dx.doi.org/10.1016/j.ucl.2015.08.004
0094-0143/16/$ – see front matter © 2016 Elsevier Inc. All rights reserved.

LIMITATIONS IN PROSTATE-SPECIFIC ANTIGEN–BASED SCREENING FOR PROSTATE CANCER

The National Comprehensive Cancer Network supports the continued use of PSA testing for the early detection of prostate cancer[8] based on randomized trials confirming its efficacy to diminish prostate cancer mortality.[9,10] However, despite the survival benefits associated with PSA-based screening, the concern regarding the overdetection of insignificant prostate cancers remains.[11,12] Aggressive PSA-based screening decreases mortality by maximizing the early detection of both indolent and aggressive cancers. Overdetection is the diagnosis of screen-detected indolent prostate cancer that, left untreated, would otherwise not diminish overall or prostate cancer–specific survival. The rate of overdetection within the European Randomized Study of Screening for Prostate Cancer (ERSPC) was estimated to be approximately 50%.[13,14]

Overtreatment of screen-detected indolent cancers with surgery and radiation may unnecessarily expose patients to substantial risks that diminish health-related quality of life without affecting long-term oncologic outcomes. Overtreatment of prostate cancer in the United States is a momentous concern as 90% of US men diagnosed undergo treatment, and approximately 66% of those treated will be confirmed to have indolent disease.[12]

The lack of specificity and low positive predictive value of PSA contribute to the overdetection and, thus, overtreatment of prostate cancer.[9,10,15,16] PSA is an organ-specific rather than prostate cancer–specific biomarker.[16–18] No single PSA cutoff threshold has particularly good test performance characteristics in prostate cancer screening,[16,18,19] with a particularly low predictive accuracy in the gray zone of elevated PSA (3 ng/mL to 10 ng/mL).[20] Although higher PSA is associated with a higher stage and Gleason sum among men with cancer,[21,22] a prostate biopsy is positive for cancer in only around 25% of men with a PSA between 2 and 10 ng/mL and no prior diagnosis.[10,23] Moreover, some men with a low PSA may have clinically significant cancer.[24]

It is clear that blanket cessation of all screening for prostate cancer, as recommended by the US Preventative Services Task Force,[25] fails to acknowledge the biological heterogeneity of prostate cancer. Without screening, the 20% to 30% of men diagnosed with aggressive prostate cancer at presentation would potentially lose an opportunity for cure.[26] One potential solution is to focus on the detection of clinically significant prostate cancer by using tests with enhanced specificity.[27]

HUMAN KALLIKREINS

Human tissue kallikreins are a family of 15 secreted serine proteases, the regulatory functions of which are linked with the development of malignancy, respiratory disease, neurodegeneration, schizophrenia, and inflammation.[28] Kallikreins have received focused investigation over the past decade after the clinical applicability of human kallikrein 3 (hK3, or PSA) in prostate cancer screening was discovered.[28]

Most of the kallikreins are coexpressed in the prostate in varying amounts, although PSA (hK3) expression is restricted to the prostate and is almost exclusively produced by prostate epithelial cells.[28] PSA is produced under androgen regulation[29] and acts to liquefy semen after ejaculation.[30] PSA is present in several molecular forms within blood and prostatic fluid and is normally found at low concentrations in serum compared with that found in ejaculate. Most of the PSA in blood is complexed to protease inhibitors and is catalytically inactive.[16] The noncomplexed form, free PSA (fPSA), has several molecular forms (nicked, intact, and pro-PSA).[28,31] In proportion to total PSA (tPSA), fPSA is lower in men with prostate cancer than in men with benign prostate hyperplasia[32]; the percentage of fPSA has been used in an attempt to improve PSA specificity.[23]

Pro-PSA is an inactive precursor of PSA, which is cleaved by the protease action of human kallikrein 2 (hK2) rendering the mature form of PSA. The hK2 has several structural and functional similarities to PSA, although the concentration of hK2 in serum is lower than PSA.[17] The development of accurate assays for hK2 suggested that it may be useful in prostate cancer detection[33,34] and was subsequently found to be strongly expressed in high-grade prostate cancer.[35,36] Intact PSA (iPSA) and nicked PSA have also been found to be useful in discriminating men with benign from malignant prostatic disease.[37] Similar to hK2, iPSA increases as prostate cancer becomes more aggressive.[38,39]

KALLIKREIN PANEL

Combining other kallikreins with PSA in a screening panel enhances its performance characteristics. Multiple studies have observed that a panel of 4 serum kallikrein markers combined (the 4K panel) (tPSA, fPSA, single-chain iPSA, and hK2) improves the prediction of biopsy-detectable cancer compared with PSA alone. Assays for tPSA and fPSA are currently widely available; however, iPSA and hK2 require sophisticated assay calibration, which is not readily available.[40,41]

Method for Evaluating the 4 Kallikrein Panel

Diagnostic and prognostic models that predict the accuracy of a test may not address the relevance of such a test on actual clinical outcomes. Most studies on the 4K panel have assessed the predictive accuracy of adding kallikreins to a comparison base model of PSA alone and reported the results as the area under the receiver operating characteristic curve (**Table 1**). High-grade cancer was defined as biopsy Gleason sum 7 or higher.[42,43]

To evaluate whether the panel would improve clinical decision making, all relevant studies use a *decision curve analysis*.[44] This analytical method was first described in 2006 and estimates the net benefit of using a prediction model by summing the benefits (true positives) and subtracting the harms (false positives), whereby the latter is weighted by a factor related to the relative harm of a missed disease or event compared with an unnecessary intervention.[44]

When used in 4K analyses, the weighting is derived from the threshold probability of prostate cancer at which a patient would choose to be biopsied, and the net benefit is calculated across a range of probabilities. The model incorporating the 4K panel was deemed to be of clinical value if it had the highest net benefit across the full range of threshold probabilities at which a patient would choose to be biopsied.[42,44,45]

FOUR KALLIKREIN STUDIES IN MEN BEFORE BIOPSY
Unscreened Men

The 4K panel was initially evaluated in 2008 among 740 previously unscreened men who underwent a 6 core biopsy for a PSA of 3 ng/mL or greater in the Göteborg cohort of the ERSPC.[43] The panel was found to increase the predictive accuracy of diagnosing Gleason 7 or greater prostate cancer when added to a base model, including age, digital rectal examination (DRE), and tPSA. The area under the curve (AUC) for detecting high-grade cancer for the base model increased from 0.87 to 0.90 when the full kallikrein panel was added. These investigators concluded that using the full kallikrein panel would reduce biopsy rates by 60% for men with elevated PSA while missing only a small number of cancers (31 of 152 low-grade and 1 of 40 high-grade cancers).[43]

The 4 kallikrein proteins were subsequently evaluated in several additional European cohorts of unscreened men. The full panel, including age, DRE, tPSA, fPSA, intact PSA, and hK2, was assessed among 2914 unscreened men from the Rotterdam arm of the ERSPC.[46] Similar improvement in predictive accuracy for high-grade cancers was observed (AUC improved from 0.81 to 0.84); a reduction of biopsy rates was reported as 513 per 1000 men with elevated PSA and only missing a small number of high-grade cancers (12 per 100 men).[46]

In the Göteborg and Rotterdam ERSPC cohorts, all men with an elevated PSA were referred for biopsy per ERSPC protocol. In usual clinical practice, men with elevated PSA usually undergo clinical work-up before making the decision to proceed with biopsy. This work-up commonly includes an assessment of prior prostatitis, prostate hypertrophy, and family history of prostate cancer. This type of work-up can affect biomarker properties[47] and potentially the properties of a predictive model for prostate cancer. In an independent validation study, Benchikh and colleagues[45] determined whether a statistical model based on patients in the Rotterdam arm of ERPSC,[46] who underwent biopsy secondary to elevated PSA alone, would lose its predictive utility in a cohort of men who underwent a biopsy based on elevated PSA as well as clinical judgment, such as men biopsied in the Tarn, France arm of ERSPC.[45] In the France protocol, the decision to biopsy based on clinical judgment following DRE or repeat PSA test.[48] The kallikrein panel had a significantly higher predictive accuracy for any grade of cancer than the base model, with an AUC increase from 0.63 to 0.78, which was similar for high-grade cancer (0.77–0.87). Using a threshold of 20% or greater risk as indication for biopsy, 492 out of 1000 men would avoid biopsy and 61 men with cancer would be missed, of whom 12 would have high-grade disease. Individual contribution of each kallikrein to the panel was also assessed; fPSA was found to have the greatest contribution, although removing intact PSA and hK2 also led to a reduction in AUC, supporting the use of all 4 kallikreins in the panel. The investigators concluded the 4K panel can predict the result of prostate biopsy in men with elevated PSA and retains its value in men who underwent additional clinical evaluation before biopsy.

Screened Men

The predictive accuracy of PSA is lower in men who have been previously screened.[49,50] Initial reports of the kallikrein panel were based on the first round of the ERSPC, in which a small proportion had been previously screened with PSA (~3%). To assess whether the 4K panel retains its value in men with a recent PSA testing, Vickers and colleagues[50] applied the panel to 1241 men with an initial PSA less than 3 who, in subsequent rounds

Table 1
Review of 4K panel and 4Kscore studies

Study, Year	Study Population	Study Sample	Outcome Assessed	AUC Increase HG Cancers[a]	Set Threshold Risk	Clinical Outcome Reduction (%)	HG Cancers Missed
Vickers, 2008	Göteborg ERSPC	740 Unscreened men	6 Core bx	0.04	20% Any cancer	60 bx	2.5% (1 of 40)
Vickers, 2010	Rotterdam ERSPC	2914 Unscreened men	6 Core bx	0.03	20% Any cancer	51 bx	12% (12 of 100)
Benchikh, 2010	Tarn, France ERSPC	262 Unscreened men	10–12[b] Core bx	0.10	20% Any cancer	49 bx	6.8% (12 of 175)
Vickers, 2010	Göteborg ERSPC	1241 Screened men	6 Core bx	0.11	20% Any cancer	41 bx	2.3% (1 of 43)
Vickers, 2010	Rotterdam ERSPC	1501 Screened men	6 Core bx	0.09	20% Any cancer	44 bx	4.4% (4 of 91)
Gupta, 2010	Rotterdam ERSPC	925 Men with prior neg bx	6 Core bx	0.11	15% Any cancer	71 bx	16.7% (3 of 18)
Carlsson, 2013	Rotterdam ERSPC	392 Men after RP	RP pathology	0.03	30% Aggressive[c] cancer at RP	33 RP insignificant disease	3.9% (26 of 666)[c]
Parekh, 2014	US prospective trial	1012 Men referred for bx	10 Core bx	0.08[d]	9% HG cancer	43 bx	10.4% (24 of 231)

Abbreviations: AUC, area under the curve; bx, biopsy; HG, high grade; neg, negative; RP, radical prostatectomy.
[a] Area-under-the-curve increase of full kallikrein model compared with the base clinical model.
[b] Decision to biopsy based on clinical judgment following digital rectal examination or repeat PSA.
[c] Aggressive radical prostatectomy pathology defined as pT3-T4, extracapsular extension, tumor volume greater than 0.5 cm³, or any Gleason grade of 4 or greater.
[d] An 4Kscore area-under-the-curve increase compared with modified Prostate Cancer Prevention Trial Risk Calculator 2.0.

of the Göteborg arm of ERSPC, were found to have PSA greater than 3 and, therefore, underwent biopsy. The previously published model was poorly calibrated and missed many cancers. The investigators observed findings similar to those in unscreened men; a significant number of biopsies could be avoided (413 per 1000 men) and delay the diagnosis of only 1 high-grade cancer per 1000 men with elevated PSA.

The model was subsequently applied to 1501 previously screened men in the Rotterdam section of ERSPC in order to determine if findings could be replicated.[42] The AUC of high-grade cancer in the base model increased from 0.71 to 0.80 when the kallikrein panel was added. When the biopsy threshold was set at 20% risk of any cancer, the decrease in biopsy rate was deemed to be 362 for every 1000 men with elevated PSA and delayed 47 cancers, which would predominately be low grade. The investigators noted that a new model for recently screened men was necessary with the Göteborg cohort but not with the Rotterdam cohort. Newer assays were used to measure iPSA and hK2 for Rotterdam measurements.

FOUR KALLIKREIN STUDIES IN MEN WITH PRIOR NEGATIVE BIOPSY

The ability of PSA to predict the outcomes of repeat biopsy after initial negative biopsy is low.[51,52]

Men diagnosed with prostate cancer after a previous negative biopsy tend to have lower-risk disease with favorable outcomes.[53,54] Of the 3056 screened men with an initial negative biopsy in the Rotterdam division of the ERSPC, after a median follow-up of 11 years, 0.6% of cancers found on repeat biopsy resulted in death, compared with a 4.2% mortality rate of those cancers found at first biopsy.[53] Repeat biopsy in all men with continued elevated PSA and prior negative biopsy will lead to a substantial number of unnecessary biopsies and many potentially indolent cancers.[54] Thus, a strategy to decrease the number of unnecessary repeat biopsies is crucial.

The predictive accuracy of the kallikrein panel in men who underwent a second biopsy because of persistently elevated PSA after initial negative biopsy in the Rotterdam section of the ERSPC was assessed.[54] These investigators found that the full model including age, DRE, and 4K panel improved AUC from 0.76 to 0.87. When the decision for biopsy was set at a risk threshold of 15%, the biopsy rate would be decreased by 712 per 1000 men, missing 53 cancers—of which 3 would be Gleason 7.

SURGICAL PATHOLOGY PREDICTION

It has also been questioned as to whether a patient found to have pathologically insignificant disease of radical prostatectomy (RP) specimen should have instead undergone active surveillance. Recent data from randomized trials have suggested there is little or no difference in prostate cancer mortality between men with low-risk cancer who underwent radical therapy versus those who were observed.[55,56] Currently available prediction tools based on RP pathology demonstrate AUCs that from 0.70 to 0.80.[6]

Panel prognostication on pathologic examination of RP specimens was assessed in 392 screened men in the Rotterdam arm of ERSPC diagnosed with prostate cancer secondary to a PSA of 3 or greater and treated with RP from 1994 and 2004.[57] Clinical predictors (age, stage, PSA, biopsy findings) were assessed with and without levels of the 4 kallikreins. The AUC for predicting aggressive disease (pT3-T4, extracapsular extension, tumor volume $>0.5cm^3$, or any Gleason ≥ 4) with the clinical model was 0.81, which increased to 0.84 with the 4K panel. Clinical application of the model with the 4K panel would reduce rates of surgery by 110 out of 334 patients with pathologically insignificant disease.[57]

DEVELOPMENT OF THE 4K PROBABILITY SCORE

Samples from the ERSPC have been stored for years and may have previously been thawed and refrozen. Long-term storage and repeated freezing and rethawing degrade kallikreins.[58] Incorporating the 4K panel into the United States for investigation required modifications. The PSA and fPSA assays used in European studies are not approved by the Food and Drug Administration; therefore, different US assays are used.[59] Based on ERSPC studies and the Prostate Testing for Cancer and Treatment algorithm,[60] the 4 kallikreins were combined with age, DRE, and history of prior prostate biopsy into a single plasma test that assigns a probability score from less than 1% to greater than 95% of having biopsy-detectable, clinically significant prostate cancer (Gleason ≥ 7); 100% minus the score provides the negative predictive value or probability that a patient will not have Gleason 7 or greater cancer on biopsy.[61]

United States Prospective Validation

Before 2014, all reports of the 4K panel were consequent of retrospective European cohorts, sextant biopsy schemes, and noncontemporary Gleason grading. Parekh and colleagues[61] conducted the first multi-institutional prospective trial in the United States that evaluated the 4K panel among 1312 men referred to 26 urology centers for prostate biopsy. Referral for biopsy was per urologist discretion; no standard criteria were used, although a 10 core minimum prostate biopsy was included. Discrimination in predicting the probability of a clinically significant tumor was similar to previous reports. Analysis was performed with the threshold for biopsy set at 9% or greater probability of Gleason 7 or greater cancer revealed that 434 (43%) biopsies could be avoided and delay diagnosis of 24 (24%) of high-grade cancers. The investigators also compared the 4-kallikrein probability score with a modified Prostate Cancer Prevention Trial Risk Calculator 2.0 and showed a superior ability to predict Gleason 7 or greater prostate cancer with an AUC of 0.82 versus 0.74.

THE ECONOMIC IMPACT OF THE 4 KALLIKREIN PANEL AND 4KSCORE

The cost-effectiveness of the 4K panel in the setting of ambiguous PSA results (3 ng/mL–10 ng/mL) with or without prior PSA screening and with or without prior biopsy for a cancer-detection risk threshold of 20% or higher was examined in a meta-analysis.[6] These investigators determined the 4K panel provided a significant 8% to 13% improvement in predictive accuracy and resulted in a potential reduction in the number of biopsies by 48% to 56%, resulting in an annual US savings of $19 million to nearly $1 billion, depending on the test adoption and actual cost of the test. The 4Kscore Test is not readily available and currently only available in the United States through a single laboratory. The 4K panel does not require a novel clinical procedure, such as collection of urine after prostatic massage; however, the out-of-pocket cost to patients is currently $1185.00.[62]

SUMMARY

The 4K panel potentially informs care by providing an individualized prediction of clinically significant prostate cancer regardless of prior screening or previous biopsy.[61] This test may aid clinicians and patients in a process of shared decision for prostate biopsy and early detection of prostate cancer. In all cohorts, the proportion of biopsies that could have been avoided ranged from 41% to 71%, although the likelihood of potential delayed diagnosis of significant prostate cancer

was minimal. The model outcomes were replicated in independent validation studies with similar concordance between reported AUCs and biopsy reduction, although prospective studies focused on a younger population of men are needed. The threshold for biopsy will vary by patient and provider and is potentially lower for younger, healthier patients.[61] In order for such a panel to be useful among a large screening population it will need to become readily available and without a significant financial burden on patients.

REFERENCES

1. Siegel RL, Miller KD, Jemal A. Cancer statistics, 2015. CA Cancer J Clin 2015;65:5–29.
2. Jhaveri FM, Klein EA, Kupelian PA, et al. Declining rates of extracapsular extension after radical prostatectomy: evidence for continued stage migration. J Clin Oncol 1999;17:3167–72.
3. Etzioni R, Gulati R, Tsodikov A, et al. The prostate cancer conundrum revisited: treatment changes and prostate cancer mortality declines. Cancer 2012;118:5955–63.
4. Siegel R, Naishadham D, Jemal A. Cancer statistics, 2013. CA Cancer J Clin 2013;63:11–30.
5. Wilt TJ, Brawer MK, Jones KM, et al. Radical prostatectomy versus observation for localized prostate cancer. N Engl J Med 2012;367:203–13.
6. Voigt JD, Zappala SM, Vaughan ED, et al. The Kallikrein panel for prostate cancer screening: its economic impact. Prostate 2014;74:250–9.
7. Nam RK, Diamandis EP, Toi A, et al. Serum human glandular kallikrein-2 protease levels predict the presence of prostate cancer among men with elevated prostate-specific antigen. J Clin Oncol 2000;18:1036–42.
8. Carroll PR, Parsons JK, Andriole G, et al. Prostate cancer early detection, version 1.2014. Featured updates to the NCCN guidelines. J Natl Compr Canc Netw 2014;12:1211–9 [quiz: 1219].
9. Andriole GL, Crawford ED, Grubb RL 3rd, et al. Mortality results from a randomized prostate-cancer screening trial. N Engl J Med 2009;360:1310–9.
10. Schroder FH, Hugosson J, Roobol MJ, et al. Screening and prostate-cancer mortality in a randomized European study. N Engl J Med 2009;360: 1320–8.
11. Welch HG, Albertsen PC. Prostate cancer diagnosis and treatment after the introduction of prostate-specific antigen screening: 1986-2005. J Natl Cancer Inst 2009;101:1325–9.
12. Jalloh M, Myers F, Cowan JE, et al. Racial variation in prostate cancer upgrading and upstaging among men with low-risk clinical characteristics. Eur Urol 2015;67:451–7.

13. Draisma G, Boer R, Otto SJ, et al. Lead times and overdetection due to prostate-specific antigen screening: estimates from the European Randomized Study of Screening for Prostate Cancer. J Natl Cancer Inst 2003;95:868–78.

14. Draisma G, Etzioni R, Tsodikov A, et al. Lead time and overdiagnosis in prostate-specific antigen screening: importance of methods and context. J Natl Cancer Inst 2009;101:374–83.

15. Hugosson J, Carlsson S, Aus G, et al. Mortality results from the Goteborg randomised population-based prostate-cancer screening trial. Lancet Oncol 2010;11:725–32.

16. Lilja H, Ulmert D, Vickers AJ. Prostate-specific antigen and prostate cancer: prediction, detection and monitoring. Nat Rev Cancer 2008;8:268–78.

17. Bryant RJ, Lilja H. Emerging PSA-based tests to improve screening. Urol Clin North Am 2014;41: 267–76.

18. Punglia RS, D'Amico AV, Catalona WJ, et al. Impact of age, benign prostatic hyperplasia, and cancer on prostate-specific antigen level. Cancer 2006;106: 1507–13.

19. Ulmert D, Serio AM, O'Brien MF, et al. Long-term prediction of prostate cancer: prostate-specific antigen (PSA) velocity is predictive but does not improve the predictive accuracy of a single PSA measurement 15 years or more before cancer diagnosis in a large, representative, unscreened population. J Clin Oncol 2008;26:835–41.

20. Gilligan T. The new data on prostate cancer screening: what should we do now? Cleve Clin J Med 2009;76:446–8.

21. Stamey TA, Yang N, Hay AR, et al. Prostate-specific antigen as a serum marker for adenocarcinoma of the prostate. N Engl J Med 1987;317:909–16.

22. Pinsky PF, Andriole G, Crawford ED, et al. Prostate-specific antigen velocity and prostate cancer Gleason grade and stage. Cancer 2007;109:1689–95.

23. Catalona WJ, Partin AW, Slawin KM, et al. Use of the percentage of free prostate-specific antigen to enhance differentiation of prostate cancer from benign prostatic disease: a prospective multicenter clinical trial. JAMA 1998;279:1542–7.

24. Thompson IM, Pauler DK, Goodman PJ, et al. Prevalence of prostate cancer among men with a prostate-specific antigen level < or =4.0 ng per milliliter. N Engl J Med 2004;350:2239–46.

25. Moyer VA, U.S. Preventive Services Task Force. Screening for prostate cancer: U.S. Preventive Services Task Force recommendation statement. Ann Intern Med 2012;157:120–34.

26. Punnen S, Cooperberg MR. The epidemiology of high-risk prostate cancer. Curr Opin Urol 2013;23:331–6.

27. Prensner JR, Rubin MA, Wei JT, et al. Beyond PSA: the next generation of prostate cancer biomarkers. Sci Transl Med 2012;4:127rv3.

28. Prassas I, Eissa A, Poda G, et al. Unleashing the therapeutic potential of human kallikrein-related serine proteases. Nat Rev Drug Discov 2015;14: 183–202.

29. Young CY, Montgomery BT, Andrews PE, et al. Hormonal regulation of prostate-specific antigen messenger RNA in human prostatic adenocarcinoma cell line LNCaP. Cancer Res 1991;51:3748–52.

30. Lilja H. A kallikrein-like serine protease in prostatic fluid cleaves the predominant seminal vesicle protein. J Clin Invest 1985;76:1899–903.

31. Lilja H, Christensson A, Dahlen U, et al. Prostate-specific antigen in serum occurs predominantly in complex with alpha 1-antichymotrypsin. Clin Chem 1991;37:1618–25.

32. Christensson A, Bjork T, Nilsson O, et al. Serum prostate specific antigen complexed to alpha 1-antichymotrypsin as an indicator of prostate cancer. J Urol 1993;150:100–5.

33. Kumar A, Mikolajczyk SD, Goel AS, et al. Expression of pro form of prostate-specific antigen by mammalian cells and its conversion to mature, active form by human kallikrein 2. Cancer Res 1997;57:3111–4.

34. Martin BJ, Finlay JA, Sterling K, et al. Early detection of prostate cancer in African-American men through use of multiple biomarkers: human kallikrein 2 (hK2), prostate-specific antigen (PSA), and free PSA (fPSA). Prostate Cancer Prostatic Dis 2004;7:132–7.

35. Darson MF, Pacelli A, Roche P, et al. Human glandular kallikrein 2 (hK2) expression in prostatic intraepithelial neoplasia and adenocarcinoma: a novel prostate cancer marker. Urology 1997;49:857–62.

36. Tremblay RR, Deperthes D, Tetu B, et al. Immunohistochemical study suggesting a complementary role of kallikreins hK2 and hK3 (prostate-specific antigen) in the functional analysis of human prostate tumors. Am J Pathol 1997;150:455–9.

37. Steuber T, Nurmikko P, Haese A, et al. Discrimination of benign from malignant prostatic disease by selective measurements of single chain, intact free prostate specific antigen. J Urol 2002;168:1917–22.

38. Nam RK, Zhang WW, Trachtenberg J, et al. Single nucleotide polymorphism of the human kallikrein-2 gene highly correlates with serum human kallikrein-2 levels and in combination enhances prostate cancer detection. J Clin Oncol 2003;21:2312–9.

39. Denmeade SR, Sokoll LJ, Dalrymple S, et al. Dissociation between androgen responsiveness for malignant growth vs. expression of prostate specific differentiation markers PSA, hK2, and PSMA in human prostate cancer models. Prostate 2003;54: 249–57.

40. Vaisanen V, Peltola MT, Lilja H, et al. Intact free prostate-specific antigen and free and total human glandular kallikrein 2. Elimination of assay interference by enzymatic digestion of antibodies to F(ab')2 fragments. Anal Chem 2006;78:7809–15.

41. Haese A, Vaisanen V, Finlay JA, et al. Standardization of two immunoassays for human glandular kallikrein 2. Clin Chem 2003;49:601–10.

42. Vickers AJ, Cronin AM, Roobol MJ, et al. A four-kallikrein panel predicts prostate cancer in men with recent screening: data from the European Randomized Study of Screening for Prostate Cancer, Rotterdam. Clin Cancer Res 2010;16:3232–9.

43. Vickers AJ, Cronin AM, Aus G, et al. A panel of kallikrein markers can reduce unnecessary biopsy for prostate cancer: data from the European Randomized Study of Prostate Cancer Screening in Goteborg, Sweden. BMC Med 2008;6:19.

44. Vickers AJ, Elkin EB. Decision curve analysis: a novel method for evaluating prediction models. Med Decis Making 2006;26:565–74.

45. Benchikh A, Savage C, Cronin A, et al. A panel of kallikrein markers can predict outcome of prostate biopsy following clinical work-up: an independent validation study from the European Randomized Study of Prostate Cancer screening, France. BMC Cancer 2010;10:635.

46. Vickers A, Cronin A, Roobol M, et al. Reducing unnecessary biopsy during prostate cancer screening using a four-kallikrein panel: an independent replication. J Clin Oncol 2010;28:2493–8.

47. Vickers AJ, Cronin AM, Roobol MJ, et al. The relationship between prostate-specific antigen and prostate cancer risk: the Prostate Biopsy Collaborative Group. Clin Cancer Res 2010;16:4374–81.

48. Villers A, Malavaud B, Rebillard X, et al. ERSPC: features and preliminary results of France. BJU Int 2003;92(Suppl 2):27–9.

49. Eggener SE, Yossepowitch O, Roehl KA, et al. Relationship of prostate-specific antigen velocity to histologic findings in a prostate cancer screening program. Urology 2008;71:1016–9.

50. Vickers AJ, Cronin AM, Aus G, et al. Impact of recent screening on predicting the outcome of prostate cancer biopsy in men with elevated prostate-specific antigen: data from the European Randomized Study of Prostate Cancer Screening in Gothenburg, Sweden. Cancer 2010;116:2612–20.

51. Roobol MJ, Schroder FH, Kranse R, et al. A comparison of first and repeat (four years later) prostate cancer screening in a randomized cohort of a symptomatic men aged 55-75 years using a biopsy indication of 3.0 ng/mL (results of ERSPC, Rotterdam). Prostate 2006;66:604–12.

52. Walz J, Graefen M, Chun FK, et al. High incidence of prostate cancer detected by saturation biopsy after previous negative biopsy series. Eur Urol 2006;50:498–505.

53. Schroder FH, van den Bergh RC, Wolters T, et al. Eleven-year outcome of patients with prostate cancers diagnosed during screening after initial negative sextant biopsies. Eur Urol 2010;57:256–66.

54. Gupta A, Roobol MJ, Savage CJ, et al. A four-kallikrein panel for the prediction of repeat prostate biopsy: data from the European Randomized Study of Prostate Cancer screening in Rotterdam, Netherlands. Br J Cancer 2010;103:708–14.

55. Wilt TJ. The Prostate Cancer Intervention Versus Observation Trial: VA/NCI/AHRQ Cooperative Studies Program #407 (PIVOT): design and baseline results of a randomized controlled trial comparing radical prostatectomy with watchful waiting for men with clinically localized prostate cancer. J Natl Cancer Inst Monogr 2012;2012:184–90.

56. Bill-Axelson A, Holmberg L, Garmo H, et al. Radical prostatectomy or watchful waiting in early prostate cancer. N Engl J Med 2014;370:932–42.

57. Carlsson S, Maschino A, Schroder F, et al. Predictive value of four kallikrein markers for pathologically insignificant compared with aggressive prostate cancer in radical prostatectomy specimens: results from the European Randomized Study of Screening for Prostate Cancer section Rotterdam. Eur Urol 2013;64:693–9.

58. Ulmert D, Becker C, Nilsson JA, et al. Reproducibility and accuracy of measurements of free and total prostate-specific antigen in serum vs plasma after long-term storage at −20 degrees C. Clin Chem 2006;52:235–9.

59. Punnen S, Pavan N, Parekh DJ. Finding the wolf in sheep's clothing: the 4Kscore is a novel blood test that can accurately identify the risk of aggressive prostate cancer. Rev Urol 2015;17:3–13.

60. Donovan J, Hamdy F, Neal D, et al. Prostate Testing for Cancer and Treatment (ProtecT) feasibility study. Health Technol Assess 2003;7:1–88.

61. Parekh DJ, Punnen S, Sjoberg DD, et al. A multi-institutional prospective trial in the USA confirms that the 4Kscore accurately identifies men with high-grade prostate cancer. Eur Urol 2015;68(3):464–70.

62. OPKO Health, Inc. Available at: http://4kscore.opko.com. Accessed July 28, 2015.

Current Status of Urinary Biomarkers for Detection and Surveillance of Bladder Cancer

Aurélie Mbeutcha, MD[a,b], Ilaria Lucca, MD[a,c], Romain Mathieu, MD[a,d], Yair Lotan, MD[e], Shahrokh F. Shariat, MD[a,e,f,*]

KEYWORDS

- Bladder cancer • Transitional cell carcinoma • Urothelial carcinoma • Urinary biomarkers • Urine
- Detection • Surveillance • Follow-up

KEY POINTS

- Due to its high rate of recurrence, bladder cancer (BC) requires a close follow-up that includes regular cytologic and cystoscopy examinations and leads to expensive lifetime health care expenditures.
- Urinary cytology has a low sensitivity especially for low grade tumors, whereas cystoscopy remains an invasive examination. Therefore, urine-based biomarkers should be considered good alternatives for the detection and follow-up of BC.
- Many biomarkers have shown a higher sensitivity than cytology. Most of them, however, failed to reach its specificity. A combination of biomarkers may increase their performance.
- A standardization of the techniques used for their detection followed by multicenter and prospective analysis needs to be performed before any assessment in large controlled clinical trials.

INTRODUCTION

With an estimated 74,000 new cases and 16,000 deaths for 2015, BC is the fifth most frequent malignancy in the United States.[1] Urothelial carcinoma of the bladder (UCB) constitutes the most common histologic type and is the dominant histology in more than 90% of cases of BC.[2] Approximately 75% of newly diagnosed BCs are non–muscle-invasive BCs (NMIBCs), of which 70% are Ta, 20% T1, and 10% carcinoma in situ.[3] These lesions are usually treated with

Funding Sources: Bourse des Amis de la Faculté de Médecine de Nice (A. Mbeutcha); Nil (I. Lucca, R. Mathieu, Y. Lotan, and S.F. Shariat).

Conflict of Interest: Nil (A. Mbeutcha, I. Lucca, R. Mathieu, and S.F. Shariat); Research with Abbott, Pacific Edge, Cepheid, MDxHealth, and Nucleix (Y. Lotan).

[a] Department of Urology, Comprehensive Cancer Center, Vienna General Hospital, Medical University of Vienna, Währinger Gürtel 18-20, Vienna 1090, Austria; [b] Department of Urology, Hôpital Archet 2, Centre Hospitalier Universitaire de Nice, University of Nice Sophia-Antipolis, 151 Route de Saint-Antoine, Nice 06200, France; [c] Department of Urology, Centre Hospitalier Universitaire Vaudois, Rue du Bugnon 46, Lausanne 1010, Switzerland; [d] Department of Urology, Rennes University Hospital, 2 Rue Henri le Guilloux, Rennes 35000, France; [e] Department of Urology, University of Texas Southwestern Medical Center, 5303 Harry Hines Boulevard #110, Dallas, TX 75235, USA; [f] Department of Urology, Weill Cornell Medical College, Cornell University, 525 E 68th St, New York, NY 10011, USA

* Corresponding author. Department of Urology, Comprehensive Cancer Center, Vienna General Hospital, Medical University of Vienna, Währinger Gürtel 18-20, Vienna A-1090, Austria.

E-mail address: sfshariat@gmail.com

urologic.theclinics.com

transurethral resection of the bladder with or without intravesical instillation therapies according to guidelines.[4,5] The remaining 25% of BCs are muscle-invasive BCs (MIBCs) and the standard of care is radical cystectomy and bilateral lymph node dissection with or without perioperative chemotherapy.[6] Although the prognosis of MIBC is poor (5-year mortality rate of 38%),[7] the main issue with NMIBCs is that more than half of the patients experience disease recurrence within a period of 5 years and up to 30% of them experience disease progression to an MIBC despite therapy with curative intent.[8]

This high recurrence rate is the primary reason that BCs have the highest lifetime treatment cost per person of all cancers.[9,10] After initial treatment, patients with NMIBC are committed to a lifelong surveillance to identify recurrence early, with the goal of preventing disease progression to invasive disease. Depending on initial stage and grade, surveillance is of varying intensity but the current recommendation for high-grade tumors is cystoscopy and voided urine cytology every 3 months for 2 years, then every 6 months for 5 years, then yearly.[4,5] Unfortunately, each recurrence restarts the scheduling scheme such that with 50% to 70% recurrence for high-grade tumors, many patients have ever more cystoscopic procedures.

With a sensitivity of 90%, standard white light cystoscopy is the gold standard for detection of BC, but it remains an invasive and costly examination, limiting the compliance of patients for the follow-up.[11] Voided urine cytology is a highly specific test (99% specificity) but is limited by its low sensitivity (34%), especially in low-grade tumors[12,13] and by interobserver variations.[14]

Thus, to improve the management and the quality of life of patients with BC and to decrease the morbidity associated with current diagnostic and follow-up tests, many investigators have searched for a noninvasive, highly sensitive and specific marker of BC. Because urine is in contact with BC and can be collected noninvasively and in large amounts, urine-based assays are a natural and promising source for these biomarkers.

The assessment of a good biomarker should follow international guidelines.[15,16] Guidelines edited by the International Bladder Cancer Network define biomarkers according to their clinical use: detection (screening and assessment of patients with hematuria) and follow-up of patients with BC.[17] For each purpose, the required characteristics of biomarkers are different. To avoid unnecessary investigations and limit cystoscopies, a good diagnostic biomarker should have a low false-positive rate, whereas a good surveillance marker should have a high sensitivity and negative predictive value (NPV).[18]

To date, 6 tests (BTA stat [Polymedco, Cortlandt Manor, New York], BTA TRAK [Polymedco], NMP22 BC test kit [Matritech, Newton, Massachusetts], NMP22 BladderChek Test [Alere, Waltham, MA], uCyt+ [Scimedx, Denville, New Jersey], and UroVysion Bladder Cancer Kit [Abbott Molecular, Des Plaines, Illinois]) have been approved by the Food and Drug Administration (FDA) and are commercially available for clinical use. A multitude of newer markers, however, using genetic testing are currently undergoing validation and have the potential to change clinical practice.

This nonsystematic review summarizes the current data on commercially available and emerging urinary biomarkers for detection and surveillance of BC. Screening for BC is not discussed because this is a complex subject requiring its own review.[19–21]

MATERIAL AND METHOD

The authors performed a Pubmed/Medline search on articles published in English from 2000 to June 2015 using a combination of the following keywords: bladder cancer, urothelial carcinoma, transitional cell carcinoma, urine, urinary biomarker, marker, surveillance, detection, diagnosis, follow-up, recurrence, and progression.

COMMERCIALLY AVAILABLE BIOMARKERS
Food and Drug Administration–Approved Biomarkers

Nuclear matrix protein 22
Nuclear matrix proteins (NMPs) are a family of proteins that play an important role in the structural framework of nucleus and are involved in every step of its function, from DNA replication to regulation of gene expression. NMP22 is specifically involved in mitosis by enabling a correct distribution of chromatin to daughter cells.[22] The urinary concentration of NMP22 is 5-fold higher in patients with BC compared with healthy patients.[23]

Two assays have been developed to detect NMP22 in voided urine. The original assay is the NMP22 BC test kit, a laboratory-based quantitative sandwich ELISA test using 2 antibodies. The NMP22 BladderChek Test is a qualitative immunochromatic assay designed as a point of care (POC) test. A few drops of urine on the cartridge containing NMP22 detection and reporter antibodies provide results within 30 minutes. Both tests have been approved by the FDA for BC surveillance, and the NMP22 BladderChek Test is also approved for detection of BC in patients at risk or presenting suspicious symptoms.

Pooled data analysis, including 41 studies and enrolling 13,885 patients, reported that NMP22 outperformed cytology with a sensitivity of 68% versus 44%.[24] This high sensitivity was mainly due to a better detection rate of low-grade tumors compared with cytology.[25] But NMP22 failed to reach the level of cytology for specificity (79% vs 95%) due a high rate of false-positive results.[24] Because NMP22 is a ubiquitous nuclear protein, any aggression of the urinary epithelium (infection, inflammation, hematuria, urolithiasis, or instrumentation) can increase the release of NMP22 in the urine.[26,27]

The clinical accuracy of NMP22 BladderChek has been evaluated in 2 large multicenter studies conducted by Grossman and colleagues.[28,29] As a detection tool in patients with hematuria, NMP22 had a better sensitivity than urinary cytology (56% vs 16%) but its specificity remained lower (86% vs 99%).[28] In a surveillance setting, the sensitivity and specificity of NMP22 were 50% and 87%, respectively.[29] But in combination with cystoscopy, NMP22 increased significantly the detection rate of recurrence, up to 99% compared with cystoscopy alone (91%).[29] The lower sensitivity of NMP22 test in a surveillance setting could be explained by the larger size and more advanced stage of tumors at the time of diagnosis compared with those detected during follow-up.[30]

Tested in a large cohort of 1328 patients who were referred with hematuria to urologists, the overall positive predictive value (PPV) was 20% and the NPV was 97%.[31]

The reliability and clinical utility of NMP22 have been questioned due to its low specificity compared with cytology and because the initial studies were performed with the laboratory-based assay that prevented the heterogeneity of widespread application.[32] Decision curve analyses have suggested that its clinical benefit could be in decision making between immediate and delayed cystoscopy depending on a clinician's threshold for conduction of cystoscopy.[33,34] When compared with cytology-based nomograms, the accuracy of NMP22-based nomograms was higher (area under the curve–receiver operating characteristic curve [AUC-ROC] 82% versus 75%, $P = .006$).[35,36]

In the detection setting, the use of a nomogram incorporating clinical factors (age, gender, and smoking) and BladderChek was validated prospectively in a multicenter cohort of 381 patients with a predictive accuracy of the BC detection nomogram of 80%.[36]

At this time there is no current test to risk stratify patients with hematuria for referral to urology and there is a significant problem associated with lack of referral of patients with hematuria to urology.[37–40] There is a potential role for a urine marker to benefit in this clinical scenario and validation studies, such as the one performed for BladderChek, are needed prior to incorporation into clinical care.

Bladder tumor antigen

The bladder tumor antigen (BTA) is a human complement factor H-related protein produced by BC cells and is similar to human complement factor H. By interrupting the complement cascade activation, BTA confers a selective growth advantage and allows tumor cells to evade the host immune system.[41,42]

The BTA test exists in 2 assays, both designed to detect BTA in voided urine. BTA TRAK is a quantitative, laboratory-based ELISA assay, whereas BTA stat is a qualitative and immunochromatic POC device. Its design enables its use in a clinical setting. Both tests have been approved by FDA only for surveillance in complement of cystoscopy.

The reported overall sensitivity and specificity of BTA TRAK were 66% and 65%, respectively, whereas BTA stat had a sensitivity of 70% and a specificity of 75%.[43,44] For both tests, sensitivity improved with increasing histologic stage and grade, but specificity remained lower than cytology and the improvement of accuracy in sensitivity for low-grade, low-stage tumors remained modest.[45,46]

These high rates of specificity have to be balanced by the fact that many studies excluded patients with benign genitourinary conditions. When including these patients, specificity dropped to 56%.[47] Most of the false-positive results were due to hematuria, benign prostatic hyperplasia, urolithiasis, infection, inflammation, history of bacille Calmette-Guérin (BCG) instillations, and bowel interpositions.[47–52] BTA has today a limited clinical value with only few centers using it for any clinical decision making.

ImmunoCyt/uCyt+

The uCyt+ assay (formerly called ImmunoCyt) is a combination of cytology and immunofluorescence. It detects exfoliated BC cells in the urine by using 3 fluorescent monoclonal antibodies targeting 3 specific antigens of BC cells: M344 is a high-molecular-weight form of carcinoembryonic antigen, and LDQ10 and 19A11 are bladder tumor cell–associated mucins. The test requires trained cytopathologists and is performed under microscopy. A large number of exfoliated cells (more than 500 per slide) is required to perform an accurate test. The test is scored positive when the presence of either 1 red or green fluorescent cell is observed, but the manufacturer recommends that all positive cells should be correlated to morphology.[53,54] The test is approved by the FDA for monitoring of patients with a history of BC, as an adjunct to cystoscopy.

In a systematic review, including 10 studies and 4199 patients, the reported overall sensitivity was 84% and specificity was 75%.[24] In low-grade and low-stage tumors, uCyt+ had a superior sensitivity compared with cytology alone. In a study including 2217 patients, when combined with cytology, uCyt+ reached an overall sensitivity of 73%, with 59% for grade 1, 77% for grade 2, and 90% for grade 3 tumors, but specificity of combined assays remained lower than cytology alone (72% vs 98%, respectively).[55] In a study including 870 patients, the NPVs of cytology, uCyt+, and both analyses were 88%, 93%, and 95%, respectively, and the PPVs were 70%, 26%, and 29%, respectively.[56]

As a cell-based assay, uCyt was less impacted by hematuria and inflammatory conditions compared with other urinary assays.[57] In a multicenter prospective study that enrolled 1182 patients without a history of BC and presenting with painless hematuria, uCyt+ was a strong predicator of BC. Decision curve analyses on multivariable models, including uCyt+, achieved the highest predictive accuracy (91%).[58] Nevertheless, the limited evidence and the user dependency of this assay had led to infrequent use in clinical care.

UroVysion

The UroVysion Bladder Cancer Kit is a multitarget fluorescence in situ hybridization (FISH) assay that identifies the most common urothelial carcinoma–related chromosomal alterations in exfoliated cells in urine: aneuploidy for chromosomes 3, 7, and 17 and the loss of the 9p21 locus of the p16 tumor suppressor gene. With a fluorescent microscope, the cytopathologist needs to count the 4-color fluorescent signals that assess the copy number of each target in the nuclei. To date, there are no uniform criteria for positive UroVysion, but the test is generally considered positive when a minimum of 25 abnormal cells is observed, including at 4 cells with a gain of 1 or more chromosome, or 12 or more cells with an homozygous loss of the 9p21 locus.[59] The test is FDA approved for use in conjunction with current standard procedures for detection of BC in patients with hematuria and surveillance of patients with history of BC.

A pooled data analysis performed on 14 studies involving 2477 FISH tests found that UroVysion outperformed cytology (AUC-ROC 87% vs 63%) and had overall sensitivity of 72%, but a lower specificity than cytology (83%). When excluding Ta tumors, the sensitivity of UroVysion reached 86% compared with 61% for cytology, but the overall test performance almost disappeared when excluding this population, suggesting that UroVysion has a better sensitivity in low-grade tumors.[60]

Due to its laboratory cell-based nature, UroVysion accuracy is dependent on several technical aspects, such as laboratory staff experience with performing FISH and sample quality with a sufficient number of tumor cells. The use of automatic scanning systems combining FISH and cellular morphology analysis improves the accuracy for BC detection.[61,62]

Several follow-up studies reported that almost half of the patients with initial false-positive FISH tests and negative cystoscopy results experienced disease recurrence within the year after the test, suggesting that the detection of chromosomal abnormalities anticipated the diagnostic of recurrence by cystoscopy or urinary cytology. Therefore, an abnormal UroVysion test could constitute an accurate surveillance assay by anticipating disease recurrence.[63] Some other studies promoted a reflex FISH in cases of atypical cystoscopy or cytology to assess tumor recurrence.[59,64,65] This type of strategy may reduce number of unnecessary biopsies and may be cost effective.[66] Finally, UroVysion could also be useful in monitoring patients treated with intravesical BCG.[67,68] Further studies are necessary to validate these indications. The cost-effectiveness of such labor-intensive tests need to be assessed in different health care settings.

Non–Food and Drug Administration–Approved Biomarkers

CxBladder

Cxbladder Detect (Pacific Edge, Hummelstown, PA) is based on the detection 4 mRNAs significantly increased in voided urine and patients with BC (IGFBP5, HOXA13, MDK, and CDK1) and another mRNA (CXCR2) that is associated with nonmalignant inflammatory conditions to reduce false-positive results. The expression of these mRNAs is assessed with real-time reverse transcription polymerase chain reaction (RT-qPCR). In a prospective study, including 485 patients with hematuria and without history of BC, CxBladder reached a sensitivity of 82% when the cutoff was prespecified to give a specificity of 85%. CxBladder seemed to be able to distinguish between low-grade Ta tumors and other detected urothelial carcinoma with a sensitivity of 91% and a specificity of 90%.[69] These data need to be confirmed by further studies.

Survivin

Survivin is an antiapoptotic protein that is almost exclusively expressed by malignant epithelium. Several techniques and assays have been used to detect mRNA or the protein level of survivin, but the commercially available assay is a dot-blot technique (BioDot assay, Fujirebio Diagnostics [Malvern, PA]).[70]

A meta-analysis, including 2051 subjects, reported a sensitivity of 77% and a specificity of 92% and an AUC-ROC of 94%.[71] Nevertheless, these results need to be balanced by the lack of standardization of assay and cutoff values that yield the interpretation of the data difficult.[72]

Cytokeratin fragment 21.1

Cytokeratin is a family of marker of epithelium differentiation and some members have been related to BC. Cytokeratin fragment 21.1 (CYFRA 21.1) is an ELISA assay that detects fragments of cytokeratin 19.

In a pooled data analysis, including 2495 patients, the sensitivity was 82% and the specificity was 80%. The AUC-ROC was 87%.[73] When including patients with benign conditions, such as urolithiasis, infection, history of BCG, and radiotherapy, the high rate of false-positive results led to a lower specificity, making CYFRA 21.1 not useful as a surveillance tool anymore.[74,75]

Bladder cancer rapid test

Cytokeratin 8 and 18 can be detected by the urinary BC test (UBC, IDL Biotech, Bromma,

Sweden) with a POC assay (UBC Rapid test [IDL Biotech]) or an ELISA assay. The POC assay can provide qualitative results within 10 minutes, whereas ELISA provides quantitative results.

In a study including 112 patients, the reported sensitivity and specificity for the UBC Rapid test were both 64%.[76] When including potential false-positive confounders in cohorts, such as other urinary tract malignancies or benign conditions, the sensitivity was 79% and the specificity 49%. In these cases, the UBC Rapid test performed worse than BTA tests.[77] The false-positive rate reached 20% for patients with benign urologic diseases and 44% for patients with other urinary tract malignancies.[78] Most of the side-by-side comparisons with other biomarkers were not in favor of the UBC Rapid test[79,80] but, when combined with the POC reader instead of visual reading, the diagnostic accuracy seemed to improve.[81]

Table 1 summarizes commercially available biomarkers.

INVESTIGATIONAL BIOMARKERS
Protein-Based and Cell-Based Biomarkers

Apoptosis markers

Soluble Fas (sFas) isoforms are antiapoptotic proteins produced and released by BC cells, protecting them from host antitumor immunity and are measurable by ELISA. Urinary levels of sFas have been shown an independent predictor of BC recurrence.[82] In a study, including 191 patients, reported sensitivity and specificity for sFas

---

Table 1
Commercially available urinary biomarkers

Marker	Assay Type	Sensitivity (%)	Specificity (%)	Food and Drug Administration Approved	Ref.
Cytology	Giemsa or hematoxylin-eosin staining	34	99	Diagnostic and follow-up	13,140
NMP22	ELISA	40	99	Follow-up	141
NMP22	POC device	68 (62–74)	79 (74–84)	Diagnosis and follow-up of high risks	24
BTA stat	Dipstick immunoassay	70	75	Diagnosis and follow-up	43,44
BTA TRAK	Sandwich ELISA	66	65	Diagnosis and follow-up	43,44
uCyt+	Immunocytochemistry	84 (77–91)	75 (68–83)	Follow-up in adjunct to cystoscopy	24
UroVysion	Multicolored and multiprobed FISH	72 (69–75)	83 (82–85)	Diagnosis and follow-up	60
CxBladder	RT-qPCR	82	85	Not approved	69
Survivin	BioDot test	77 (75–80)	92 (90–93)	Not approved	71
CYFRA 21.1	Immunoradiometric assay or ELISA	82 (70–90)	80 (73–86)	Not approved	73
UBC test	Sandwich ELISA or POC	64	64	Not approved	76

were 88% and 89%, respectively.[83] When compared with NMP22, sFas seemed a better predictor of BC and invasiveness with an AUC-ROC of 76%, outperforming NMP22 (70%).[84]

Clusterin is a multifunctional secretory glycoprotein that has a potential role in development and progression of several human cancers[85,86] and is measurable by ELISA. Urinary levels of clusterin were significantly higher in patients with BC.[87] Reported sensitivity rates were between 70% and 87%. Reported specificity was between 83% and 97%.[88,89]

Angiogenesis markers

Vascular endothelial growth factor (VEGF) is a key mediator of angiogenesis produced by BC cells and measurable by ELISA in voided urine. Mean levels of VEGF were significantly associated with presence of BC and increased with tumor stage.[90] The reported sensitivity and specificity ranged from 68% to 83% and from 62% to 93%, respectively.[91–93] The AUC-ROC was 89%.[93]

Interleukins (ILs) are small signaling proteins secreted by white blood cells and involved in the inflammatory process of the immune system. They are measurable by ELISA. Urinary levels of IL-8 were significantly higher in patients with BC and were correlated with tumor stage.[94] In a detection setting, IL-8 showed a high accuracy with an AUC-ROC at 79%.[95] In a post-BCG surveillance setting, urinary levels of IL-8 were greater in patients who experienced disease recurrence[94,96]: at a cutoff of 112 pg/mL, IL-8 measured 2 hours after BCG instillation predicted recurrence with a sensitivity of 53%, specificity of 89%, PPV of 73%, and NPV of 77%.[97] IL-6 was also an independent predictor of BCG response,[98] and the ratio IL-6/IL-10 has been shown to predict both recurrence after BCG response and recurrence in patients at intermediate risk, with a sensitivity of 83% and a specificity of 76%.[99,100]

Although angiogenesis and inflammation are definite hallmarks of cancer, they are relatively nonspecific and, therefore, unlikely to help in BC diagnosis or surveillance.

Proliferation and invasion

Telomerase is a ribonucleoprotein enzyme that synthetizes telomeres (repeated sequences of TTAGGG) at the ends of chromosomes to ensure genome stability. Several malignant cell types, including BC cells, acquire immortality by hyperactivating telomerase. Telomerase activity can be measured by different assays: the telomeric repeat amplification test is a PCR-based technique, or measuring the activity by RT-qPCR of human telomerase RNA the telomerase reverse transcriptase (hTERT).[101–103] The most accurate method seemed to be hTERT, with an overall reported sensitivity from 75% to 96%, specificity from 69% to 96%, NPV of 91%, and PPV of 96%. From grades 1 to 3, reported sensitivity was 52%, 80%, and 94%, respectively.[104–109] The assays still need to be standardized and validated before widespread use. Moreover, the lack of specificity of telomerase activity makes it a biomarker of little value with a high rate of false-positive.

Hyaluronic acid (HA) is a glycosaminoglycan constitutive of the extracellular matrix and is involved in cell adhesion and proliferation. It is degraded by hyaluronidase (HAase) into small fragments that promote angiogenesis. Both components are increased in urine of patients with BC. HA-HAase is measurable by ELISA, and HAase can be assessed by RT-qPCR. When combined, the performance of the test was better than either test alone, reaching a sensitivity of 92%, specificity of 85%, accuracy of 88%, PPV of 64% to 92%, and NPV of 67% to 91%. The levels of HA/Hases were correlated with tumor grade.[49,110,111] Further research is needed to assess and establish the clinical relevance of this biomarker.

Fibronectin is a structural glycoprotein widely present in cells, plasma, and extracellular tissue matrix that is implicated in cell migration and adhesion. When tumors are present, the components of the extracellular matrix are degraded by proteases resulting from metastatic or invasive conditions. In a meta-analysis, including 5 studies involving 649 patients and 291 controls, urine levels of fibronectin had a pooled sensitivity of 81% and specificity of 80%. The AUC-ROC was 86%.[112] These results are interesting but early because the clinical scenario needs to be identified and tested.

CD44 antigen is a cell-surface glycoprotein involved in cell adhesion, proliferation, and migration. Among CD44 variants, the variant 6 (CD44v6) expression is measurable in the urine by RT-qPCR and was significantly increased in patients with BC, with a reported sensitivity between 50% and 86%, specificity between 72% and 79%, and PPV of 78%.[91,113] Here also, a valid, reliable, and reproducible assay is far from development.

Metabolomics

Like genomics and proteomics, metabolomics is another "omics" science that has emerged in recent years. It aims to identify a biological signature of BC based on the analysis of metabolites produced in an abnormal quantity by BC cells compared with normal cells. Various analytical platforms based on liquid chromatography and mass spectrophotometry are currently used to analyze these metabolites. More than 10,000 compounds have been identified so far, but when reduced to a panel of 3 to 15 metabolites, the reported sensitivity, specificity, and AUC-ROC are 91% to 100%, 93% to 100%, and 90% to 94%, respectively. Their detection seems correlated with cancer-specific survival.[114–119] The domain of research is preliminary and further studies are needed to assess the clinical relevance of such techniques.

Table 2 summarizes investigational biomarkers.

Gene-Based Biomarkers

Aurora A kinase
Aurora A kinase (AURKA) is a serine/threonine kinase implicated in the regulation of gene stability during the mitosis. Overexpression of AURKA gene can be assessed by FISH, with a sensitivity of 87%, specificity of 97%, and AUC-ROC of 94%.[120] It can also be measured through AURKA mRNA expression with RT-qPCR, providing an overall sensitivity of 84% and specificity of 65%. When compared with cytology, accuracy of AURKA was particularly evident in patients with low-grade tumors, with a predictive accuracy of 73 versus 59%.[121] This biomarker holds much promise, and further studies are awaited.

Fibroblast growth factor 3 receptor
Mutations in fibroblast growth factor 3 receptor (FGFR3) are present in more than 50% of voided urine of BC patients and are more common in low-grade (70%) and low-stage BC (60%).[122] A multiplex PCR (SNaPshot [Applied Biosystems, Foster City, CA]) has been used to assess it.[123] FGFR3 mutations were an independent factor of BC recurrence.[124] In a surveillance setting for low-grade tumors, the sensitivity of the assay

was 58%, which was higher than cytology.[125] Moreover, when combined with cytology, the sensitivity reached 76%.[126] In a detection setting in patients with hematuria, sensitivity, specificity, PPV, and NPV were 25%, 99%, 17% and 99%, respectively.[127] A cost-effectiveness study has shown that surveillance in which cystoscopy was partly replaced by mutation analysis of urine seemed safe, effective, and cost effective.[128] This biomarker has high potential because it may have several roles, including cancer detection, therapeutic target, and tool for monitoring for treatment response.

Microsatellite/loss of heterozygosity detection
Microsatellites are highly polymorphic short tandem DNA repeats found through the genome resulting from a failure of the DNA mismatch repair and playing an important role in tumor cell transformation. This loss of heterozygosity could be a marker of carcinogenesis. It has been established that microsatellite changes in urine samples matched DNA extracts from tumor tissue.[129] The reported overall sensitivity ranged from 79% to 84%, increasing with tumor grades 1 to 3 from 75% to 96%; specificity ranged from 85% to 100%.[129–134] The accuracy of the test is too low to use it in a surveillance setting (sensitivity 58% and specificity 73%)[135] and would not be cost effective.[136] This biomarker may have a specific role in upper tract urothelial carcinoma rather than BC.[137]

DNA methylation
Table 3 summarizes some of the genes investigated for methylation epigenetic changes. In a detection setting, reported sensitivity ranged from 65% to 100% and specificity from 77% to 100% (see **Table 3**). Few studies explored DNA

Table 2
Investigational protein and cell-based urinary biomarkers

Marker	Assay Type	Sensitivity (%)	Specificity (%)	Ref.
sFas	ELISA	88	89	83
Clusterin	ELISA	70–87	83–97	88,89
VEGF	ELISA	68–83	62–93	91–93
Telomerase	RT-qPCR PCR	75–96	69–96	104–109
HA HAase	ELISA RT-qPCR	92	85	110
Fibronectin	IEMA	81	80	112
CD44v6	RT-qPCR	50–86	72–79	91,113
AURKA	RT-qPCR	84	65	121
FGFR3	Snapshot analysis	25–58	99	125,127

Abbreviation: IEMA, immunoenzymatic assay.

Table 3
Investigational methylation DNA-based urine biomarkers

Gene Profiled	Assay Type	Cohort Size		Clinical Setting	Sensitivity (%)	Specificity (%)	Ref.
		Patients	Controls				
TWIST1 and NID2	qMSP	209	—	Detection	67	78	142
CCND2, CCNA1, and CALCA	qMSP	148	56	Surveillance	73	70	143
SOX1, LINE-1, and IRAK3	Pyrosequencing	90	—	Surveillance	89	97	144
TWIST1 and NID2	qMSP	111	—	Surveillance	75	71	145
OSR1, SIM2, OTX1, MEIS1, and ONECUT2	Bisulfite-PCR	54	115	Detection	82	82	146
SOX1 and VAMP8	Pyrosequencing	73	18	Detection	100	100	147
APC_a, TERT_a, TERT_b, and EDNRB	MS-MLPA	385	—	Screening	25	90	127
APC_a, TERT_a, TERT_b, and EDNRB	MS-MLPA	49	60	Surveillance	63–72	55–58	148
BCL2, CDKN2A, and NID2	qMSP	42	21	Detection	81	86	149
EOMES, HOXA9, POU4F2, TWIST1, VIM, and ZNF154	qMSP	184	35	Surveillance	82–89	94–100	138
APC, RARβ; and Survivin	MSP	32	—	Detection	94	—	150
VAX1, KCNV1, TAL1, PPOX1, and CFTR	methylCap/seq	212	190	Detection	89	87	151
RAR-β2	qMSP	100	116	Detection	65	90	152
IRF8, p14 or sFRP1	qMSP	30	19	Detection	87	95	153
MYO3A, CA10, NKX6-2, DBC1, and SOX11 or PENK	qMSP	128	110	Detection	85	95	154
GDF15, TMEFF2, and VIM	qMSP	51	59	Detection	94	90	155
BCL2 and hTERT	qMSP	108	105	Detection	76	98	156
IFNA, MBP, ACTBP2, D9S162 and of RASSF1A, and WIF1	qMSP	40	—	Surveillance	86	8	157
CDKN2A, ARF, MGMT, and GSTP1	qMSP	175	94	Detection	69	100	158
DAPK, BCL2, and TERT	MSP	37	20	Detection	78	100	159
DAPK, RARβ, E-cadherin, and p16	MSP	22	17	Detection	91	77	160

Abbreviations: MS-MLPA, custom methylation-specific multiplex ligation-dependent probe amplification; qMSP, real-time methylation-specific PCR.

Table 4
Investigational microRNA urine biomarkers

	Cohort Size					
microRNA	Bladder Cancer	Controls	Sensitivity (%)	Specificity (%)	AUC-ROC (%)	Ref.
Ratio of miRNA-126: miRNA-152	29	18	82	72	77	161
miR-96	78	74	71	89	—	162
miR-183			74	77		
miR-125n and miR-126	8	3	80	100	—	163
miRs-135b/15b/1224-3p	68	53	94	51	77	164
miR-1224-3p			76	83		
miR-145 NMIBC	207	144	78	61	73	165
MIBC			84	61	79	
miR-187, miR-18a, miR-25, miR-142-3p, miR-140-5p, miR-204	151	126	85	87	92	166
miR-92a and miR-125b			85	74	83	
miR-106b	112	78	77	72	80	167
miR-99a and miR-125b	50	21	87	81	—	168

methylation in a surveillance setting. In a study including 184 patients, Reinert and colleagues[138] reported a sensitivity of 82% to 89% and a specificity of 94% to 100% when studying a panel of 6 genes. Further studies, with standardized techniques should be performed to assess the role of DNA methylation detection in voided urine and its potential integration in detection and follow-up of patients with BC. Methylation biomarkers could also serve as a target for epigenetic modifiers that would enhance the efficacy of other therapies.

MicroRNA

MicroRNAs (miRNAs) are small noncoding RNA that regulate post-transcription of genes by binding mRNA. Alteration of expression of miRNA can induce carcinogenesis and are measurable by RT-qPCR. Several studies investigated miRNA produced by BC cells and excreted in urine, constituting a miRNA signature. **Table 4** summarizes the main miRNA studies in urine. The overall sensitivity was 71% to 94%, specificity 51% to 100%, and AUC-ROC 73% to 92% (see **Table 4**). Some epigenetic changes silencing of miRNAs have been shown involved in development of BC. Methylation study of miR-137, miR-124-2, miR-124-3, and miR-9-3 enabled BC detection with sensitivity of 81%, specificity of 89%, and AUC-ROC of 92%.[139] These are stable and biologically sound biomarkers would measure a broader picture than single biomarkers.

SUMMARY

Many urinary biomarkers are able to assess BC, and many more are going to be developed through the output of high-frequency analysis methods, such as proteomics, metabolomics, and genomics. A combination of biomarkers seems to increase their performance. But their clinical relevance is not obvious enough to enable a widespread use because most of them have not yet reached quality criteria established by guidelines for development of accurate biomarkers yet.[15,18] Before testing them in clinical trials, a standardization of detection techniques followed by multicenter prospective analysis needs to be performed in different settings, requiring different performance characteristics.

REFERENCES

1. Siegel RL, Miller KD, Jemal A. Cancer statistics, 2015. CA Cancer J Clin 2015;65:5–29.
2. Eble JN, Sauter G, Epstein JI, et al. World Health Organization Classification of Tumours. Pathology and Genetics of Tumours of the Urinary System and Male Genital Organs. IARC Press: Lyon 2004.
3. Burger M, Catto JWF, Dalbagni G, et al. Epidemiology and risk factors of urothelial bladder cancer. Eur Urol 2013;63:234–41.
4. Babjuk M, Burger M, Zigeuner R, et al. EAU guidelines on non-muscle-invasive urothelial carcinoma of the bladder: update 2013. Eur Urol 2013;64:639–53.

5. Hall MC, Chang SS, Dalbagni G, et al. Guideline for the management of nonmuscle invasive bladder cancer (stages Ta, T1, and Tis): 2007 update. J Urol 2007;178:2314–30.

6. Witjes JA, Compérat E, Cowan NC, et al. EAU guidelines on muscle-invasive and metastatic bladder cancer: summary of the 2013 guidelines. Eur Urol 2014;65:778–92.

7. Nuhn P, May M, Sun M, et al. External validation of postoperative nomograms for prediction of all-cause mortality, cancer-specific mortality, and recurrence in patients with urothelial carcinoma of the bladder. Eur Urol 2012;61:58–64.

8. Sylvester RJ, van der Meijden APM, Oosterlinck W, et al. Predicting recurrence and progression in individual patients with stage Ta T1 bladder cancer using EORTC risk tables: a combined analysis of 2596 patients from seven EORTC trials. Eur Urol 2006;49. 466–7. [discussion: 475–7].

9. Sievert KD, Amend B, Nagele U, et al. Economic aspects of bladder cancer: what are the benefits and costs? World J Urol 2009;27:295–300.

10. Mossanen M, Gore JL. The burden of bladder cancer care. Curr Opin Urol 2014;24:487–91.

11. Schrag D, Hsieh LJ, Rabbani F, et al. Adherence to surveillance among patients with superficial bladder cancer. J Natl Cancer Inst 2003;95:588–97.

12. Karakiewicz PI, Benayoun S, Zippe C, et al. Institutional variability in the accuracy of urinary cytology for predicting recurrence of transitional cell carcinoma of the bladder. BJU Int 2006;97:997–1001.

13. Lotan Y, Roehrborn CG. Sensitivity and specificity of commonly available bladder tumor markers versus cytology: results of a comprehensive literature review and meta-analyses. Urology 2003;61:109–18 [discussion: 118].

14. Reid MD, Osunkoya AO, Siddiqui MT, et al. Accuracy of grading of urothelial carcinoma on urine cytology: an analysis of interobserver and intraobserver agreement. Int J Clin Exp Pathol 2012;5:882–91.

15. Bensalah K, Montorsi F, Shariat SF. Challenges of cancer biomarker profiling. Eur Urol 2007;52:1601–9.

16. Kamat AM, Hegarty PK, Gee JR, et al. ICUD-EAU international consultation on bladder cancer 2012: screening, diagnosis, and molecular markers. Eur Urol 2013;63:4–15.

17. Goebell PJ, Groshen SL, Schmitz-Dräger BJ. Guidelines for development of diagnostic markers in bladder cancer. World J Urol 2008;26:5–11.

18. Shariat SF, Lotan Y, Vickers A, et al. Statistical consideration for clinical biomarker research in bladder cancer. Urol Oncol 2010;28:389–400.

19. Schmitz-Dräger BJ, Droller M, Lokeshwar VB, et al. Molecular markers for bladder cancer screening, early diagnosis, and surveillance: the WHO/ICUD consensus. Urol Int 2015;94:1–24.

20. Xylinas E, Kluth LA, Rieken M, et al. Urine markers for detection and surveillance of bladder cancer. Urol Oncol 2014;32:222–9.

21. Larré S, Catto JW, Cookson MS, et al. Screening for bladder cancer: rationale, limitations, whom to target, and perspectives. Eur Urol 2013;63:1049–58.

22. Berezney R, Coffey DS. Identification of a nuclear protein matrix. Biochem Biophys Res Commun 1974;60:1410–7.

23. Jamshidian H, Kor K, Djalali M. Urine concentration of nuclear matrix protein 22 for diagnosis of transitional cell carcinoma of bladder. Urol J 2008;5:243–7.

24. Mowatt G, Zhu S, Kilonzo M, et al. Systematic review of the clinical effectiveness and cost-effectiveness of photodynamic diagnosis and urine biomarkers (FISH, ImmunoCyt, NMP22) and cytology for the detection and follow-up of bladder cancer. Health Technol Assess 2010;14:1–331.

25. Hwang EC, Choi HS, Jung SI, et al. Use of the NMP22 BladderChek test in the diagnosis and follow-up of urothelial cancer: a cross-sectional study. Urology 2011;77:154–9.

26. Behrens T, Stenzl A, Brüning T. Factors influencing false-positive results for nuclear matrix protein 22. Eur Urol 2014;66:970–2.

27. Miyake M, Goodison S, Giacoia EG, et al. Influencing factors on the NMP-22 urine assay: an experimental model. BMC Urol 2012;12:23.

28. Grossman HB, Messing E, Soloway M, et al. Detection of bladder cancer using a point-of-care proteomic assay. JAMA 2005;293:810–6.

29. Grossman HB, Soloway M, Messing E, et al. Surveillance for recurrent bladder cancer using a point-of-care proteomic assay. JAMA 2006;295:299–305.

30. Boman H, Hedelin H, Jacobsson S, et al. Newly diagnosed bladder cancer: the relationship of initial symptoms, degree of microhematuria and tumor marker status. J Urol 2002;168:1955–9.

31. Lotan Y, Shariat SF. Impact of risk factors on the performance of the nuclear matrix protein 22 point-of-care test for bladder cancer detection. BJU Int 2008;101:1362–7.

32. Shariat SF, Marberger MJ, Lotan Y, et al. Variability in the performance of nuclear matrix protein 22 for the detection of bladder cancer. J Urol 2006;176:919–26 [discussion: 926].

33. Barbieri CE, Cha EK, Chromecki TF, et al. Decision curve analysis assessing the clinical benefit of NMP22 in the detection of bladder cancer: secondary analysis of a prospective trial. BJU Int 2012;109:685–90.

34. Shariat SF, Savage C, Chromecki TF, et al. Assessing the clinical benefit of nuclear matrix protein 22

in the surveillance of patients with nonmuscle-invasive bladder cancer and negative cytology: a decision-curve analysis. Cancer 2011;117:2892–7.

35. Lotan Y, Capitanio U, Shariat SF, et al. Impact of clinical factors, including a point-of-care nuclear matrix protein-22 assay and cytology, on bladder cancer detection. BJU Int 2009;103:1368–74.

36. Lotan Y, Svatek RS, Krabbe L-M, et al. Prospective external validation of a bladder cancer detection model. J Urol 2014;192:1343–8.

37. Buteau A, Seideman CA, Svatek RS, et al. What is evaluation of hematuria by primary care physicians? Use of electronic medical records to assess practice patterns with intermediate follow-up. Urol Oncol 2014;32:128–34.

38. Singh R, Saleemi A, Walsh K, et al. Near misses in bladder cancer – an airline safety approach to urology. Ann R Coll Surg Engl 2003;85:378–81.

39. Nieder AM, Manoharan M, Vyas S, et al. Evaluation and work-up of hematuria among primary care physicians in Miami-Dade County: an anonymous questionnaire-based survey. J Urol 2007;177:357. [abstract: 1082].

40. Johnson E, Daignault S, Zhang Y, et al. Gender disparities in urologic referral of hematuria. J Urol 2006;175(4 Suppl):286. [abstract 887].

41. Kinders R, Jones T, Root R, et al. Complement factor H or a related protein is a marker for transitional cell cancer of the bladder. Clin Cancer Res 1998;4: 2511–20.

42. Malkowicz SB. The application of human complement factor H-related protein (BTA TRAK) in monitoring patients with bladder cancer. Urol Clin North Am 2000;27:63–73, ix.

43. Glas AS, Roos D, Deutekom M, et al. Tumor markers in the diagnosis of primary bladder cancer. A systematic review. J Urol 2003;169:1975–82.

44. Guo A, Wang X, Gao L, et al. Bladder tumour antigen (BTA stat) test compared to the urine cytology in the diagnosis of bladder cancer: a meta-analysis. Can Urol Assoc J 2014;8:E347–52.

45. Poulakis V, Witzsch U, De Vries R, et al. A comparison of urinary nuclear matrix protein-22 and bladder tumour antigen tests with voided urinary cytology in detecting and following bladder cancer: the prognostic value of false-positive results. BJU Int 2001;88:692–701.

46. Thomas L, Leyh H, Marberger M, et al. Multicenter trial of the quantitative BTA TRAK assay in the detection of bladder cancer. Clin Chem 1999;45: 472–7.

47. Raitanen M-P. The role of BTA stat test in follow-up of patients with bladder cancer: results from Finn-Bladder studies. World J Urol 2008;26:45–50.

48. Miyake M, Goodison S, Rizwani W, et al. Urinary BTA: indicator of bladder cancer or of hematuria. World J Urol 2012;30:869–73.

49. Lokeshwar VB, Schroeder GL, Selzer MG, et al. Bladder tumor markers for monitoring recurrence and screening comparison of hyaluronic acid-hyaluronidase and BTA-Stat tests. Cancer 2002; 95:61–72.

50. Oge O, Kozaci D, Gemalmaz H. The BTA stat test is nonspecific for hematuria: an experimental hematuria model. J Urol 2002;167:1318–9 [discussion: 1319–20].

51. Mahnert B, Tauber S, Kriegmair M, et al. Measurements of complement factor H-related protein (BTA-TRAK assay) and nuclear matrix protein (NMP22 assay)–useful diagnostic tools in the diagnosis of urinary bladder cancer? Clin Chem Lab Med 2003;41:104–10.

52. Nasuti JF, Gomella LG, Ismial M, et al. Utility of the BTA stat test kit for bladder cancer screening. Diagn Cytopathol 1999;21:27–9.

53. Fradet Y, Lockhard C. Performance characteristics of a new monoclonal antibody test for bladder cancer: immunocyt trade mark. Can J Urol 1997;4: 400–5.

54. Mian C, Pycha A, Wiener H, et al. Immunocyt: a new tool for detecting transitional cell cancer of the urinary tract. J Urol 1999;161:1486–9.

55. Comploj E, Mian C, Ambrosini-Spaltro A, et al. uCyt+/ImmunoCyt and cytology in the detection of urothelial carcinoma: an update on 7422 analyses. Cancer Cytopathol 2013;121:392–7.

56. Têtu B, Tiguert R, Harel F, et al. ImmunoCyt/uCyt+ improves the sensitivity of urine cytology in patients followed for urothelial carcinoma. Mod Pathol 2005; 18:83–9.

57. Todenhöfer T, Hennenlotter J, Tews V, et al. Impact of different grades of microscopic hematuria on the performance of urine-based markers for the detection of urothelial carcinoma. Urol Oncol 2013;31: 1148–54.

58. Cha EK, Tirsar LA, Schwentner C, et al. Immunocytology is a strong predictor of bladder cancer presence in patients with painless hematuria: a multicentre study. Eur Urol 2012;61:185–92.

59. Lotan Y, Bensalah K, Ruddell T, et al. Prospective evaluation of the clinical usefulness of reflex fluorescence in situ hybridization assay in patients with atypical cytology for the detection of urothelial carcinoma of the bladder. J Urol 2008;179: 2164–9.

60. Hajdinjak T. UroVysion FISH test for detecting urothelial cancers: meta-analysis of diagnostic accuracy and comparison with urinary cytology testing. Urol Oncol 2008;26:646–51.

61. Daniely M, Rona R, Kaplan T, et al. Combined morphologic and fluorescence in situ hybridization analysis of voided urine samples for the detection and follow-up of bladder cancer in patients with benign urine cytology. Cancer 2007;111:517–24.

62. Daniely M, Rona R, Kaplan T, et al. Combined analysis of morphology and fluorescence in situ hybridization significantly increases accuracy of bladder cancer detection in voided urine samples. Urology 2005;66:1354–9.

63. Seideman C, Canter D, Kim P, et al. Multicenter evaluation of the role of UroVysion FISH assay in surveillance of patients with bladder cancer: does FISH positivity anticipate recurrence? World J Urol 2015;33(9):1309–13.

64. Kim PH, Sukhu R, Cordon BH, et al. Reflex fluorescence in situ hybridization assay for suspicious urinary cytology in patients with bladder cancer with negative surveillance cystoscopy. BJU Int 2014; 114:354–9.

65. Schlomer BJ, Ho R, Sagalowsky A, et al. Prospective validation of the clinical usefulness of reflex fluorescence in situ hybridization assay in patients with atypical cytology for the detection of urothelial carcinoma of the bladder. J Urol 2010;183: 62–7.

66. Gayed BA, Seideman C, Lotan Y. Cost-effectiveness of fluorescence in situ hybridization in patients with atypical cytology for the detection of urothelial carcinoma. J Urol 2013;190:1181–6.

67. Whitson J, Berry A, Carroll P, et al. A multicolour fluorescence in situ hybridization test predicts recurrence in patients with high-risk superficial bladder tumours undergoing intravesical therapy. BJU Int 2009;104:336–9.

68. Savic S, Zlobec I, Thalmann GN, et al. The prognostic value of cytology and fluorescence in situ hybridization in the follow-up of nonmuscle-invasive bladder cancer after intravesical Bacillus Calmette-Guérin therapy. Int J Cancer 2009;124: 2899–904.

69. O'Sullivan P, Sharples K, Dalphin M, et al. A multigene urine test for the detection and stratification of bladder cancer in patients presenting with hematuria. J Urol 2012;188:741–7.

70. Shariat SF, Casella R, Khoddami SM, et al. Urine detection of survivin is a sensitive marker for the noninvasive diagnosis of bladder cancer. J Urol 2004;171:626–30.

71. Ku JH, Godoy G, Amiel GE, et al. Urine survivin as a diagnostic biomarker for bladder cancer: a systematic review. BJU Int 2012;110:630–6.

72. Jeon C, Kim M, Kwak C, et al. Prognostic role of survivin in bladder cancer: a systematic review and meta-analysis. PLoS One 2013;8:e76719.

73. Huang YL, Chen J, Yan W, et al. Diagnostic accuracy of cytokeratin-19 fragment (CYFRA 21-1) for bladder cancer: a systematic review and meta-analysis. Tumour Biol 2015;36:3137–45.

74. Nisman B, Yutkin V, Peretz T, et al. The follow-up of patients with non-muscle-invasive bladder cancer by urine cytology, abdominal ultrasound and urine CYFRA 21-1: a pilot study. Anticancer Res 2009;29: 4281–5.

75. Fernandez-Gomez J, Rodriguez-Martinez JJ, Barmadah SE, et al. Urinary CYFRA 21.1 is not a useful marker for the detection of recurrences in the follow-up of superficial bladder cancer. Eur Urol 2007;51:1267–74.

76. Hakenberg OW, Fuessel S, Richter K, et al. Qualitative and quantitative assessment of urinary cytokeratin 8 and 18 fragments compared with voided urine cytology in diagnosis of bladder carcinoma. Urology 2004;64:1121–6.

77. Babjuk M, Kostirova M, Mudra K, et al. Qualitative and quantitative detection of urinary human complement factor H-related protein (BTA stat and BTA TRAK) and fragments of cytokeratins 8, 18 (UBC rapid and UBC IRMA) as markers for transitional cell carcinoma of the bladder. Eur Urol 2002; 41:34–9.

78. Sánchez-Carbayo M, Herrero E, Megías J, et al. Initial evaluation of the new urinary bladder cancer rapid test in the detection of transitional cell carcinoma of the bladder. Urology 1999;54:656–61.

79. Lüdecke G, Pilatz A, Hauptmann A, et al. Comparative analysis of sensitivity to blood in the urine for urine-based point-of-care assays (UBC rapid, NMP22 BladderChek and BTA-stat) in primary diagnosis of bladder carcinoma. Interference of blood on the results of urine-based POC tests. Anticancer Res 2012;32:2015–8.

80. Schroeder GL, Lorenzo-Gomez M-F, Hautmann SH, et al. A side by side comparison of cytology and biomarkers for bladder cancer detection. J Urol 2004;172:1123–6.

81. Ritter R, Hennenlotter J, Kuhs U, et al. Evaluation of a new quantitative point-of-care test platform for urine-based detection of bladder cancer. Urol Oncol 2014;32:337–44.

82. Yang H, Li H, Wang Z, et al. Is urinary soluble Fas an independent predictor of non-muscle-invasive bladder cancer? A prospective chart study. Urol Int 2013;91:456–61.

83. Srivastava AK, Singh PK, Singh D, et al. Clinical utility of urinary soluble Fas in screening for bladder cancer. Asia Pac J Clin Oncol 2014. [Epub ahead of print].

84. Svatek RS, Herman MP, Lotan Y, et al. Soluble Fas–a promising novel urinary marker for the detection of recurrent superficial bladder cancer. Cancer 2006;106:1701–7.

85. Miyake H, Gleave M, Kamidono S, et al. Overexpression of clusterin in transitional cell carcinoma of the bladder is related to disease progression and recurrence. Urology 2002;59:150–4.

86. Pucci S, Bonanno E, Sesti F, et al. Clusterin in stool: a new biomarker for colon cancer screening? Am J Gastroenterol 2009;104:2807–15.

87. Stejskal D, Fiala RR. Evaluation of serum and urine clusterin as a potential tumor marker for urinary bladder cancer. Neoplasma 2006;53:343–6.

88. Hazzaa SM, Elashry OM, Afifi IK. Clusterin as a diagnostic and prognostic marker for transitional cell carcinoma of the bladder. Pathol Oncol Res 2010;16:101–9.

89. Shabayek MI, Sayed OM, Attaia HA, et al. Diagnostic evaluation of urinary angiogenin (ANG) and clusterin (CLU) as biomarker for bladder cancer. Pathol Oncol Res 2014;20:859–66.

90. Sankhwar M, Sankhwar SN, Abhishek A, et al. Clinical significance of the VEGF level in urinary bladder carcinoma. Cancer Biomarkers 2015; 15(4):349–55.

91. Sun Y, He D, Ma Q, et al. Comparison of seven screening methods in the diagnosis of bladder cancer. Chin Med J (Engl) 2006;119:1763–71.

92. Eissa S, Salem AM, Zohny SF, et al. The diagnostic efficacy of urinary TGF-beta1 and VEGF in bladder cancer: comparison with voided urine cytology. Cancer Biomark 2007;3:275–85.

93. Urquidi V, Goodison S, Kim J, et al. Vascular endothelial growth factor, carbonic anhydrase 9, and angiogenin as urinary biomarkers for bladder cancer detection. Urology 2012;79:1185.e1–6.

94. Sheryka E, Wheeler MA, Hausladen DA, et al. Urinary interleukin-8 levels are elevated in subjects with transitional cell carcinoma. Urology 2003;62:162–6.

95. Urquidi V, Chang M, Dai Y, et al. IL-8 as a urinary biomarker for the detection of bladder cancer. BMC Urol 2012;12:12.

96. Kumar A, Dubey D, Bansal P, et al. Urinary interleukin-8 predicts the response of standard and low dose intravesical bacillus Calmette-Guerin (modified Danish 1331 strain) for superficial bladder cancer. J Urol 2002;168:2232–5.

97. Sagnak L, Ersoy H, Ozok U, et al. Predictive value of urinary interleukin-8 cutoff point for recurrences after transurethral resection plus induction bacillus Calmette-Guérin treatment in non-muscle-invasive bladder tumors. Clin Genitourin Cancer 2009;7: E16–23.

98. Rigaud J, Leger A, Devilder M-C, et al. Development of predictive value of urinary cytokine profile induced during intravesical bacillus calmette-guérin instillations for bladder cancer. Clin Genitourin Cancer 2015;13(4):e209–15.

99. Cai T, Nesi G, Mazzoli S, et al. Prediction of response to bacillus Calmette-Guérin treatment in non-muscle invasive bladder cancer patients through interleukin-6 and interleukin-10 ratio. Exp Ther Med 2012;4:459–64.

100. Cai T, Mazzoli S, Meacci F, et al. Interleukin-6/10 ratio as a prognostic marker of recurrence in patients with intermediate risk urothelial bladder carcinoma. J Urol 2007;178:1902–6.

101. Muller M. Telomerase: its clinical relevance in the diagnosis of bladder cancer. Oncogene 2002;21: 650–5.

102. Sanchini MA, Gunelli R, Nanni O, et al. Relevance of urine telomerase in the diagnosis of bladder cancer. JAMA 2005;294:2052–6.

103. Lamarca A, Barriuso J. Urine telomerase for diagnosis and surveillance of bladder cancer. Adv Urol 2012;2012:693631.

104. Neves M, Ciofu C, Larousserie F, et al. Prospective evaluation of genetic abnormalities and telomerase expression in exfoliated urinary cells for bladder cancer detection. J Urol 2002;167:1276–81.

105. Isurugi K, Suzuki Y, Tanji S, et al. Detection of the presence of catalytic subunit mRNA associated with telomerase gene in exfoliated urothelial cells from patients with bladder cancer. J Urol 2002; 168:1574–7.

106. Melissourgos N, Kastrinakis NG, Davilas I, et al. Detection of human telomerase reverse transcriptase mRNA in urine of patients with bladder cancer: evaluation of an emerging tumor marker. Urology 2003;62:362–7.

107. Weikert S, Krause H, Wolff I, et al. Quantitative evaluation of telomerase subunits in urine as biomarkers for noninvasive detection of bladder cancer. Int J Cancer 2005;117:274–80.

108. Eissa S, Swellam M, Ali-Labib R, et al. Detection of telomerase in urine by 3 methods: evaluation of diagnostic accuracy for bladder cancer. J Urol 2007;178:1068–72.

109. Eissa S, Motawi T, Badr S, et al. Evaluation of urinary human telomerase reverse transcriptase mRNA and scatter factor protein as urine markers for diagnosis of bladder cancer. Clin Lab 2013;59:317–23.

110. Lokeshwar VB, Block NL. HA-HAase urine test. A sensitive and specific method for detecting bladder cancer and evaluating its grade. Urol Clin North Am 2000;27:53–61.

111. Hautmann S, Toma M, Lorenzo Gomez MF, et al. Immunocyt and the HA-HAase urine tests for the detection of bladder cancer: a side-by-side comparison. Eur Urol 2004;46:466–71.

112. Yang X, Huang H, Zeng Z, et al. Diagnostic value of bladder tumor fibronectin in patients with bladder tumor: a systematic review with meta-analysis. Clin Biochem 2013;46:1377–82.

113. Hattori S, Kojima K, Minoshima K, et al. Detection of bladder cancer by measuring CD44v6 expression in urine with real-time quantitative reverse transcription polymerase chain reaction. Urology 2014; 83:1443.e9–15.

114. Shen C, Sun Z, Chen D, et al. Developing urinary metabolomic signatures as early bladder cancer diagnostic markers. OMICS 2015;19:1–11.

115. Wittmann BM, Stirdivant SM, Mitchell MW, et al. Bladder cancer biomarker discovery using global

metabolomic profiling of urine. PLoS One 2014;9: e115870.

116. Jin X, Yun SJ, Jeong P, et al. Diagnosis of bladder cancer and prediction of survival by urinary metabolomics. Oncotarget 2014;5:1635–45.

117. Putluri N, Shojaie A, Vasu VT, et al. Metabolomic profiling reveals potential markers and bioprocesses altered in bladder cancer progression. Cancer Res 2011;71:7376–86.

118. Pasikanti KK, Esuvaranathan K, Ho PC, et al. Noninvasive urinary metabonomic diagnosis of human bladder cancer. J Proteome Res 2010;9: 2988–95.

119. Issaq HJ, Nativ O, Waybright T, et al. Detection of bladder cancer in human urine by metabolomic profiling using high performance liquid chromatography/mass spectrometry. J Urol 2008;179: 2422–6.

120. Park H-S, Park WS, Bondaruk J, et al. Quantitation of Aurora kinase A gene copy number in urine sediments and bladder cancer detection. J Natl Cancer Inst 2008;100:1401–11.

121. De Martino M, Shariat SF, Hofbauer SL, et al. Aurora A Kinase as a diagnostic urinary marker for urothelial bladder cancer. World J Urol 2014; 33:105–10.

122. Knowles MA. Role of FGFR3 in urothelial cell carcinoma: biomarker and potential therapeutic target. World J Urol 2007;25:581–93.

123. Van Oers JM, Lurkin I, van Exsel AJ, et al. A simple and fast method for the simultaneous detection of nine fibroblast growth factor receptor 3 mutations in bladder cancer and voided urine. Clin Cancer Res 2005;11:7743–8.

124. Miyake M, Sugano K, Sugino H, et al. Fibroblast growth factor receptor 3 mutation in voided urine is a useful diagnostic marker and significant indicator of tumor recurrence in non-muscle invasive bladder cancer. Cancer Sci 2010;101:250–8.

125. Zuiverloon TC, van der Aa MN, van der Kwast TH, et al. Fibroblast growth factor receptor 3 mutation analysis on voided urine for surveillance of patients with low-grade non-muscle-invasive bladder cancer. Clin Cancer Res 2010;16:3011–8.

126. Zuiverloon TC, Beukers W, van der Keur KA, et al. Combinations of urinary biomarkers for surveillance of patients with incident nonmuscle invasive bladder cancer: the European FP7 UROMOL project. J Urol 2013;189:1945–51.

127. Bangma CH, Loeb S, Busstra M, et al. Outcomes of a bladder cancer screening program using home hematuria testing and molecular markers. Eur Urol 2013;64:41–7.

128. Van Kessel KE, Kompier LC, de Bekker-Grob EW, et al. FGFR3 mutation analysis in voided urine samples to decrease cystoscopies and cost in non-muscle invasive bladder cancer surveillance: a comparison of 3 strategies. J Urol 2013;189: 1676–81.

129. Frigerio S, Padberg BC, Strebel RT, et al. Improved detection of bladder carcinoma cells in voided urine by standardized microsatellite analysis. Int J Cancer 2007;121:329–38.

130. Schneider A, Borgnat S, Lang H, et al. Evaluation of microsatellite analysis in urine sediment for diagnosis of bladder cancer. Cancer Res 2000;60: 4617–22.

131. Seripa D, Parrella P, Gallucci M, et al. Sensitive detection of transitional cell carcinoma of the bladder by microsatellite analysis of cells exfoliated in urine. Int J Cancer 2001;95:364–9.

132. Bartoletti R, Dal Canto M, Cai T, et al. Early diagnosis and monitoring of superficial transitional cell carcinoma by microsatellite analysis on urine sediment. Oncol Rep 2005;13:531–7.

133. Bartoletti R, Cai T, Dal Canto M, et al. Multiplex polymerase chain reaction for microsatellite analysis of urine sediment cells: a rapid and inexpensive method for diagnosing and monitoring superficial transitional bladder cell carcinoma. J Urol 2006; 175:2032–7 [discussion: 2037].

134. Dal Canto M, Bartoletti R, Travaglini F, et al. Molecular urinary sediment analysis in patients with transitional cell bladder carcinoma. Anticancer Res 2003;23:5095–100.

135. Van der Aa MN, Zwarthoff EC, Steyerberg EW, et al. Microsatellite analysis of voided-urine samples for surveillance of low-grade non-muscle-invasive urothelial carcinoma: feasibility and clinical utility in a prospective multicenter study (Cost-Effectiveness of Follow-Up of Urinary Bladder Cancer trial [CEFUB]. Eur Urol 2009;55:659–67.

136. De Bekker-Grob EW, van der Aa MN, Zwarthoff EC, et al. Non-muscle-invasive bladder cancer surveillance for which cystoscopy is partly replaced by microsatellite analysis of urine: a cost-effective alternative? BJU Int 2009;104:41–7.

137. Ho CL, Tzai TS, Chen JC, et al. The molecular signature for urothelial carcinoma of the upper urinary tract. J Urol 2008;179:1155–9.

138. Reinert T, Borre M, Christiansen A, et al. Diagnosis of bladder cancer recurrence based on urinary levels of EOMES, HOXA9, POU4F2, TWIST1, VIM, and ZNF154 hypermethylation. PLoS One 2012;7:e46297.

139. Shimizu T, Suzuki H, Nojima M, et al. Methylation of a panel of microRNA genes is a novel biomarker for detection of bladder cancer. Eur Urol 2013;63: 1091–100.

140. Shariat SF, Karam JA, Raman JD. Urine cytology and urine-based markers for bladder urothelial carcinoma detection and monitoring: developments and future prospects. Biomark Med 2008;2:165–80.

141. Hatzichristodoulou G, Kubler H, Schwaibold H, et al. Nuclear matrix protein 22 for bladder cancer

detection: comparative analysis of the Bladder-Chek(R) and ELISA. Anticancer Res 2012;32:5093–7.

142. Fantony JJ, Abern MR, Gopalakrishna A, et al. Multi-institutional external validation of urinary TWIST1 and NID2 methylation as a diagnostic test for bladder cancer. Urol Oncol 2015;33(9): 387e1–6.

143. Maldonado L, Brait M, Michailidi C, et al. An epigenetic marker panel for recurrence risk prediction of low grade papillary urothelial cell carcinoma (LGPUCC) and its potential use for surveillance after transurethral resection using urine. Oncotarget 2014;5:5218–33.

144. Su SF, de Castro Abreu AL, Chihara Y, et al. A panel of three markers hyper- and hypomethylated in urine sediments accurately predicts bladder cancer recurrence. Clin Cancer Res 2014;20: 1978–89.

145. Abern MR, Owusu R, Inman BA. Clinical performance and utility of a DNA methylation urine test for bladder cancer. Urol Oncol 2014;32:51.e21–6.

146. Beukers W, Kandimalla R, van Houwelingen D, et al. The use of molecular analyses in voided urine for the assessment of patients with hematuria. PLoS One 2013;8:e77657.

147. Chihara Y, Kanai Y, Fujimoto H, et al. Diagnostic markers of urothelial cancer based on DNA methylation analysis. BMC Cancer 2013;13:275.

148. Zuiverloon TCM, Beukers W, van der Keur KA, et al. A methylation assay for the detection of non-muscle-invasive bladder cancer (NMIBC) recurrences in voided urine. BJU Int 2012;109:941–8.

149. Scher MB, Elbaum MB, Mogilevkin Y, et al. Detecting DNA methylation of the BCL2, CDKN2A and NID2 genes in urine using a nested methylation specific polymerase chain reaction assay to predict bladder cancer. J Urol 2012;188:2101–7.

150. Berrada N, Amzazi S, Ameziane El Hassani R, et al. Epigenetic alterations of adenomatous polyposis coli (APC), retinoic acid receptor beta (RARβ) and survivin genes in tumor tissues and voided urine of bladder cancer patients. Cell Mol Biol (Noisy-le-grand) 2012;(Suppl 58):OL1744–51.

151. Zhao Y, Guo S, Sun J, et al. Methylcap-seq reveals novel DNA methylation markers for the diagnosis and recurrence prediction of bladder cancer in a Chinese population. PLoS One 2012;7:e35175.

152. Eissa S, Zohny SF, Shehata HH, et al. Urinary retinoic acid receptor-beta2 gene promoter methylation and hyaluronidase activity as noninvasive tests for diagnosis of bladder cancer. Clin Biochem 2012;45:402–7.

153. Chen PC, Tsai MH, Yip SK, et al. Distinct DNA methylation epigenotypes in bladder cancer from different Chinese sub-populations and its implication in cancer detection using voided urine. BMC Med Genomics 2011;4:45.

154. Chung W, Bondaruk J, Jelinek J, et al. Detection of bladder cancer using novel DNA methylation biomarkers in urine sediments. Cancer Epidemiol Biomarkers Prev 2011;20:1483–91.

155. Costa VL, Henrique R, Danielsen SA, et al. Three epigenetic biomarkers, GDF15, TMEFF2, and VIM, accurately predict bladder cancer from DNA-based analyses of urine samples. Clin Cancer Res 2010;16:5842–51.

156. Vinci S, Giannarini G, Selli C, et al. Quantitative methylation analysis of BCL2, hTERT, and DAPK promoters in urine sediment for the detection of non-muscle-invasive urothelial carcinoma of the bladder: a prospective, two-center validation study. Urol Oncol 2011;29:150–6.

157. Rouprêt M, Hupertan V, Yates DR, et al. A comparison of the performance of microsatellite and methylation urine analysis for predicting the recurrence of urothelial cell carcinoma, and definition of a set of markers by Bayesian network analysis. BJU Int 2008;101:1448–53.

158. Hoque MO, Begum S, Topaloglu O, et al. Quantitation of promoter methylation of multiple genes in urine DNA and bladder cancer detection. J Natl Cancer Inst 2006;98:996–1004.

159. Friedrich MG, Weisenberger DJ, Cheng JC, et al. Detection of methylated apoptosis-associated genes in urine sediments of bladder cancer patients. Clin Cancer Res 2004;10:7457–65.

160. Chan MW, Chan LW, Tang NL, et al. Hypermethylation of multiple genes in tumor tissues and voided urine in urinary bladder cancer patients. Clin Cancer Res 2002;8:464–70.

161. Hanke M, Hoefig K, Merz H, et al. A robust methodology to study urine microRNA as tumor marker: microRNA-126 and microRNA-182 are related to urinary bladder cancer. Urol Oncol 2010;28: 655–61.

162. Yamada Y, Enokida H, Kojima S, et al. MiR-96 and miR-183 detection in urine serve as potential tumor markers of urothelial carcinoma: correlation with stage and grade, and comparison with urinary cytology. Cancer Sci 2011;102: 522–9.

163. Snowdon J, Boag S, Feilotter H, et al. A pilot study of urinary microRNA as a biomarker for urothelial cancer. Can Urol Assoc J 2013;7(1–2):28–32.

164. Miah S, Dudziec E, Drayton RM, et al. An evaluation of urinary microRNA reveals a high sensitivity for bladder cancer. Br J Cancer 2012;107: 123–8.

165. Yun SJ, Jeong P, Kim WT, et al. Cell-free microRNAs in urine as diagnostic and prognostic biomarkers of bladder cancer. Int J Oncol 2012;41: 1871–8.

166. Mengual L, Lozano JJ, Ingelmo-Torres M, et al. Using microRNA profiling in urine samples to develop

a non-invasive test for bladder cancer. Int J Cancer 2013;133:2631–41.

167. Zhou X, Zhang X, Yang Y, et al. Urinary cell-free microRNA-106b as a novel biomarker for detection of bladder cancer. Med Oncol 2014;31:197.

168. Zhang DZ, Lau KM, Chan ES, et al. Cell-free urinary microRNA-99a and microRNA-125b are diagnostic markers for the non-invasive screening of bladder cancer. PLoS One 2014; 9:e100793.

Emerging Bladder Cancer Biomarkers and Targets of Therapy

George J. Netto, MD[a,b,c],*, Laura J. Tafe, MD[d,e]

KEYWORDS

- Urothelial carcinoma ● Bladder cancer ● Genomics ● Targeted therapy ● Clinical trials ● Biomarkers

KEY POINTS

- Bladder cancer is a heterogeneous disease, and recent genomic studies have identified several potential therapeutic targets.
- Alterations in tyrosine kinase receptors, intracellular signaling pathways, such as the PI3K/AKT/mTOR pathway, cell-cycle regulators, chromatin remodeling, and immune mediation, are significant in disease progression, and therapies targeting many of these alterations are currently in clinical trials.
- Novel noninvasive strategies are being developed, using identification of genomic, epigenetic, and proteomic markers, for early detection and surveillance in urine and serum.

GENETIC AND MOLECULAR BIOMARKERS

Deciphering the molecular pathways of bladder cancer has accelerated the identification of prognostic and theranostic markers, allowed for the development of novel noninvasive early detection and surveillance strategies, and elucidated new targets of therapy in bladder cancer.[1–26] Although widespread clinical adoption of novel biomarkers has been limited due to lack of validation by multi-institutional randomized prospective trials, recent genomic studies[27–30] have spurred efforts to evaluate these therapies, and such trials are finally being launched.

GENOMICS OF BLADDER CANCER

Recent genomic studies have validated and expanded on previously identified genetic pathways

of bladder cancer development and have unmasked additional crucial driver genetic alterations. Although earlier array-based gene expression studies highlighted differentially expressed genetic signatures capable of predicting recurrence and progression,[7–9,21,23,31–40] recent integrated genomic and protein analysis studies have better defined clinically relevant molecular subtypes of bladder cancer. By integrating genomic data from aCGH, gene expression arrays, targeted mutation sequencing analysis, and protein analyses, Lindgren and colleagues[29,38] brought to light 2 main genomic molecular circuits in urothelial carcinoma: the first characterized by FGFR3 alterations, overexpression of CCND1, and deletions in 9q and CDKN2A; and the second by E2F3 amplifications, RB1 and PTEN deletions, gains of 5p, and overexpression of CDKN2A (p16). Alterations in TP53/MDM2 were

Disclosure Statement: The authors have nothing to disclose.
a Department of Pathology, The Johns Hopkins Medical Institutes, Baltimore, MD, USA; b Department of Oncology, The Johns Hopkins Medical Institutes, Baltimore, MD, USA; c Department of Urology, The Johns Hopkins Medical Institutes, Baltimore, MD, USA; d Department of Pathology, Dartmouth-Hitchcock Medical Center, One Medical Center Drive, Lebanon, NH 03756, USA; e Geisel School of Medicine at Dartmouth, 1 Rope Ferry Rd, Hanover, NH 03755, USA
* Corresponding author. Department of Pathology, Johns Hopkins University School of Medicine, 401 North Broadway Weinberg 2242, Baltimore, MD 21231.
E-mail address: gnetto1@jhmi.edu

Urol Clin N Am 43 (2016) 63–76
http://dx.doi.org/10.1016/j.ucl.2015.08.006
0094-0143/16/$ – see front matter © 2016 Elsevier Inc. All rights reserved.

demonstrated in advanced tumors in both groups. Lindgren and colleagues[29] first recognized the significantly worse prognosis associated with a gene expression profile of a keratinized/squamous phenotype; this molecular subtype was further validated by Choi and colleagues[27] (**Fig. 1**). Termed basallike and characterized by p63 activation, squamous differentiation, positive CK5/6, epidermal growth factor receptor (EGFR), and cluster of differentiation (CD)44 expression and lack of cytokeratin (CK)20, this subtype is clinically aggressive but potentially sensitive to neoadjuvant chemotherapy. Choi and colleagues[27] also characterized a luminal subtype typically enriched for activating *FGFR3*

mutations, active estrogen receptor pathway, and ERBB2 and PPARγ expression profile, and a third subtype, characterized by wild-type TP53 gene expression and strongly associated with resistance to neoadjuvant methotrexate, vinblastine, adriamycin/doxorubicin, and cisplatin (MVAC) therapy. Interestingly, upon resistance to chemotherapy, tumors from the basallike and luminal subtypes also displayed the TP53 wild-type expression.[27]

Finally, The Cancer Genome Atlas (TCGA) project's comprehensive molecular characterization of bladder cancer[28] provided a genomic analysis of 131 high-grade muscle-invasive bladder cancers (MI-BC), which revealed a staggering 302

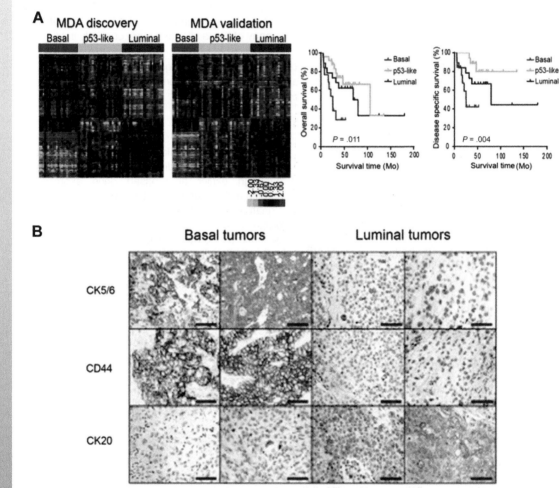

Fig. 1. (*A*) Three molecular subtype signatures (basal, luminal, and p53 wild-type signature) on whole genome mRNA expression (Illumina's DASL [cDNA-mediated Annealing, Selection, extension, and Ligation] platform). Corresponding Kaplan-Meier plots of overall survival and DSS are depicted. (*B*) Immunohistochemical analysis (CK5/6, CD44, and CK20) of basal and luminal marker expression. Representative basal (*left*) and luminal (*right*) tumors, as defined by gene expression profiling, are displayed. (*Adapted from* Choi W, Porten S, Kim S, et al. Identification of distinct basal and luminal subtypes of muscle-invasive bladder cancer with different sensitivities to frontline chemotherapy. Cancer Cell 2014;25(2):152–65; with permission.)

mutations, 204 segmental copy number alterations (CNA), and 22 rearrangements on average per tumor. Recurrent "driver" mutations in 32 genes were found, which include genes involved in cell-cycle regulation, chromatin regulation, kinase signaling pathways, and 9 additional genes not previously shown to have recurrent mutational pattern in other tumors. Based on integration of mRNA/miRNA sequencing data and protein expression analysis, 4 major expression clusters were identified (**Fig. 2**). Among them, papillarylike cluster (cluster I), enriched for *FGFR3* gene alterations, together with cluster II share expression of luminal urothelial differentiations markers (activated expression of ER, GATA3, Uroplakin, and ERBB2) and cluster III

basal/squamouslike, as in the Choi and colleagues study,[27] characterized by CK5/6 and EGFR expression (**Table 1**).[28,29] When compared with the TCGA profiles of several other tumor types, bladder cancer clusters I and II are very similar to luminal A breast cancer subtype, whereas cluster III is similar to basallike breast cancer, and squamous cell carcinoma of the head and neck and lung.[28]

BIOMARKERS AND PATHWAY TARGETS
Receptor Tyrosine Kinases and Cell-Cycle Markers

Numerous studies suggest a prognostic value for receptor tyrosine kinases, such as *FGFR3*, *EGFR*,

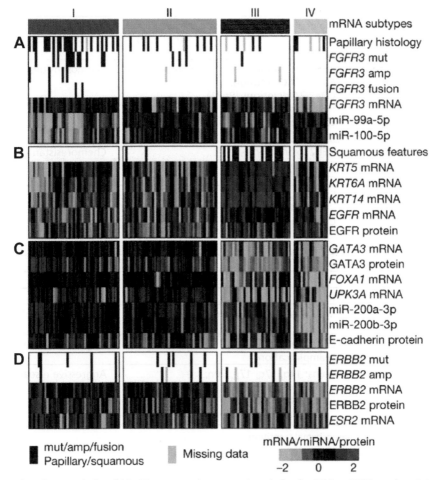

Fig. 2. Expression characteristics of bladder cancer. Integrated analysis of mRNA, miRNA, and protein data led to identification of distinct subsets of urothelial carcinoma. Data from RNA, miRNA, and protein were z-normalized, and samples were organized in the horizontal direction by mRNA clustering. (*A*) Papillary histology, FGFR3 alterations, FGFR3 expression, and reduced FGFR3-related miRNA expression are enriched in cluster I. (*B*) Expression of epithelial lineage genes and stem/progenitor cytokeratins are generally high in cluster III, some of which show variant squamous histology. (*C*) Luminal breast and urothelial differentiation factors are enriched in clusters I and II. (*D*) ERBB2 mutation and estrogen receptor β(ESR2) expression are enriched in clusters I and II. (*Adapted from* Cancer Genome Atlas Research Network. Comprehensive molecular characterization of urothelial bladder carcinoma. Nature 2014;507(7492):315–22; with permission.)

Table 1
Genomic characteristics of non-muscle-invasive and muscle-invasive bladder cancer and micropapillary and plasmacytoid variants

Subtype/Cluster	Molecular Characteristics	Histology (General)	Noteworthy Clinical Features
Non-muscle-invasive bladder cancer			
Papillary	*FGFR3* mutations 9q deletions *CDKN2A* deletions (9p21)	Papillary	*Low grade:* Recurrence risk ~50% Risk of progression (~5–10%) *High grade:* Recurrence risk >50% Risk of progression (15%–40%)
Muscle-invasive bladder cancer			
Subtype/TCGA cluster based on RNA sequencing	Molecular characteristics	Histology (general)	Noteworthy clinical features
Luminal (I) (similar to luminal A breast cancer subtype)	*FGFR3* mutations *FGFR3-TACC3* fusions *CDKN2A* deletions (9p21) HER2 expression ESR2 expression miR-200 family (EMT)	Papillary-like	Chemosensitive
P53-like (II) (similar to luminal A breast cancer subtype)	HER2 expression ESR2 expression miR-200 family (EMT)		Chemoresistant
Basal/squamous-like (III) (similar to basal-like breast cancer, squamous cell carcinoma of head and lung)	Express cytokeratins (KRT14, KRT5) *CCND1* amplification	Squamous-like; sarcomatoid	Chemosensitive
Claudin-low (IV)	—	—	Uncertain
Special variant histology of note			
	Molecular characteristics	—	Noteworthy clinical features
Micropapillary	*ERBB2* mutations and amplification	—	Aggressive disease
Plasmacytoid	Gains: 11q, 17q, 17p, 20q; losses on 4q and 6q; CCND1 and CDH1 deletions (25087089)	—	Aggressive disease

Abbreviation: EMT, epithelial mesenchymal transition.
  Data from Refs.[27,29,115–118]

ERBB2, and *ERBB3* in bladder cancer[13,41–52]; for instance, *FGFR3* mutations correlate with a favorable outcome.[42,53] An elevated tumor proliferation index, measured by ki67 or Monoclonal Anti-Human Ki-67 Antigen, Clone MIB-1 (MIB-1) immunohistochemistry, consistently predicts a worse outcome in bladder cancer.[42,53–59] A molecular grade (mG), initially proposed by Van Rhijn and colleagues,[42,53] combining *FGFR3* gene mutation status and MIB-1 index, was found to be superior to the NBI-BC risk calculator of the European Organization for Research and Treatment of Cancer.[60] mG independently predicts disease-specific survival (DSS), and when added to the multivariable model for progression, increases the predictive accuracy to 81.7%. Proliferation index is also prognostic in MI-BC[55]; a large cystectomy cohort from the bladder consortium multi-institutional trial confirmed the role of Ki67 in predicting progression-free survival (PFS) and DSS.[56] In addition, a synergistic prognostic role for combining p53 expression status with other cell-cycle control elements, such as pRb, cyclin E1, p21, and p27, has been repeatedly shown in non-muscle-invasive bladder cancer (NMI-BC) as well as MI-BC (**Fig. 3**).[16,18,61–63]

Epigenetic Markers

Both gene methylation and miRNAs have been successfully analyzed in patients with bladder cancer, demonstrating their potential utility as tools for early detection and prognosis.[37,64–76] Epigenetic profiles, specifically, promoter methylation of *RASSF1A*, *DAPK*, *CDH1* (encodes for E-cadherin), *TNFSR25*, *EDNRB*, and *APC* genes,

have been shown to predict disease progression and possibly death from disease independent of tumor stage.[71,76]

MONITORING/DETECTION METHODS

With the goal of early detection and improved surveillance, less invasive techniques are being investigated in order to develop the "liquid biopsy" to measure biomarkers in either blood or urine. Urovysion, which is US Food and Drug Administration (FDA) approved for surveillance as well as screening and early detection in high-risk patients with hematuria, exploits recurrent chromosomal alterations (gains of chromosomes 3q, 7p, and 17q, and 9p21 deletions [*CDKN2A*/p16 locus]) in a urine-based multitarget interphase fluorescence in situ hybridization (FISH) assay.[77–79] When used as a reflex test in combination with routine urine cytology, a sensitivity of 69% to 87% and specificity of 89% to 96% are achieved.[80,81] In

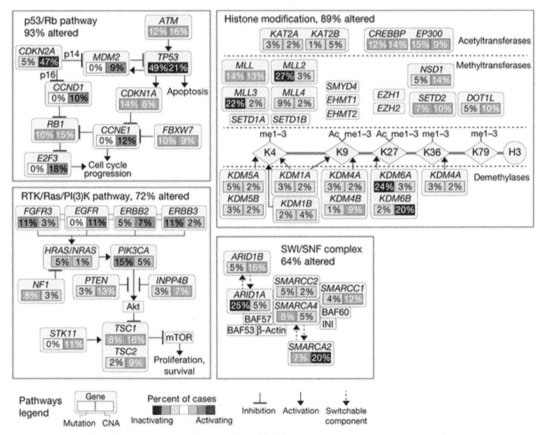

Fig. 3. Altered molecular pathways and networks in bladder cancer. Somatic mutations and CNA in components of the p53/Rb pathway, RTK/RAS/PI(3)K pathway, histone modification system, and SWI/SNF complex. (*Red*) Activating genetic alterations; (*blue*) inactivating genetic alterations. Percentages shown denote activation or inactivation of at least one allele. (*Adapted from* Cancer Genome Atlas Research Network. Comprehensive molecular characterization of urothelial bladder carcinoma. Nature 2014;507(7492):315–22; with permission.)

addition, up to two-thirds of patients with positive FISH but clinically absent disease have been shown to develop cancer within 29 months,[82] suggesting a lead time value for molecular early detection.[83–86]

More recently, urine-based assays for *FGFR3* mutation, given the high prevalence in NMI-BC, and *TERT* promotor mutations, either as a single marker or in combination with other alterations,

are being evaluated.[30,87,88] **Table 2** further elucidates these and some other biomarker assays that are currently available and are in development for this purpose.

CLINICAL TRIALS

The TCGA[28] and preceding comprehensive genomic studies have identified a spectrum of

Table 2
Noninvasive strategies for identification of genomic, epigenetic, and proteomic biomarkers for the purpose of early detection and surveillance of bladder cancer in urine and serum samples

Product	Methodology/Target	Sensitivity/Specificity	Reference
Commercially available products (representative)			
Multicolor FISH (FDA approved; Urovysion; Abbott Molecular, Abbott Park, IL, USA)	FISH for 4 chromosomal markers: gains of 3, 7, and 17 and loss of 9p21	Sensitivity of 69%–87% Specificity of 89%–96% when combined with urine cytology	77–81
ImmunoCyt (FDA approved; Scimedx, Denville, NJ, USA)	Detects 3 different proteins: M344, 19A211, and LDQ10 on the surface of voided cells (fluorescence immunohistochemistry)	Sensitivity 50%–100% for early stage disease Overall sensitivity 62% Overall specificity 79%	118,119
Developing methods			
Circulating tumor cells mutation analysis/ detection • Serum • Urine	*FGFR3* mutation in combination with methylation markers (PCR based)	Sensitivity 62% (urine) Specificity 100%	37
	TERT promoter mutation (PCR based)	Variable according to clinical indication, tumor grade and methodology	30,120–122
	Urine cytology	Sensitivity 48% Specificity 86% (Sensitivity for LG, 16%; HG, 84%)	119
Cell-free DNA/circulating tumor DNA/epigenetic markers • Serum • Urine	DNA-based; RNA-based; DNA methylation; miRNA; long noncoding RNA	—	123,124
Proteomics • Serum • Urine	Upregulation of calgranulin A (S100A8), calgranulin B (S100A9), calcium binding protein (S100A4), carbonic anhydrase I, and downregulation of calcium-dependent phospholipid-binding protein (annexin V) (MALDI-TOF-MS)	Sensitivity 80% (serum) Specificity 81%	125
	An 8-biomarker panel: IL-8, MMP-9, PAI-1, VEGF, ANG, CA-9, APOE, MMP-10 (ELISA)	Sensitivity 92% (urine) Specificity 97%	126

Abbreviations: ELISA, enzyme-linked immunosorbent assay; FISH, Florescence in situ hybridization; HG, high grade; LG, low grade; MALDI-TOF-MS, matrix-assisted laser desorption/ionization-time of flight-mass spectrometry; PCR, Polymerase chain reaction.

therapeutic targets that are present in the majority (>70%) of MI-BC.[27–29] Clinical trials investigating such targeted therapeutic strategies along with identification and validation of predictive markers that correlate with response to therapy are underway.[89–92] Key targets include members of the *PI3KCA/AKT/mTOR*,[93–96] *RTK/MAPK* (including *EGFR, FGFR3,* and *ERBB2*), and estrogen receptor (*ER*) pathways, immune response check point modulators,[97,98] and chromatin regulation and remodeling targets[99–101] (**Table 3**).

Receptor tyrosine kinase–targeted therapies under investigation include small molecule pan-FGFR inhibitors, which have demonstrated encouraging results in patients with bladder cancer harboring activating *FGFR* mutations or translocations (luminal/papillarylike subtypes). Trials of EGFR inhibitors may be effective in chemotherapy-naive bladder cancer with EGFR or ERBB2 overexpression.[102] Preclinical results with trastuzumab conjugated with a cytotoxic agent, DM1 (derivative of maytansine 1) (T-DM1), are promising in ERBB2-positive tumors.[103–105] Currently, evidence of tumor ERBB2 positivity by either immunohistochemistry or FISH could determine eligibility for ERBB2 targeted trials.[106] Interestingly, in contrast to breast cancer, there is a higher rate of *ERBB2* mutations in bladder cancer, and ERBB2 overexpression is typically not associated with *ERBB2* gene amplification.[107]

Molecular biomarkers to predict response to neoadjuvant chemotherapy is another crucial area of development because only 20% to 30% of patients will achieve pathologic complete response.[108–111] Molecular signatures (basallike/squamous, luminal, and papillarylike)[27,28] can be used to define subsets of patients that will respond to and achieve a higher survival rate with a particular therapeutic regimen while preventing unnecessary drug exposure and toxicity and delay of cystectomy in others (p53 wild-type signature).[108–111] In 2014, SWAG (Southwest Oncology Group) launched a clinical trial (NCT02177695) stratifying patients to 2 frontline chemotherapy regimens (gemcitabine plus cisplatin vs MVAC) to determine the ability of a treatment-specific COXEN score (based on a novel gene expression profiling-based algorithm {COXEN (Co-eXpression ExtrapolatioN)}) to predict complete pathologic response.[111]

Other trials are examining the utility of mTOR pathway inhibitors in combination with MEK inhibitors[89] and inhibitors of cell-cycle regulators (aurora kinase [AURKA],[112,113] PLK1, and cyclin-dependent kinase 4 [CDK4])[114] in combination with chemotherapy.

Preliminary positive responses with anti-CTLA4 and anti-PDL1, novel immune modulating agents,[97] are promising. In fact, in 2014, the FDA granted MPDL3280A, a PDL1 monoclonal antibody inhibitor, a breakthrough therapy designation based on the results phase I trial of patients with metastatic bladder cancer that showed up to a 43% response rate in patients with 2 to 3+ PDL1 positivity by immunohistochemistry.[97] A large phase II study with 2 cohorts, one for treatment-naive and the other for pretreated patients (NCT02108652), is currently enrolling patients with metastatic bladder cancer.

As the genomic landscape advances, a paradigm shift is seen in the design and execution of clinical trials and an emergence of so-called basket trials that are designed based on tumor genotype independent of tumor site of origin and histology. These trials assign patients in a nonrandomized fashion to a specific treatment arm. The National Cancer Institute (NCI) Molecular Analysis for Therapy Choice (NCI-MATCH) trials are a series of multiple single-arm phase II clinical trials initially focused on single-agent therapies that match a patient's tumor molecular genotype to a targeted agent. Currently, eligibility criteria include (1) solid tumors or lymphomas that have progressed following standard therapy (at least one line); (2) presence of tumor accessible for biopsy and patient agreeable to biopsy (biopsy must have >50% tumor content); (3) 18 years of age and older; (4) ECOG (Eastern Cooperative Oncology Group) 0 to 2 performance status or better; and (5) adequate organ function. For these trials, centralized sequencing will be performed on the Ion Torrent Ion Personal Genome Machine using a custom Ampliseq panel of 200 to 300 actionable genes. If and when patients progress on these protocols, tumors will be rebiopsied and resequenced to better characterize resistance mechanisms; if additional targetable mutations are identified, alternative targeted therapies will be offered. For each mutation-drug match, the dual primary endpoints are overall response rate 5% versus 25% or PFS 6 months 15% versus 35%.[127,128]

In addition, an NCI-led initiative to identify and characterize individuals that are exceptional responders to therapy is currently underway (NCT02243592). It is hoped that characterizing the genotypes of these individuals can better inform the design of clinical trials and the identification of other individuals who may benefit from similar targeted therapies.

In summary, bladder cancer is a heterogeneous disease characterized by complex networks of molecular alterations and gene expression. Recent genomic studies have identified several potential therapeutic targets, including tyrosine kinase receptors, intracellular signaling pathways, cell-cycle regulators, chromatin remodeling, and

Table 3
Alterations in the following pathways/genes are potential therapeutic targets in bladder cancer; many of these targeted therapeutics are currently in clinical trials

Altered Gene/Protein	Drug Category	Drug Examples	Clinical Trial Examples (Phase)
RTK/RAS pathway			
KRAS, HRAS, NRAS, BRAF, EGFR	MEK inhibitor	Selumetinib	NCT00749892 (2)
	EGFR inhibitor or antibody	Cetuximab; erlotinib	NCT00380029 (2)
FGFR1, FGFR2, FGFR3	pan-FGFR inhibitor	BGJ398; dovitinib	NCT01004224 (1) NCT01928459 (1) NCT01732107 (2)
ERBB2, ERBB3	ERBB2 inhibitor	Trastuzumab; lapatinib[a]; neratinib[a]; DN24-02; T-DM1	NCT02342587 (2) NCT01353222 (2) NCT01953926 (2)
VEGF	VEGF inhibitor	Bevacizumab; sorafenib; pazomanib	NCT01108055 (2)
MET	MET inhibitor	Cabozantinib (XL184)	NCT02496208 (1)
PI3K/AKT/mTOR pathway			
PIK3CA, AKT1, AKT3, TSC1, TSC2, PTEN	AKT inhibitor mTOR inhibitor pan-PI3K inhibitor	MK2206; AZD5363 Everolimus; temsirolimus; AZD2014 BKM120 (buparlisib); BYL719	— NCT01259063 (1) NCT01470209 (1) (combined with everolimus)
Cell-cycle regulation			
AURKA, PLK1, CDK4, CCND1/CCND3, CDKN2A	Cdk4/6 inhibitor	LEE011; Palbociclib (PD-0332991)	NCT02187783 (2) NCT02334527 (2)

Chromatin remodeling/histone modification

ARID1A, MLL2, KDM6A, EP300	Agents that bind to acetyl-lysine binding motifs (bromodomains)	BMS-986158; OTX015; TEN-010	
Hormonal therapies			
ESR2 upregulation (estrogen receptor)	Estrogen receptor modulator	Tamoxifen; raloxifene	
Immune modulators			
CTLA4	Anti-CTLA4	Ipilimumab; tremelimumab	
PDL1 (CD274)	Anti-PDL1	MPDL3280A; MED14736;	NCT02450331 (3) NCT02108652 (2) NCT02302807 (3)
PD1	Anti-PD1	Pembrolizumab (MK-3475)	NCT02335424 (2) NCT02256436 (3)
Stress response			
HSP upregulation	HSP90 inhibitor HSP27 inhibitor	Ganetespib OGX-427	NCT01780545 (2)
Cancer stem-cell expression			
KRT14, KRT5	—	—	NCT02027649 (NA) (KRT14 detection)
Basket trials			
NCI-MATCH	—	—	Many
Signature trials	—	—	Many

Abbreviation: NA, nonapplicable.

^a Lapatinib and neratinib are dual inhibitors of human EGFR 2 (Her2/ERBB2) and EGFR kinases.

Data from US National Institutes of Health. ClinicalTrials.gov. Available at: https://clinicaltrials.gov/. Accessed July 24, 2015.

immune mediators. Noninvasive techniques to evaluate biomarkers in patients' urine and serum for early detection and surveillance are being developed. Multiple clinical trials targeting the genomic alterations in bladder cancer are underway.

REFERENCES

1. Netto GJ. Molecular diagnostics in urologic malignancies: a work in progress. Arch Pathol Lab Med 2011;135(5):610–21.
2. Netto GJ, Epstein JI. Theranostic and prognostic biomarkers: genomic applications in urological malignancies. Pathology 2010;42(4):384–94.
3. Netto GJ. Molecular biomarkers in urothelial carcinoma of the bladder: are we there yet? Nat Rev Urol 2011;9(1):41–51.
4. Netto GJ, Cheng L. Emerging critical role of molecular testing in diagnostic genitourinary pathology. Arch Pathol Lab Med 2012;136(4):372–90.
5. van der Kwast TH, Bapat B. Predicting favourable prognosis of urothelial carcinoma: gene expression and genome profiling. Curr Opin Urol 2009;19(5):516–21.
6. Rabbani F, Koppie TM, Charytonowicz E, et al. Prognostic significance of p27(Kip1) expression in bladder cancer. BJU Int 2007;100(2):259–63.
7. Sanchez-Carbayo M, Socci ND, Lozano J, et al. Defining molecular profiles of poor outcome in patients with invasive bladder cancer using oligonucleotide microarrays. J Clin Oncol 2006;24(5):778–89.
8. Sanchez-Carbayo M, Socci ND, Charytonowicz E, et al. Molecular profiling of bladder cancer using cDNA microarrays: defining histogenesis and biological phenotypes. Cancer Res 2002;62(23):6973–80.
9. Sanchez-Carbayo M, Cordon-Cardo C. Applications of array technology: identification of molecular targets in bladder cancer. Br J Cancer 2003;89(12):2172–7.
10. Ioachim E, Michael M, Salmas M, et al. Hypoxia-inducible factors HIF-1alpha and HIF-2alpha expression in bladder cancer and their associations with other angiogenesis-related proteins. Urol Int 2006;77(3):255–63.
11. Ioachim E, Michael MC, Salmas M, et al. Thrombospondin-1 expression in urothelial carcinoma: prognostic significance and association with p53 alterations, tumour angiogenesis and extracellular matrix components. BMC Cancer 2006;6:140.
12. Lascombe I, Clairotte A, Fauconnet S, et al. N-cadherin as a novel prognostic marker of progression in superficial urothelial tumors. Clin Cancer Res 2006;12(9):2780–7.
13. Rotterud R, Nesland JM, Berner A, et al. Expression of the epidermal growth factor receptor family in normal and malignant urothelium. BJU Int 2005;95(9):1344–50.
14. Highshaw RA, McConkey DJ, Dinney CP. Integrating basic science and clinical research in bladder cancer: update from the first bladder Specialized Program of Research Excellence (SPORE). Curr Opin Urol 2004;14(5):295–300.
15. Clairotte A, Lascombe I, Fauconnet S, et al. Expression of E-cadherin and alpha-, beta-, gamma-catenins in patients with bladder cancer: identification of gamma-catenin as a new prognostic marker of neoplastic progression in T1 superficial urothelial tumors. Am J Clin Pathol 2006;125(1):119–26.
16. Chatterjee SJ, Datar R, Youssefzadeh D, et al. Combined effects of p53, p21, and pRb expression in the progression of bladder transitional cell carcinoma. J Clin Oncol 2004;22(6):1007–13.
17. Beekman KW, Bradley D, Hussain M. New molecular targets and novel agents in the treatment of advanced urothelial cancer. Semin Oncol 2007;34(2):154–64.
18. Shariat SF, Ashfaq R, Sagalowsky AI, et al. Predictive value of cell cycle biomarkers in nonmuscle invasive bladder transitional cell carcinoma. J Urol 2007;177(2):481–7 [discussion: 487].
19. Miyamoto H, Kubota Y, Fujinami K, et al. Infrequent somatic mutations of the p16 and p15 genes in human bladder cancer: p16 mutations occur only in low-grade and superficial bladder cancers. Oncol Res 1995;7(7–8):327–30.
20. Miyamoto H, Kubota Y, Shuin T, et al. Analyses of p53 gene mutations in primary human bladder cancer. Oncol Res 1993;5(6–7):245–9.
21. Birkhahn M, Mitra AP, Williams AJ, et al. Predicting recurrence and progression of noninvasive papillary bladder cancer at initial presentation based on quantitative gene expression profiles. Eur Urol 2010;57(1):12–20.
22. Cheng L, Davidson DD, Maclennan GT, et al. The origins of urothelial carcinoma. Expert Rev Anticancer Ther 2010;10(6):865–80.
23. Mengual L, Burset M, Ribal MJ, et al. Gene expression signature in urine for diagnosing and assessing aggressiveness of bladder urothelial carcinoma. Clin Cancer Res 2010;16(9):2624–33.
24. Shariat SF, Ashfaq R, Sagalowsky AI, et al. Association of cyclin D1 and E1 expression with disease progression and biomarkers in patients with nonmuscle-invasive urothelial cell carcinoma of the bladder. Urol Oncol 2007;25(6):468–75.
25. Bolenz C, Lotan Y. Translational research in bladder cancer: from molecular pathogenesis to useful tissue biomarkers. Cancer Biol Ther 2010;10(5):407–15.

26. Bensalah K, Montorsi F, Shariat SF. Challenges of cancer biomarker profiling. Eur Urol 2007;52(6): 1601–9.

27. Choi W, Porten S, Kim S, et al. Identification of distinct basal and luminal subtypes of muscle-invasive bladder cancer with different sensitivities to frontline chemotherapy. Cancer Cell 2014; 25(2):152–65.

28. Cancer Genome Atlas Research Network. Comprehensive molecular characterization of urothelial bladder carcinoma. Nature 2014; 507(7492):315–22.

29. Lindgren D, Sjodahl G, Lauss M, et al. Integrated genomic and gene expression profiling identifies two major genomic circuits in urothelial carcinoma. PLoS One 2012;7(6):e38863.

30. Kinde I, Munari E, Faraj SF, et al. TERT promoter mutations occur early in urothelial neoplasia and are biomarkers of early disease and disease recurrence in urine. Cancer Res 2013;73(24): 7162–7.

31. Cheng L, Zhang S, Maclennan GT, et al. Bladder cancer: translating molecular genetic insights into clinical practice. Hum Pathol 2011;42(4):455–81.

32. Miyamoto H, Brimo F, Schultz L, et al. Low-grade papillary urothelial carcinoma of the urinary bladder: a clinicopathologic analysis of a post-World Health Organization/International Society of Urological Pathology classification cohort from a single academic center. Arch Pathol Lab Med 2010;134(8):1160–3.

33. Mitra AP, Pagliarulo V, Yang D, et al. Generation of a concise gene panel for outcome prediction in urinary bladder cancer. J Clin Oncol 2009;27(24): 3929–37.

34. Mitra AP, Datar RH, Cote RJ. Molecular pathways in invasive bladder cancer: new insights into mechanisms, progression, and target identification. J Clin Oncol 2006;24(35):5552–64.

35. Rothman N, Garcia-Closas M, Chatterjee N, et al. A multi-stage genome-wide association study of bladder cancer identifies multiple susceptibility loci. Nat Genet 2010;42(11):978–84.

36. Sanchez-Carbayo M, Cordon-Cardo C. Molecular alterations associated with bladder cancer progression. Semin Oncol 2007;34(2):75–84.

37. Serizawa RR, Ralfkiaer U, Steven K, et al. Integrated genetic and epigenetic analysis of bladder cancer reveals an additive diagnostic value of FGFR3 mutations and hypermethylation events. Int J Cancer 2011;129(1):78–87.

38. Lindgren D, Frigyesi A, Gudjonsson S, et al. Combined gene expression and genomic profiling define two intrinsic molecular subtypes of urothelial carcinoma and gene signatures for molecular grading and outcome. Cancer Res 2010;70(9): 3463–72.

39. Heidenblad M, Lindgren D, Jonson T, et al. Tiling resolution array CGH and high density expression profiling of urothelial carcinomas delineate genomic amplicons and candidate target genes specific for advanced tumors. BMC Med Genomics 2008;1:3.

40. Lindgren D, Liedberg F, Andersson A, et al. Molecular characterization of early-stage bladder carcinomas by expression profiles, FGFR3 mutation status, and loss of 9q. Oncogene 2006;25(18): 2685–96.

41. Wu XR. Urothelial tumorigenesis: a tale of divergent pathways. Nat Rev Cancer 2005;5(9):713–25.

42. van Rhijn BW, Zuiverloon TC, Vis AN, et al. Molecular grade (FGFR3/MIB-1) and EORTC risk scores are predictive in primary non-muscle-invasive bladder cancer. Eur Urol 2010;58(3): 433–41.

43. Mason RA, Morlock EV, Karagas MR, et al. EGFR pathway polymorphisms and bladder cancer susceptibility and prognosis. Carcinogenesis 2009; 30(7):1155–60.

44. Simonetti S, Russo R, Ciancia G, et al. Role of polysomy 17 in transitional cell carcinoma of the bladder: immunohistochemical study of HER2/neu expression and fish analysis of c-erbB-2 gene and chromosome 17. Int J Surg Pathol 2009; 17(3):198–205.

45. Latif Z, Watters AD, Dunn I, et al. HER2/neu gene amplification and protein overexpression in G3 pT2 transitional cell carcinoma of the bladder: a role for anti-HER2 therapy? Eur J Cancer 2004; 40(1):56–63.

46. Gandour-Edwards R, Lara PN Jr, Folkins AK, et al. Does HER2/neu expression provide prognostic information in patients with advanced urothelial carcinoma? Cancer 2002;95(5):1009–15.

47. Eissa S, Ali HS, Al Tonsi AH, et al. HER2/neu expression in bladder cancer: relationship to cell cycle kinetics. Clin Biochem 2005;38(2):142–8.

48. Billerey C, Chopin D, Aubriot-Lorton MH, et al. Frequent FGFR3 mutations in papillary non-invasive bladder (pTa) tumors. Am J Pathol 2001; 158(6):1955–9.

49. Leibl S, Zigeuner R, Hutterer G, et al. EGFR expression in urothelial carcinoma of the upper urinary tract is associated with disease progression and metaplastic morphology. APMIS 2008;116(1): 27–32.

50. Bolenz C, Shariat SF, Karakiewicz PI, et al. Human epidermal growth factor receptor 2 expression status provides independent prognostic information in patients with urothelial carcinoma of the urinary bladder. BJU Int 2010;106(8):1216–22.

51. Al-Ahmadie HA, Iyer G, Janakiraman M, et al. Somatic mutation of fibroblast growth factor receptor-3 (FGFR3) defines a distinct

morphological subtype of high-grade urothelial carcinoma. J Pathol 2011;224(2):270–9.

52. Ling S, Chang X, Schultz L, et al. An EGFR-ERK-SOX9 signaling cascade links urothelial development and regeneration to cancer. Cancer Res 2011;71(11):3812–21.

53. van Rhijn BW, Vis AN, van der Kwast TH, et al. Molecular grading of urothelial cell carcinoma with fibroblast growth factor receptor 3 and MIB-1 is superior to pathologic grade for the prediction of clinical outcome. J Clin Oncol 2003;21(10):1912–21.

54. Quintero A, Alvarez-Kindelan J, Luque RJ, et al. Ki-67 MIB1 labelling index and the prognosis of primary TaT1 urothelial cell carcinoma of the bladder. J Clin Pathol 2006;59(1):83–8.

55. Margulis V, Shariat SF, Ashfaq R, et al. Ki-67 is an independent predictor of bladder cancer outcome in patients treated with radical cystectomy for organ-confined disease. Clin Cancer Res 2006; 12(24):7369–73.

56. Margulis V, Lotan Y, Karakiewicz PI, et al. Multi-institutional validation of the predictive value of Ki-67 labeling index in patients with urinary bladder cancer. J Natl Cancer Inst 2009;101(2):114–9.

57. Ramos D, Ruiz A, Morell L, et al. Prognostic value of morphometry in low grade papillary urothelial bladder neoplasms. Anal Quant Cytol Histol 2004; 26(5):285–94.

58. Kruger S, Mahnken A, Kausch I, et al. P16 immunoreactivity is an independent predictor of tumor progression in minimally invasive urothelial bladder carcinoma. Eur Urol 2005;47(4):463–7.

59. Lopez-Beltran A, Luque RJ, Alvarez-Kindelan J, et al. Prognostic factors in stage T1 grade 3 bladder cancer survival: the role of G1-S modulators (p53, p21Waf1, p27kip1, Cyclin D1, and Cyclin D3) and proliferation index (ki67-MIB1). Eur Urol 2004;45(5):606–12.

60. Sylvester RJ, van der Meijden AP, Oosterlinck W, et al. Predicting recurrence and progression in individual patients with stage Ta T1 bladder cancer using EORTC risk tables: a combined analysis of 2596 patients from seven EORTC trials. Eur Urol 2006;49(3):466–75 [discussion: 475–7].

61. Garcia del Muro X, Condom E, Vigues F, et al. p53 and p21 expression levels predict organ preservation and survival in invasive bladder carcinoma treated with a combined-modality approach. Cancer 2004;100(9):1859–67.

62. Shariat SF, Karakiewicz PI, Ashfaq R, et al. Multiple biomarkers improve prediction of bladder cancer recurrence and mortality in patients undergoing cystectomy. Cancer 2008;112(2):315–25.

63. Shariat SF, Bolenz C, Godoy G, et al. Predictive value of combined immunohistochemical markers in patients with pT1 urothelial carcinoma at radical cystectomy. J Urol 2009;182(1):78–84 [discussion: 84].

64. Nishiyama N, Arai E, Chihara Y, et al. Genome-wide DNA methylation profiles in urothelial carcinomas and urothelia at the precancerous stage. Cancer Sci 2010;101(1):231–40.

65. Lin HH, Ke HL, Huang SP, et al. Increase sensitivity in detecting superficial, low grade bladder cancer by combination analysis of hypermethylation of E-cadherin, p16, p14, RASSF1A genes in urine. Urol Oncol 2010;28(6):597–602.

66. Vinci S, Giannarini G, Selli C, et al. Quantitative methylation analysis of BCL2, hTERT, and DAPK promoters in urine sediment for the detection of non-muscle-invasive urothelial carcinoma of the bladder: a prospective, two-center validation study. Urol Oncol 2011;29(2):150–6.

67. Cabello MJ, Grau L, Franco N, et al. Multiplexed methylation profiles of tumor suppressor genes in bladder cancer. J Mol Diagn 2011;13(1):29–40.

68. Vallot C, Stransky N, Bernard-Pierrot I, et al. A novel epigenetic phenotype associated with the most aggressive pathway of bladder tumor progression. J Natl Cancer Inst 2011;103(1):47–60.

69. Dudziec E, Miah S, Choudhry H, et al. Hypermethylation of CpG islands and shores around specific MicroRNAs and mirtrons is associated with the phenotype and presence of bladder cancer. Clin Cancer Res 2011;17(6):1287–96.

70. Wiklund ED, Bramsen JB, Hulf T, et al. Coordinated epigenetic repression of the miR-200 family and miR-205 in invasive bladder cancer. Int J Cancer 2011;128(6):1327–34.

71. Catto JW, Azzouzi AR, Rehman I, et al. Promoter hypermethylation is associated with tumor location, stage, and subsequent progression in transitional cell carcinoma. J Clin Oncol 2005;23(13):2903–10.

72. Friedrich MG, Weisenberger DJ, Cheng JC, et al. Detection of methylated apoptosis-associated genes in urine sediments of bladder cancer patients. Clin Cancer Res 2004;10(22):7457–65.

73. Chan MW, Chan LW, Tang NL, et al. Hypermethylation of multiple genes in tumor tissues and voided urine in urinary bladder cancer patients. Clin Cancer Res 2002;8(2):464–70.

74. Yates DR, Rehman I, Meuth M, et al. Methylational urinalysis: a prospective study of bladder cancer patients and age stratified benign controls. Oncogene 2006;25(13):1984–8.

75. Hoque MO, Begum S, Topaloglu O, et al. Quantitation of promoter methylation of multiple genes in urine DNA and bladder cancer detection. J Natl Cancer Inst 2006;98(14):996–1004.

76. Yates DR, Rehman I, Abbod MF, et al. Promoter hypermethylation identifies progression risk in bladder cancer. Clin Cancer Res 2007;13(7): 2046–53.

77. Kawauchi S, Sakai H, Ikemoto K, et al. 9p21 index as estimated by dual-color fluorescence in situ

hybridization is useful to predict urothelial carcinoma recurrence in bladder washing cytology. Hum Pathol 2009;40(12):1783–9.

78. Kruger S, Mess F, Bohle A, et al. Numerical aberrations of chromosome 17 and the 9p21 locus are independent predictors of tumor recurrence in non-invasive transitional cell carcinoma of the urinary bladder. Int J Oncol 2003;23(1):41–8.

79. Skacel M, Fahmy M, Brainard JA, et al. Multitarget fluorescence in situ hybridization assay detects transitional cell carcinoma in the majority of patients with bladder cancer and atypical or negative urine cytology. J Urol 2003;169(6):2101–5.

80. Sarosdy MF, Kahn PR, Ziffer MD, et al. Use of a multitarget fluorescence in situ hybridization assay to diagnose bladder cancer in patients with hematuria. J Urol 2006;176(1):44–7.

81. Moonen PM, Merkx GF, Peelen P, et al. UroVysion compared with cytology and quantitative cytology in the surveillance of non-muscle-invasive bladder cancer. Eur Urol 2007;51(5):1275–80 [discussion: 1280].

82. Yoder BJ, Skacel M, Hedgepeth R, et al. Reflex UroVysion testing of bladder cancer surveillance patients with equivocal or negative urine cytology: a prospective study with focus on the natural history of anticipatory positive findings. Am J Clin Pathol 2007;127(2):295–301.

83. Fritsche HM, Burger M, Dietmaier W, et al. Multicolor FISH (UroVysion) facilitates follow-up of patients with high-grade urothelial carcinoma of the bladder. Am J Clin Pathol 2010;134(4):597–603.

84. Karnwal A, Venegas R, Shuch B, et al. The role of fluorescence in situ hybridization assay for surveillance of non-muscle invasive bladder cancer. Can J Urol 2010;17(2):5077–81.

85. Schlomer BJ, Ho R, Sagalowsky A, et al. Prospective validation of the clinical usefulness of reflex fluorescence in situ hybridization assay in patients with atypical cytology for the detection of urothelial carcinoma of the bladder. J Urol 2010;183(1):62–7.

86. Ferra S, Denley R, Herr H, et al. Reflex UroVysion testing in suspicious urine cytology cases. Cancer 2009;117(1):7–14.

87. Zheng X, Zhuge J, Bezerra SM, et al. High frequency of TERT promoter mutation in small cell carcinoma of bladder, but not in small cell carcinoma of other origins. J Hematol Oncol 2014;7:47.

88. Killela PJ, Reitman ZJ, Jiao Y, et al. TERT promoter mutations occur frequently in gliomas and a subset of tumors derived from cells with low rates of self-renewal. Proc Natl Acad Sci U S A 2013;110(15):6021–6.

89. Carneiro BA, Meeks JJ, Kuzel TM, et al. Emerging therapeutic targets in bladder cancer. Cancer Treat Rev 2015;41(2):170–8.

90. Montironi R, Santoni M, Lopez-Beltran A, et al. Morphologic and molecular backgrounds for personalized management of genito-urinary cancers: an overview. Curr Drug Targets 2015;16(2):96–102.

91. Gartrell BA, Sonpavde G. Emerging drugs for urothelial carcinoma. Expert Opin Emerg Drugs 2013;18(4):477–94.

92. Bellmunt J, Teh BT, Tortora G, et al. Molecular targets on the horizon for kidney and urothelial cancer. Nat Rev Clin Oncol 2013;10(10):557–70.

93. Fahmy M, Mansure JJ, Brimo F, et al. Relevance of the mammalian target of rapamycin pathway in the prognosis of patients with high-risk non-muscle invasive bladder cancer. Hum Pathol 2013;44(9):1766–72.

94. Chaux A, Comperat E, Varinot J, et al. High levels of phosphatase and tensin homolog expression are associated with tumor progression, tumor recurrence, and systemic metastases in pT1 urothelial carcinoma of the bladder: a tissue microarray study of 156 patients treated by transurethral resection. Urology 2013;81(1):116–22.

95. Gonzalez-Roibon ND, Chaux A, Al-Hussain T, et al. Dysregulation of mammalian target of rapamycin pathway in plasmacytoid variant of urothelial carcinoma of the urinary bladder. Hum Pathol 2013;44(4):612–22.

96. Schultz L, Chaux A, Albadine R, et al. Immunoexpression status and prognostic value of mTOR and hypoxia-induced pathway members in primary and metastatic clear cell renal cell carcinomas. Am J Surg Pathol 2011;35(10):1549–56.

97. Powles T, Eder JP, Fine GD, et al. MPDL3280A (anti-PD-L1) treatment leads to clinical activity in metastatic bladder cancer. Nature 2014;515(7528):558–62.

98. Inman BA, Sebo TJ, Frigola X, et al. PD-L1 (B7-H1) expression by urothelial carcinoma of the bladder and BCG-induced granulomata: associations with localized stage progression. Cancer 2007;109(8):1499–505.

99. Hay DA, Fedorov O, Martin S, et al. Discovery and optimization of small-molecule ligands for the CBP/p300 bromodomains. J Am Chem Soc 2014;136(26):9308–19.

100. Fedorov O, Lingard H, Wells C, et al. [1,2,4]triazolo[4,3-A]phthalazines: inhibitors of diverse bromodomains. J Med Chem 2014;57(2):462–76.

101. Filippakopoulos P, Qi J, Picaud S, et al. Selective inhibition of BET bromodomains. Nature 2010;468(7327):1067–73.

102. Mooso BA, Vinall RL, Mudryj M, et al. The role of EGFR family inhibitors in muscle invasive bladder cancer: a review of clinical data and molecular evidence. J Urol 2015;193(1):19–29.

103. Hayashi T, Jaeger W, Moskalev I, et al. Targeting HER2 withtrastuzumab-DM1 (T-DM1) in HER2-overexpressing bladder cancer. J Urol 2014;191(Suppl 4):E301.

104. Richards DA, Braiteh FS, Garcia AA, et al. A phase 1 study of MM-111, a bispecific HER2/HER3 antibody fusion protein, combined with multiple treatment regimens in patients with advanced HER2-positive solid tumors. J Clin Oncol 2014;32(Suppl 15):651.

105. Bajorin DF, Gomella LG, Sharma P, et al. Preliminary product parameter and safety results from NeuACT, a phase 2 randomized, open-label trial of DN24-02 in patients with surgically resected HER2+ urothelial cancer at high risk for recurrence. J Clin Oncol 2014;32(Suppl 15):4566.

106. Hussain MH, MacVicar GR, Petrylak DP, et al. Trastuzumab, paclitaxel, carboplatin, and gemcitabine in advanced human epidermal growth factor receptor-2/neu-positive urothelial carcinoma: results of a multicenter phase II National Cancer Institute trial. J Clin Oncol 2007;25(16):2218–24.

107. Hansel DE, Swain E, Dreicer R, et al. HER2 overexpression and amplification in urothelial carcinoma of the bladder is associated with MYC coamplification in a subset of cases. Am J Clin Pathol 2008; 130(2):274–81.

108. International Collaboration of Trialists, Medical Research Council Advanced Bladder Cancer Working Party (now the National Cancer Research Institute Bladder Cancer Clinical Studies Group), European Organisation for Research and Treatment of Cancer Genito-Urinary Tract Cancer Group, et al. International phase III trial assessing neoadjuvant cisplatin, methotrexate, and vinblastine chemotherapy for muscle-invasive bladder cancer: long-term results of the BA06 30894 trial. J Clin Oncol 2011;29(16):2171–7.

109. Grossman HB, Natale RB, Tangen CM, et al. Neoadjuvant chemotherapy plus cystectomy compared with cystectomy alone for locally advanced bladder cancer. N Engl J Med 2003;349(9):859–66.

110. Zargar H, Espiritu PN, Fairey AS, et al. Multicenter assessment of neoadjuvant chemotherapy for muscle-invasive bladder cancer. Eur Urol 2015; 67(2):241–9.

111. Dinney CP, Hansel D, McConkey D, et al. Novel neoadjuvant therapy paradigms for bladder cancer: results from the National Cancer Center Institute Forum. Urol Oncol 2014;32(8):1108–15.

112. Dees EC, Cohen RB, von Mehren M, et al. Phase I study of aurora A kinase inhibitor MLN8237 in advanced solid tumors: safety, pharmacokinetics, pharmacodynamics, and bioavailability of two oral formulations. Clin Cancer Res 2012;18(17): 4775–84.

113. Dees EC, Infante JR, Cohen RB, et al. Phase 1 study of MLN8054, a selective inhibitor of Aurora A kinase in patients with advanced solid tumors. Cancer Chemother Pharmacol 2011;67(4):945–54.

114. Lin CC, Su WC, Yen CJ, et al. A phase I study of two dosing schedules of volasertib (BI 6727), an intravenous polo-like kinase inhibitor, in patients with advanced solid malignancies. Br J Cancer 2014;110(10):2434–40.

115. Damrauer JS, Hoadley KA, Chism DD, et al. Intrinsic subtypes of high-grade bladder cancer reflect the hallmarks of breast cancer biology. Proc Natl Acad Sci U S A 2014;111(8):3110–5.

116. Guancial EA, Rosenberg JE. The role of genomics in the management of advanced bladder cancer. Curr Treat Options Oncol 2015;16(1)::319.

117. Sjodahl G, Lauss M, Lovgren K, et al. A molecular taxonomy for urothelial carcinoma. Clin Cancer Res 2012;18(12):3377–86.

118. Fradet Y, Lockhard C. Performance characteristics of a new monoclonal antibody test for bladder cancer: ImmunoCyt trade mark. Can J Urol 1997;4(3): 400–5.

119. Yafi FA, Brimo F, Steinberg J, et al. Prospective analysis of sensitivity and specificity of urinary cytology and other urinary biomarkers for bladder cancer. Urol Oncol 2015;33(2):66.e25–31.

120. Hurst CD, Platt FM, Knowles MA. Comprehensive mutation analysis of the TERT promoter in bladder cancer and detection of mutations in voided urine. Eur Urol 2014;65(2):367–9.

121. Wang K, Liu T, Ge N, et al. TERT promoter mutations are associated with distant metastases in upper tract urothelial carcinomas and serve as urinary biomarkers detected by a sensitive castPCR. Oncotarget 2014;5(23):12428–39.

122. Allory Y, Beukers W, Sagrera A, et al. Telomerase reverse transcriptase promoter mutations in bladder cancer: high frequency across stages, detection in urine, and lack of association with outcome. Eur Urol 2014;65(2):360–6.

123. Ralla B, Stephan C, Meller S, et al. Nucleic acid-based biomarkers in body fluids of patients with urologic malignances. Crit Rev Clin Lab Sci 2014;51(4):200–31.

124. Ellinger J, Muller SC, Dietrich D. Epigenetic biomarkers in the blood of patients with urological malignancies. Expert Rev Mol Diagn 2015;15(4): 505–16.

125. Bansal N, Gupta A, Sankhwar SN, et al. Low- and high-grade bladder cancer appraisal via serum-based proteomics approach. Clin Chim Acta 2014;436:97–103.

126. Goodison S, Chang M, Dai Y, et al. A multi-analyte assay for the non-invasive detection of bladder cancer. PLoS One 2012;7(10):e47469.

127. Available at: http://www.cancer.gov/about-cancer/treatment/clinical-trials/nci-supported/nci-match. Accessed July 18, 2015.

128. Available at: http://deainfo.nci.nih.gov/advisory/ncab/164_1213/Conley.pdf. Accessed July 18, 2015.

Pharmacogenomics
Biomarker-Directed Therapy for Bladder Cancer

Robert T. Jones, BS[a,b], Kenneth M. Felsenstein, MS[a,b],
Dan Theodorescu, MD, PhD[a,b],*

KEYWORDS

- Bladder cancer • Pharmacogenomics • Personalized medicine • Immunotherapy • Clinical trials
- Molecular subtype • Predictive biomarker • Precision medicine

KEY POINTS

- Predictive biomarkers that can identify patients most likely to respond to a given therapy will be of critical importance in advancing bladder cancer management.
- Genome-wide DNA and RNA sequencing efforts have revealed bladder cancer to be a heterogeneous disease that harbors alterations conferring sensitivity to targeted agents commonly used in other cancer types.
- Bladder cancers have recently been described as having shared properties with several other tumor types, such as lung and breast, and are composed of molecularly distinct subtypes that might predict therapeutic sensitivity.
- Immunotherapies targeting the PD-1/PD-L1 axis along with CTLA-4, have shown promising results in recent early phase clinical trials.
- Emerging clinical trials that use molecularly guided therapy selection will determine the clinical efficacy of using predictive biomarkers to guide therapeutic decision-making.

INTRODUCTION AND AIMS

It is estimated that 74,000 people in the United States and roughly 386,000 people globally will be newly diagnosed with bladder cancer in 2015.[1,2] Bladder cancer represents a significant global health problem, not only because of its high frequency of occurrence, but also because of high rates of recurrence and the need for routine monitoring via transurethral cystoscopy, which result in significant economic impact.[3] By far the most common type of bladder cancer is urothelial (transitional) cell carcinoma (UCC), which accounts for greater than 90% of all bladder cancer cases.[4] The advent of genomic technologies has led to major advances in molecular testing in cancer medicine for many cancer types with demonstrated clinical benefit in many cases. However, bladder cancer has yet to significantly benefit from these new technologies and its clinical management has changed minimally in the last 30 years.

This article discusses predictive UCC biomarker discovery efforts, and the problems that have impeded their application toward clinical use, while speculating regarding possible future directions that may allow for improved treatment. We emphasize key original articles (and some reviews)

[a] University of Colorado Cancer Center, Aurora, CO, USA; [b] Medical Scientist Training Program, University of Colorado School of Medicine, Aurora, CO, USA
* Corresponding author. University of Colorado Cancer Center, An NCI Designated, Consortium Comprehensive Cancer Center, Member Center, National Comprehensive Cancer Network (NCCN), 13001 East 17th Place, MS #F-434, Aurora, CO 80045.
E-mail address: dan.theodorescu@ucdenver.edu

Urol Clin N Am 43 (2016) 77–86
http://dx.doi.org/10.1016/j.ucl.2015.08.007
0094-0143/16/$ – see front matter © 2016 Elsevier Inc. All rights reserved.

and current views, rather than being all-inclusive and thus apologize to authors whose work was not cited. The article discusses the following topics: (1) the clinical need for predictive biomarkers, (2) emerging opportunities for personalized bladder cancer therapy, (3) individual biomarkers of response, (4) new approaches to the classification of bladder cancer, (5) immunotherapy, and (6) clinical trials using molecularly guided therapy selection.

THE CLINICAL NEED AND PROMISE OF PREDICTIVE BIOMARKERS

Standard clinical management for nonmuscle invasive bladder cancers consists of transurethral resection of the bladder, with bacille Calmette-Guérin (BCG) immunotherapy being used in cases with a high risk of progression. For muscle-invasive disease, the current standard of care is radical cystectomy along with lymphadenectomy or radiotherapy. Platinum-based chemotherapy is often recommended, because gemcitabine and cisplatin combination therapy has shown response rates of approximately 38% and 50% in the neoadjuvant and metastatic settings, respectively.[5,6] These responses are not durable, however, because the overall 5-year survival benefit associated with this neoadjuvant cisplatin-based therapy is a modest 5%.[7] In the adjuvant setting, this survival benefit may be as high as 25%, when compared with patients receiving surgery alone, although these values have been subject to debate.[8] These survival benefits are viewed by many as modest and have led to low use of neoadjuvant treatments clinically.[9] The ability to reliably predict response to platinum-based therapies and other therapies would be incredibly beneficial and would likely result in a change of this current paradigm, increasing the number of patients that are most likely to respond to a given treatment while sparing most unnecessary toxicity.

Predictive biomarkers are molecular or other tumor characteristics that can predict the likelihood of an individual's response to a given therapy. Several large-scale studies published within the last few years have revealed that bladder cancer is a significantly heterogeneous disease in terms of its genetic drivers, RNA expression profiles, and chemoresponsiveness.[10–12] The use of genetic profiling has historically been limited to small gene panels and costly molecular diagnostics; however, with the increasing incorporation of next-generation sequencing and other high-throughput technologies in molecular diagnostic laboratories, physicians increasingly have the ability to obtain a more comprehensive understanding of the molecular alterations driving an individual patient's disease.[13,14] These molecular characterization techniques have long been used in other cancers, such as breast, lung, and melanoma, to guide therapeutic selection. However, when targeted agents have been trialed in bladder cancer the results have been mixed.

This has resulted in few Food and Drug Administration–approved targeted agents for bladder cancer treatment.[15] Part of the issue with the use of targeted or personalized approaches to bladder cancer treatment is that few clinical trials have enrolled patients based on genomic or RNA expression based biomarkers. A recent review found that of 96 drug-based clinical trials for urothelial carcinoma from January 2012 to January 2015, only 37 (39%) included targeted agents, and of these only 11 (12%) sought to enroll patients based on the appropriate matched molecular or genomic biomarkers.[16] These results highlight the need for increased use of predictive biomarkers in the design of future clinical trials in bladder cancer.

The following sections discuss recent studies that have revealed that most bladder cancers harbor potentially actionable mutations that are likely to respond to existing targeted therapies and molecular profiles that can predict not only untreated patient outcome (prognostic), but also an individual's responsiveness to specific therapy.

EMERGING OPPORTUNITIES FOR PERSONALIZED THERAPEUTIC REGIMENS

In recent years, several large-scale studies have dramatically expanded on the understanding of the molecular and biochemical underpinnings of bladder cancer. The Cancer Genome Atlas (TCGA) project performed integrative analyses on 131 bladder cancer specimens including whole-exome and whole-genome sequencing, mRNA and miRNA sequencing, and total and phosphorylated protein expression studies.[10] This study, in combination with several others,[11,12] has provided a more comprehensive picture of the complex molecular landscape underlying bladder cancer development and progression. Perhaps the most important and exciting clinical implication of TCGA data is that it is rapidly being used to redefine how bladder cancers are classified.[17–20] These new classifications hold tremendous promise to revolutionize the way bladder cancers are treated and how to better predict which patients will respond to various therapeutic options. Newly identified biomarkers will be integral in providing clinicians with the information needed to significantly expand their therapeutic armamentarium for the first time in more than 30 years. TCGA identified potentially actionable alterations in 69% of tumors analyzed. Of these, alterations in the PI3K-Akt-mTOR pathway were seen in 42% of cases and 45% of cases had an alteration in RTK-MAPK pathways.[10]

The complex and heterogeneous array of alterations underlying bladder cancer makes it all the more critical that molecular screening techniques be used in bladder cancer diagnostics. There are already several promising examples of the clinical utility of genomic biomarkers in the treatment of patients with bladder cancer. Genomic biomarker-based clinical trials and promising retrospective studies are discussed next.

INDIVIDUAL BIOMARKERS OF RESPONSE
DNA Repair Pathway Alterations: ERCC1 and ERCC2

Platinum-based therapies are the current mainstay of bladder cancer care, with a subset of patients having remarkable responses. Platinum-based chemotherapies function by forming adducts to DNA and introducing crosslinks. These alterations result in inhibition of DNA replication, leading to cell cycle arrest and the induction of apoptosis.[21] ERCC1 and ERCC2 are members of the nucleotide excision repair (NER) family of proteins, which function to repair DNA damage in the cell. It is therefore not surprising that cancers with high levels of expression of NER genes have been shown to be more resistant to these platinum-based therapies.[22,23] Conversely, low expression of ERCC1 and ERCC2 has been correlated with responsiveness to cisplatin in bladder cancer.[24] Recently, another study performed whole-exome sequencing on 50 patients before receiving neoadjuvant cisplatin and identified a strong association between responders and ERCC2 mutations. The study authors further show that these mutations could result in increased cisplatin sensitivity *in vitro*, whereas overexpression of wild-type ERCC2 resulted in increased therapeutic resistance.[25]

TP53

The transcription factor p53 has long been known to play an important role in DNA repair and other cellular processes including the promotion of apoptosis and cell cycle regulation.[26,27] TCGA described the inactivation of functional TP53 in 76% of samples through a constellation of mutations in TP53 itself, combined with amplifications and overexpression of MDM2.[10] TP53 currently remains an elusive drug target,[28] but there are ongoing clinical trials examining the use of Wee-

1 inhibitors, which are thought to sensitize chemoresistant tumors to platinum-based therapies (NCT01827384).[16,29] That being said, there have been several studies suggesting that p53 expression and mutational status may be predictive of therapeutic response. These studies have produced somewhat confounding results, however, with different studies showing that p53 mutations can confer chemosensitivity or chemoresistance depending on the specific alteration.[30,31] In the context of bladder cancer, there has been some difficulty defining the role of p53 in therapeutic sensitivity. One retrospective analysis, using immunohistochemistry, showed that patients who had elevated p53 expression and received adjuvant cisplatin saw a survival benefit.[32] Conversely, in a phase III trial that sought to explore the use of p53 expression as a predictive biomarker (again determined by immunohistochemistry) no significant association was shown between p53 expression and methotrexate, vinblastine, doxorubicin, and cisplatin sensitivity.[33] Although TP53 seems to be a major contributor to the development of bladder cancer, more investigation is needed to determine its clinical use as a predictive marker.

PI3-kinase pathway

PI3-kinase pathway alterations were observed in 42% of samples analyzed by TCGA. The alterations seen in this pathway include PIK3CA mutations (17%), TSC1 or TSC2 alterations (9%), and overexpression of AKT1 (9%).[10] Other studies have described cases where TSC1 mutations may confer exceptional sensitivity to targeted therapy, describing the first bladder cancer case of complete response to treatment with everolimus, an MTOR inhibitor.[34] Another recent study described exceptional response in a patient with advanced metastatic bladder cancer to treatment with everolimus and the multitarget receptor tyrosine kinase inhibitor pazopanib.[35] These papers suggest that perhaps activating mutations within the PI3K pathway could serve as biomarkers of response to targeted agents already in use in other cancers.

Receptor Tyrosine Kinases: FGFR3 and ERBB2

Mutations of FGFR3, a receptor tyrosine kinase, have been well characterized in noninvasive and invasive bladder cancers, with approximately 12% of advanced bladder cancers harboring a mutation in this gene.[10] This provides an opportunity to select patients with bladder cancer based on FGFR3 mutation status for potential use of one of the many agents designed to target this gene. One such trial, where patients were screened for FGFR3 mutation status, found that treatment with the pan-FGFR inhibitor BGJ398 saw an exceptional response in a subset of patients with bladder cancer, with four out of five responding to treatment. Tumors in these patients were reduced anywhere from 27% to 48%.[36] Another phase I trial recently found a patient with metastatic bladder cancer harboring an FGFR3-TACC3 translocation showed partial response to treatment with JNJ-42756493, another pan-FGFR targeted agent that has shown promising results in patient-derived explant models harboring various FGFR alterations.[37] It is worth noting that these fusions have been identified as actionable targets across other cancers[38] and in bladder cancer,[39] with TCGA identifying recurrent FGFR3-TACC3 translocations in 3 out of 114 tumors analyzed. Although these studies are currently being expanded, the prospect of using FGFR3 as a biomarker of therapeutic response is promsing.[10]

HER2 is another receptor tyrosine kinase that has been used as a predictive biomarker of response to targeted agents and conventional chemotherapies in urothelial cancers and other cancer types. The role of HER2 in the promotion of bladder cancer has also been explored in several studies and has been associated with increased sensitivity to chemotherapy. Recently, it has been shown that ERBB2 mutations are associated with pathologic complete response (P0) following treatment with platinum-based therapies.[40] This study suggests that ERBB2 could serve as a good genomic biomarker and could provide a basis for selecting patients. Preclinical studies and phase I trials have shown high response rates to HER2-targeted therapies and there are currently phase II trials underway for trastuzumab (NCT01828736) and lapatinib (NCT00949455) in the treatment of bladder cancer.

NEW APPROACHES TO THE CLASSIFICATION OF BLADDER CANCER

Molecular analysis has clearly shown that cancers of specific histologic types are rarely genomically monolithic; infrequently are they defined by a single characteristic mutation or universally predictable in terms of therapeutic sensitivity based on a single genotypic change.[41] Although individual biomarkers may predict response in a single patient or small subset of patients, no single biomarker has the ability to predict every individual's responsiveness to a given therapy. Patients typically have many co-occurring alterations that can modify their sensitivity to a given compound and may benefit from personalized combination therapies.[41] To better predict the effects these

co-occurring events might have on therapeutic sensitivity, several recent studies have aimed to classify tumors across cancer types, describing novel "pan-cancer" subtypes based on shared genetic, molecular, and biochemical features. One of these studies has uncovered remarkable similarities across many cancer types, with bladder cancer standing out as a uniquely heterogeneous and divergently clustered disease type.[17] In this study they evaluated 3527 samples across 12 cancer types, performing integrative analyses across five genome-wide platforms including whole-exome sequencing, DNA copy number analysis, methylation profiling, mRNA sequencing, and microRNA sequencing. Furthermore, data from reverse phase protein array provided proteomic characterization of 131 proteins. Interestingly, bladder cancer primarily clustered into three distinct pan-cancer subtypes, the most divergent classification of any of the cancer types analyzed. Of the 12 cancer types analyzed, five clustered into groups corresponding to their tissues of origin, whereas seven had features that could be clustered into pan-cancer subtypes based on shared molecular characteristics with other cancer types. One of these pan-cancer groups included a subset of bladder tumors, along with samples from the squamous lung and head and neck cancer cohorts. The authors noted that this squamous-like subtype was characterized by p53 mutations, along with amplifications of p63 and enrichment of immune and proliferation pathway features. Aside from the squamous-like subtype, most other bladder tumors clustered into either a group comprised of mostly lung adenocarcinomas, or another bladder cancer–specific subtype, which was comprised primarily of tumors originating in the bladder.[17] These results, suggest that bladder cancer might be looked at through the lens of other cancer types, such as lung, where there is a wealth of data focused on predicting therapeutic response. These sorts of analyses promise to inspire a new wave of clinical trials in which therapeutic decisions are made based on molecular classification rather than traditional pathologic/histologic classification.

Another series of papers has recently been published describing intrinsic subtypes of bladder cancer based on unsupervised clustering derived from genome-wide RNA expression profiling data.[10,12,18,42,43] These independent analyses of the bladder cancer genome and transcriptome have resulted in the identification of several subtypes that share common expression profiles. The concept of intrinsic subtypes based on unsupervised clustering, has been previously established in breast cancer.[44] This concept of classifying breast tumors based on their molecular taxonomy has been reproduced by many groups independently and is commonly used clinically to inform prognosis and predict response to therapy.[45–47] Other groups have recently described molecular classification schemes in breast cancer based on normal cell types, and found these may better predict response to therapy than the existing classifications based on tumor-derived profiles.[48] This perhaps suggests that a similar taxonomic approach might be clinically informative in the context of bladder cancer. The classification of these intrinsic subtypes in bladder cancer may have remarkable implications on how patients with bladder cancer are treated and may improve the ability to predict responsiveness to various therapies. A comprehensive description of these subtypes and their role in predicting response in bladder cancer has recently been published.[20]

Immunotherapy: Promising New Horizons

A promising approach that has for years been associated with sometimes remarkable and durable response is cancer immunotherapy.[49,50] It is hypothesized that the immune system plays a natural role in the prevention of cancer. In addition to being a primary means for combatting foreign pathogens, the immune system exists as a means of surveillance for aberrant processes within one's own cells.[51] In an actively functioning immune system, when a cell becomes malignant, it displays a variety of metabolic and paracrine cell surface abnormalities that are recognized as abnormal by the innate and adaptive immune systems, causing the cell to be eliminated.[52] Cancer represents a fundamental failure of the immune system to fully execute on its duties as the sentinel to protect against malignant cellular processes, and can derive from either cancer-mediated depression of the natural immune response, or an inherent failure to recognize the cancer cells as needing to be eliminated, because fundamentally they do derive from self, and bear many similar characteristics to one's own somatic cells.[53] The concept behind cancer immunotherapy is to unleash the powerful cell-regulating potential of this system to effectively target abnormal cells within the body. The concept of immunotherapy has been attempted for many years, but with a few exceptions, until recently, there had been very few breakthroughs.

One of the immunotherapy breakthroughs before activated T-cell therapy and immune checkpoint inhibitors was the use of BCG, a bovine-derived vaccine for tuberculosis, which is injected intravesically into the bladder.[54] The notion of stimulating immune response via the introduction of potent antigens to introduce collateral damage of tumor cells, while conceptually primitive, has a long history first starting in the late 1800s when Coley's toxin (derived from *Streptococcus pyogenes*) was injected intratumorally.[55] Because the body mounts a significant innate immune response to the presence of BCG, the idea behind introducing this into the bladder was to essentially target UCC cells through a sort of bystander effect, by triggering inflammatory processes caused by the presence of BCG (the precise mechanism is not exactly understood, but BCG administration has been shown to activate the innate and adaptive immune systems, and equally targets healthy somatic bladder in addition to cancer cells).[56] Nevertheless, this approach has had significant success in treating UCC, and has been shown to be superior or equivalent to any single chemotherapeutic agent tested to date in terms of reducing progression and recurrence.[49] Associated toxicities are often manageable, because the response is mainly confined to the bladder, given the method of delivery.[57]

However, in the present age of targeted therapy, it should be possible to elicit an immune response in a more focused and specific manner, with minimal collateral damage. The most appealing aspect of targeted immunotherapy is the potential promise for a durable immune response via adaptive immune conditioning, which should prevent recurrence of malignant cells expressing the same antigenic profile. Within the last several years, there have been several breakthroughs in this area, the most successful of which use an armed cytotoxic T-lymphocyte (CTL) response. The characteristics of an effective antitumor immune response involve (1) a mechanism for cancer antigen release, uptake, and presentation by dendritic and other antigen-presenting cells; (2) the recognition of the antigens presented on these cells by appropriate T-cell clones, to prime them for clonal expansion; and (3) the creation of durable immune reserves, in the form of circulating CTLs, which recognize and destroy cells expressing markers of nonself.

One of the most exciting advances in this area has been the development of immune checkpoint inhibitors for programmed cell death protein 1 (PD-1) and its ligand PD-L1 and CTL antigen-4 (CTLA-4). PD-1 is a receptor found on CTLs and some other immune cells that interacts with two ligands, PD-L1 and PD-L2, which when triggered turns off the activated T-cell response and halts the production and release of cytokines.[58] In a healthy immune system, these signaling mechanisms exist to reestablish tissue homeostasis following successful defeat of a foreign pathogenic infection; however, with cancer, tumor cells have evolved to also engage this receptor via synthetic creation of their own PD-L1, which effectively allows them to avoid the wrath of the CTL response.[59,60]

Several drugs have entered clinical trials to target PD-L1. One of these, MPDL3280A, an anti-PD-L1 antibody, recently received breakthrough therapy status by the Food and Drug Administration because of a 43% objective response rate in patients with PD-L1$^+$ tumors in phase I trials for metastatic UCC.[61,62] Although less than half of patients saw this clinical benefit, the most exciting aspect of this trial was that even following cessation of treatment after the allotted period, the response seen in patients seemed to be sustained, and through at least the end of the data collection period, a median duration of response was not reached. Phase II trials for this drug have recently finished enrollment. Other exciting antibody-based trials to target the PD-1/PD-L1 axis are ongoing with drugs pembrolizumab, nivolumab (already approved for metastatic melanoma and squamous non–small cell lung cancer), MSB0010718C, and MEDI-4736, among others.[49]

CTLA-4 is a biomarker-based target that functions much in the same vein as PD-1/PD-L1, inhibiting activated T-cell response, via an alternative mechanism through regulation of the T-helper cell signaling that allows for the priming and expansion that ordinarily occurs to build up an army of antigen-specific reactive CTL clones.[63] Preliminary results of ipilimumab, a monoclonal antibody against CTLA-4, in bladder cancer cohorts have been promising,[64] and shown to upregulate immune response in a small cohort of patients with UCC when administered preoperatively.[65,66]

The other highly promising area of bladder cancer immunotherapy comes in the form of adoptive T-cell transfer (ACT), a proven approach in many tumor types. ACT relies on the extraction and genetic engineering of a patient's own CTLs to become reactive to tumor-based antigens, through ex vivo priming, clonal expansion, and reinfusion. These enriched CTLs can take the form of traditional α/β T-cell receptors, or be further modified to contain an extracellular domain designed as a mimetic of a tumor-specific antibody, linked to the intracellular domain of the T-cell receptor and costimulatory receptors, to generate enhanced response. This latter approach is known as chimeric antigen receptor therapy.[67] ACT is still in the fairly early stages of testing in bladder cancer, with several ongoing trials, and

a new study out of Sweden has just reported a couple of highly promising results from a small cohort of individuals with metastatic UCC, including one patient who demonstrated a complete response.[68] More research into optimizing and expanding this technology is needed to assess its potential in patients with UCC, and although it is a high-cost technology, because of the highly personalized nature of taking each individual patient's own T cells for the ex vivo modifications, that is also a large part of what makes it so appealing, at least in concept, in the current world of modern precision medicine.

CLINICAL TRIALS USING MOLECULARLY GUIDED THERAPY SELECTION

Although the previously mentioned predictive biomarkers hold great promise for improving the management of bladder cancers and the likelihood of therapeutic responsiveness on an individual patient level, more prospective clinical trials are needed to demonstrate clinical benefit of these tools (**Fig. 1**). Few trials to date have used genetic or expression-based biomarkers for patient enrollment, and as such, may have been underpowered to detect the small subset of patients most likely to respond to treatment based their individual molecular profiles. Of note, the Investigation of Serial studies to Predict Your Therapeutic Response with Imaging and Molecular Analysis trial (iSPY) has shown that use of these types of molecular analyses can improve one's ability to predict chemosensitivity and chemoresistance.[47] Moreover, the Southwest Oncology Group has another large trial intended test if CoXEN-based classification of patients can improve rates of chemoresponsiveness. There have also been a limited number of trials in bladder cancer that have enrolled patients based on specific mutations or biomarkers, but of those that have, several have seen significantly improved patient responses when compared with previous trials, most of which have failed to stratify patients based on appropriate predictive biomarkers.[16]

Recently, there have been an increasing number of prospective clinical trials wherein individuals will be matched to targeted therapies based on genomic and other molecular alterations.[69] These include several trials originated by the National Cancer Institute (NCI), such as the NCI-Molecular Profiling-based Assignment of Cancer Therapeutics (M-PAC) (NCT01827384) and the NCI-Molecular Analysis for Therapy Choice (MATCH) (NCT02465060). Others include institutional trials, such as the IMPACT2 (NCT02152254) study being conducted at the University of Texas MD

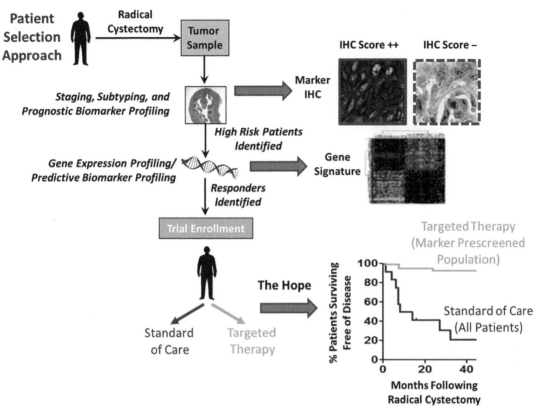

Fig. 1. Biomarker-directed therapy for bladder cancer. The paradigm for the use of precision medicine in bladder cancer therapy will involve the prescreening of individuals bearing specific relevant molecular subtypes and stratifying them into groups with therapies likely to target molecules acting as drivers in the course of their disease. It is hoped that this more rational approach leads to longer Kaplan-Meier curves and improved progression-free survival. IHC, immunohistochemistry.

Anderson Cancer Center, which aims to expand on the early promise demonstrated by the earlier IMPACT (NCT00851032) study.[70] Another exciting study that is expected to begin in late 2015, launched by the American Society for Clinical Oncology, is the Targeted Agent and Profiling Utilization Registry (TAPUR) study, which aims to facilitate the matching of patients for whom other therapeutic options are unavailable and who harbor potentially actionable genomic alterations.[71,72] In this study patients' alterations will be evaluated by a molecular tumor board, which will contain experts in genomically guided medicine, and the study will facilitate access to various targeted agents through collaborations with the pharmaceutical industry. These studies, and many others not mentioned here, represent some of the first opportunities to assess the practical utility and efficacy of precision cancer medicine. The results of these studies promise to revolutionize not only the way bladder cancer is treated, but how all cancers are managed clinically. Although the management of bladder cancer has seen little change over the last several decades, the near future promises a paradigm shift based on integration of genomics and other molecular biomarkers to guide therapeutic decisions.

ACKNOWLEDGMENTS

"RTJ and KMF are supported by the University of Colorado Medical Scientist Training Program, US National Institutes of Health training grant T32 GM008497."

REFERENCES

1. Jemal A, Bray F, Center MM, et al. Global cancer statistics. CA Cancer J Clin 2011;61(2):69–90.
2. Howlader N, Noone AM, Krapcho M, et al, editors. SEER cancer statistics review, 1975–2011. Bethesda (MD): National Cancer Institute.
3. Svatek RS, Hollenbeck BK, Holmäng S, et al. The economics of bladder cancer: costs and considerations of caring for this disease. Eur Urol 2014; 66(2):253–62.

4. Pasin E, Josephson DY, Mitra AP, et al. Superficial bladder cancer: an update on etiology, molecular development, classification, and natural history. Rev Urol 2008;10(1):31–43.

5. Grossman HB, Natale RB, Tangen CM, et al. Neoadjuvant chemotherapy plus cystectomy compared with cystectomy alone for locally advanced bladder cancer. N Engl J Med 2003;349(9):859–66.

6. von der Maase H, Hansen SW, Roberts JT, et al. Gemcitabine and cisplatin versus methotrexate, vinblastine, doxorubicin, and cisplatin in advanced or metastatic bladder cancer: results of a large, randomized, multinational, multicenter, phase III study. J Clin Oncol 2000;18(17):3068–77.

7. Vale CL. Neoadjuvant chemotherapy in invasive bladder cancer: update of a systematic review and meta-analysis of individual patient data: advanced bladder cancer (ABC) meta-analysis collaboration. Eur Urol 2005;48(2):202–6.

8. Sternberg CN, Bellmunt J, Sonpavde G, et al. ICUD-EAU international consultation on bladder cancer 2012: chemotherapy for urothelial carcinoma-neoadjuvant and adjuvant settings. Eur Urol 2013; 63(1):58–66.

9. Sfakianos JP, Galsky MD. Neoadjuvant chemotherapy in the management of muscle-invasive bladder cancer. Urol Clin North Am 2015;42(2): 181–7.

10. Cancer Genome Atlas Research Network. Comprehensive molecular characterization of urothelial bladder carcinoma. Nature 2014;507(7492):315–22.

11. Guo G, Sun X, Chen C, et al. Whole-genome and whole-exome sequencing of bladder cancer identifies frequent alterations in genes involved in sister chromatid cohesion and segregation. Nat Genet 2013;45(12):1459–63.

12. Iyer G, Al-Ahmadie H, Schultz N, et al. Prevalence and co-occurrence of actionable genomic alterations in high-grade bladder cancer. J Clin Oncol 2013;31(25):3133–40.

13. Van Allen EM, Wagle N, Stojanov P, et al. Whole-exome sequencing and clinical interpretation of formalin-fixed, paraffin-embedded tumor samples to guide precision cancer medicine. Nat Med 2014;20(6):682–8.

14. Frampton GM, Fichtenholtz A, Otto GA, et al. Development and validation of a clinical cancer genomic profiling test based on massively parallel DNA sequencing. Nat Biotechnol 2013;31(11):1023–31.

15. Sonpavde G, Sternberg CN, Rosenberg JE, et al. Second-line systemic therapy and emerging drugs for metastatic transitional-cell carcinoma of the urothelium. Lancet Oncol 2010;11(9):861–70.

16. Ikeda S, Hansel DE, Kurzrock R. Beyond conventional chemotherapy: emerging molecular targeted and immunotherapy strategies in urothelial carcinoma. Cancer Treat Rev 2015;41(8):699–706.

17. Hoadley KA, Yau C, Wolf DM, et al. Multiplatform analysis of 12 cancer types reveals molecular classification within and across tissues of origin. Cell 2014;158(4):929–44.

18. Damrauer JS, Hoadley KA, Chism DD, et al. Intrinsic subtypes of high-grade bladder cancer reflect the hallmarks of breast cancer biology. Proc Natl Acad Sci U S A 2014;111(8):3110–5.

19. Kurtoglu M, Davarpanah NN, Qin R, et al. Elevating the horizon: emerging molecular and genomic targets in the treatment of advanced urothelial carcinoma. Clin Genitourin Cancer 2015;13(5):410–20.

20. McConkey DJ, Choi W, Ochoa A, et al. Therapeutic opportunities in the intrinsic subtypes of muscle-invasive bladder cancer. Hematol Oncol Clin North Am 2015;29(2):377–94.

21. Siddik ZH. Cisplatin: mode of cytotoxic action and molecular basis of resistance. Oncogene 2003; 22(47):7265–79.

22. Rabik CA, Dolan ME. Molecular mechanisms of resistance and toxicity associated with platinating agents. Cancer Treat Rev 2007;33(1):9–23.

23. Gossage L, Madhusudan S. Current status of excision repair cross complementing-group 1 (ERCC1) in cancer. Cancer Treat Rev 2007;33(6):565–77.

24. Bellmunt J, Paz-Ares L, Cuello M, et al. Gene expression of ERCC1 as a novel prognostic marker in advanced bladder cancer patients receiving cisplatin-based chemotherapy. Ann Oncol 2007; 18(3):522–8.

25. Allen EMV, Mouw KW, Kim P, et al. Somatic ERCC2 mutations correlate with cisplatin sensitivity in muscle-invasive urothelial carcinoma. Cancer Discov 2014;4(10):1140–53.

26. Ferreira CG, Tolis C, Giaccone G. p53 and chemosensitivity. Ann Oncol 1999;10(9):1011–21.

27. Levine AJ, Oren M. The first 30 years of p53: growing ever more complex. Nat Rev Cancer 2009;9(10):749–58.

28. Morris LGT, Chan TA. Therapeutic targeting of tumor suppressor genes. Cancer 2015;121(9):1357–68.

29. Leijen S, Beijnen JH, Schellens JH. Abrogation of the G2 checkpoint by inhibition of Wee-1 kinase results in sensitization of p53-deficient tumor cells to DNA-damaging agents. Curr Clin Pharmacol 2010;5(3): 186–91.

30. Fan S, Smith ML, Rivert DJ, et al. Disruption of p53 function sensitizes breast cancer MCF-7 cells to cisplatin and pentoxifylline. Cancer Res 1995; 55(8):1649–54.

31. Fan S, El-Deiry WS, Bae I, et al. p53 gene mutations are associated with decreased sensitivity of human lymphoma cells to DNA damaging agents. Cancer Res 1994;54(22):5824–30.

32. Cote RJ, Esrig D, Groshen S, et al. p53 and treatment of bladder cancer. Nature 1997;385(6612): 123–5.

33. Stadler WM, Lerner SP, Groshen S, et al. Phase III study of molecularly targeted adjuvant therapy in locally advanced urothelial cancer of the bladder based on p53 status. J Clin Oncol 2011;29(25): 3443–9.

34. Iyer G, Hanrahan AJ, Milowsky MI, et al. Genome sequencing identifies a basis for everolimus sensitivity. Science 2012;338(6104):221.

35. Wagle N, Grabiner BC, Allen EMV, et al. Activating mTOR mutations in a patient with an extraordinary response on a phase I trial of everolimus and pazopanib. Cancer Discov 2014;4(5):546–53.

36. Sequist LV, Cassier P, Varga A, et al. Abstract CT326: phase I study of BGJ398, a selective pan-FGFR inhibitor in genetically preselected advanced solid tumors. Cancer Res 2014;74(19 Suppl): CT326.

37. Dienstmann R, Bahleda R, Adamo B, et al. Abstract CT325: first in human study of JNJ-42756493, a potent pan fibroblast growth factor receptor (FGFR) inhibitor in patients with advanced solid tumors. Cancer Res 2014;74(19 Suppl):CT325.

38. Wu Y-M, Su F, Kalyana-Sundaram S, et al. Identification of targetable FGFR gene fusions in diverse cancers. Cancer Discov 2013;3(6):636–47.

39. Williams SV, Hurst CD, Knowles MA. Oncogenic FGFR3 gene fusions in bladder cancer. Hum Mol Genet 2013;22(4):795–803.

40. Groenendijk FH, de Jong J, Fransen van de Putte EE, et al. ERBB2 mutations characterize a subgroup of muscle-invasive bladder cancers with excellent response to neoadjuvant chemotherapy. Eur Urol 2015. http://dx.doi.org/10.1016/j.eururo. 2015.01.014.

41. Kim J, Fox C, Peng S, et al. Preexisting oncogenic events impact trastuzumab sensitivity in ERBB2-amplified gastroesophageal adenocarcinoma. J Clin Invest 2014;124(12):5145–58.

42. Sjödahl G, Lauss M, Lövgren K, et al. A molecular taxonomy for urothelial carcinoma. Clin Cancer Res 2012;18(12):3377–86.

43. Choi W, Porten S, Kim S, et al. Identification of distinct basal and luminal subtypes of muscle-invasive bladder cancer with different sensitivities to frontline chemotherapy. Cancer Cell 2014;25(2): 152–65.

44. Perou CM, Sørlie T, Eisen MB, et al. Molecular portraits of human breast tumours. Nature 2000; 406(6797):747–52.

45. Prat A, Parker JS, Karginova O, et al. Phenotypic and molecular characterization of the claudin-low intrinsic subtype of breast cancer. Breast Cancer Res 2010;12(5):R68.

46. Esserman LJ, Berry DA, Cheang MCU, et al. Chemotherapy response and recurrence-free survival in neoadjuvant breast cancer depends on biomarker profiles: results from the I-SPY 1 TRIAL (CALGB 150007/150012; ACRIN 6657). Breast Cancer Res Treat 2011;132(3):1049–62.

47. Esserman LJ, Berry DA, DeMichele A, et al. Pathologic complete response predicts recurrence-free survival more effectively by cancer subset: results from the I-SPY 1 TRIAL–CALGB 150007/150012, ACRIN 6657. J Clin Oncol 2012;30(26):3242–9.

48. Santagata S, Thakkar A, Ergonul A, et al. Taxonomy of breast cancer based on normal cell phenotype predicts outcome. J Clin Invest 2014;124(2): 859–70.

49. Kim JW, Tomita Y, Trepel J, et al. Emerging immunotherapies for bladder cancer. Curr Opin Oncol 2015; 27(3):191–200.

50. Nair S, Boczkowski D, Moeller B, et al. Synergy between tumor immunotherapy and antiangiogenic therapy. Blood 2003;102(3):964–71.

51. Cohen JJ. Apoptosis: mechanisms of life and death in the immune system. J Allergy Clin Immunol 1999; 103(4):548–54.

52. Senovilla L, Vitale I, Martins I, et al. An immunosurveillance mechanism controls cancer cell ploidy. Science 2012;337(6102):1678–84.

53. Kim R, Emi M, Tanabe K. Cancer immunoediting from immune surveillance to immune escape. Immunology 2007;121(1):1–14.

54. Askeland EJ, Newton MR, O'Donnell MA, et al. Bladder cancer immunotherapy: BCG and beyond. Adv Urol 2012;2012:181987.

55. Coley WB. The treatment of malignant tumors by repeated inoculations of erysipelas. With a report of ten original cases. 1893. Clin Orthop 1991;(262): 3–11.

56. Redelman-Sidi G, Glickman MS, Bochner BH. The mechanism of action of BCG therapy for bladder cancer: a current perspective. Nat Rev Urol 2014; 11(3):153–62.

57. Gan C, Mostafid H, Khan MS, et al. BCG immunotherapy for bladder cancer: the effects of substrain differences. Nat Rev Urol 2013;10(10):580–8.

58. Herbst RS, Soria J-C, Kowanetz M, et al. Predictive correlates of response to the anti-PD-L1 antibody MPDL3280A in cancer patients. Nature 2014; 515(7528):563–7.

59. Xylinas E, Robinson BD, Kluth LA, et al. Association of T-cell co-regulatory protein expression with clinical outcomes following radical cystectomy for urothelial carcinoma of the bladder. Eur J Surg Oncol 2014;40(1):121–7.

60. Nakanishi J, Wada Y, Matsumoto K, et al. Overexpression of B7-H1 (PD-L1) significantly associates with tumor grade and postoperative prognosis in human urothelial cancers. Cancer Immunol Immunother 2007;56(8):1173–82.

61. Powles T, Eder JP, Fine GD, et al. MPDL3280A (anti-PD-L1) treatment leads to clinical activity in metastatic bladder cancer. Nature 2014;515(7528):558–62.

62. Huang Y, Zhang S-D, McCrudden C, et al. The prognostic significance of PD-L1 in bladder cancer. Oncol Rep 2015;33(6):3075–84.

63. Parry RV, Chemnitz JM, Frauwirth KA, et al. CTLA-4 and PD-1 receptors inhibit T-cell activation by distinct mechanisms. Mol Cell Biol 2005;25(21): 9543–53.

64. Schindler K, Schicher N, Kunstfeld R, et al. A rare case of primary rhabdoid melanoma of the urinary bladder treated with ipilimumab, an anti-CTLA 4 monoclonal antibody. Melanoma Res 2012;22(4): 320–5.

65. Carthon BC, Wolchok JD, Yuan J, et al. Preoperative CTLA-4 blockade: tolerability and immune monitoring in the setting of a presurgical clinical trial. Clin Cancer Res 2010;16(10):2861–71.

66. Liakou CI, Kamat A, Tang DN, et al. CTLA-4 blockade increases IFNgamma-producing CD4+ICOShi cells to shift the ratio of effector to regulatory T cells in cancer patients. Proc Natl Acad Sci U S A 2008;105(39):14987–92.

67. Rosenberg SA, Restifo NP. Adoptive cell transfer as personalized immunotherapy for human cancer. Science 2015;348(6230):62–8.

68. Sherif A, Hasan MN, Radecka E, et al. Pilot study of adoptive immunotherapy with sentinel node-derived T cells in muscle-invasive urinary bladder cancer. Scand J Urol 2015;1–10.

69. Meric-Bernstam F, Johnson A, Holla V, et al. A decision support framework for genomically informed investigational cancer therapy. J Natl Cancer Inst 2015;107(7):djv098.

70. Tsimberidou A-M, Wen S, Hong DS, et al. Personalized medicine for patients with advanced cancer in the phase I program at MD Anderson: validation and landmark analyses. Clin Cancer Res 2014;20(18):4827–36.

71. Schilsky RL. Implementing personalized cancer care. Nat Rev Clin Oncol 2014;11(7):432–8.

72. McClellan M, Daniel G, Dickson D, et al. Improving evidence developed from population-level experience with targeted agents. Clin Pharmacol Ther 2015;97(5):478–87.

Diagnostic Biomarkers in Eosinophilic Renal Neoplasms

Li Yan Khor, MD[a], Puay Hoon Tan, MD, FRCPA[a,b,c,d],*

KEYWORDS

- Renal cell carcinoma • Biopsy • Eosinophilic • Biomarkers

KEY POINTS

- CK7, S100A1, vimentin/c-KIT, and Claudin 7/8 can help to differentiate renal oncocytoma and chromophobe renal cell carcinoma (RCC).
- CAIX, CK7, racemase, CD117, and CD10 can help to differentiate oncocytoma, chromophobe RCC, clear cell RCC, and papillary RCC.
- "High-grade" nuclear features are seen in renal neoplasms with wide-ranging clinical behavior. Immunomarkers are useful in differentiating these entities.
- Unique markers and molecular tests are helpful to diagnose certain neoplasms, such as translocation-associated RCC and hereditary leiomyomatosis-related RCC.

INTRODUCTION

Immunohistochemical biomarkers are useful when diagnosing renal cell carcinomas (RCC) with less than straightforward morphology or for confirming the presence of metastatic carcinoma of renal origin.[1] They have been proven to increase the accuracy of diagnosis in limited biopsy material.[2] Incidental small renal masses identified on imaging are increasingly investigated via needle core or fine needle aspiration biopsies with limited material provided for rendering a diagnosis. These lesions are amenable to treatment by noninvasive techniques, such as ablation, instead of resection. Consequently, the readily available immunohistochemical stains take on a more significant role in current practice.

RCC with distinct morphologies do not pose much difficulty in daily diagnostic practice. Moreover, many of these have well-described immunoprofiles (**Fig. 1**, **Table 1**). The challenge lies in lesions with a prominent eosinophilic or oncocytic cell presence and where there is morphologic overlap between the well-known eosinophilic neoplasms. Additionally, with only limited biopsy material, the onus is on the pathologist to rule out an eosinophilic neoplasm with potentially aggressive behavior without the reassurance of subsequent confirmation by nephrectomy. The impact on patient care of missing such a diagnosis is not inconsequential. As such, we review the range of known benign and aggressive eosinophilic renal neoplasms and their immunoprofiles to elucidate a

Conflicts of Interest: None.
[a] Department of Pathology, Singapore General Hospital, 20 College Road, Academia, Level 7, Diagnostics Tower, Singapore 169856, Singapore; [b] Department of Anatomy, Yong Loo Lin School of Medicine, National University of Singapore, MD10, 4 Medical Drive, Singapore 117594, Singapore; [c] Department of Pathology, Yong Loo Lin School of Medicine, National University of Singapore, MD10, 4 Medical Drive, Singapore 117594, Singapore; [d] Duke-NUS Graduate Medical School Singapore, 8 College Road, Singapore 169857, Singapore
* Corresponding author. Department of Pathology, Singapore General Hospital, 20 College Road, Academia, Level 7, Diagnostics Tower, Singapore 169856, Singapore.
E-mail address: tan.puay.hoon@sgh.com.sg

urologic.theclinics.com

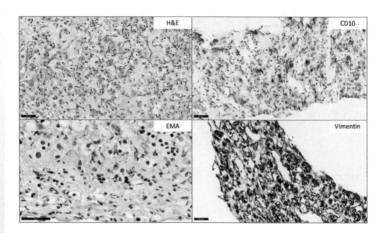

Fig. 1. A clear cell renal carcinoma with low-grade cytologic features and eosinophilic cytoplasm, showing CD10, EMA (patchy), and vimentin positivity.

useful panel of stains that could be used in this scenario.

Renal Oncocytoma Versus Chromophobe Renal Cell Carcinoma

The most commonly encountered diagnostic dilemma of a low-grade nonpapillary oncocytic renal neoplasm is between renal oncocytoma and a chromophobe RCC (ChRCC), eosinophilic type.[3] Morphologic heterogeneity can be seen in ChRCC with foci exhibiting features virtually indistinguishable from oncocytoma. Although the majority of ChRCC are regarded to have favorable prognosis, a small subset of patients show disease progression.[4] Many well-established and novel biomarkers have been tested for use in this context. However, few have been validated in more than 1 series. CK7 positivity in ChRCC is well-described and considered to be useful in differentiating ChRCC from benign renal oncocytoma, although some studies have shown similar expression in both entities[5] (**Fig. 2**). Liu and colleagues,[6] in determining a practical panel to distinguish clear cell RCC (CCRCC), ChRCC, and oncocytoma, confirmed the usefulness of CK7

Table 1
Helpful markers in the differential diagnosis of eosinophilic renal tumors

Renal Tumors	Positive Markers	Negative Markers
Clear cell RCC	Vimentin, keratin, EMA, CD10, RCCm, Pax2/8, CAIX	CK7, ksp-cadherin, parvalbumin
Papillary RCC	Keratin, CK7, AMACR, RCCm	c-KIT/CD117, ksp-cadherin, parvalbumin, WT-1
Chromophobe RCC	e-Cadherin, ksp-cadherin, c-KIT/CD117, EMA, CK, CK7	Vimentin, CAIX, AMACR
Oncocytoma	ksp-Cadherin, c-kit/CD117, parvalbumin, S100A1	CK7, moc31, EP-CAM
Translocation RCC	TFE3/TFEB, CD10, RCCm	CK
Collecting duct RCC	EMA, p63, CK7, HMWCK, Pax2/8	CD10, RCCm, CK20
Angiomyolipoma	HMB45, Melan-A, SMA	CK, CD10, RCCm, Pax2/8
Tumors with papillary architecture		
Papillary RCC	Type 1: CK7	CK20, 34BE12, ULEX-1, Type2: CK7
Collecting duct carcinoma	CK7, CK20(focal+), 34BE12, ULEX-1	CK20
Urothelial carcinoma	CK7, CK20, 34BE12, ULEX-1	—

Abbreviation: RCC, renal cell carcinoma.

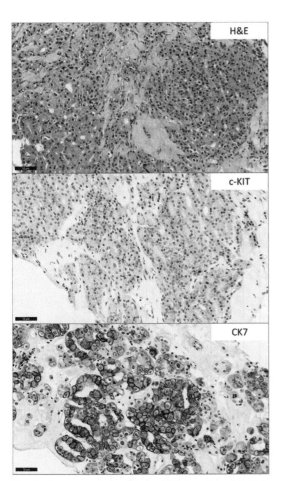

Fig. 2. An oncocytoma-like architecture is evident in this tumor characterized by nests of oncocytic cells arranged in discrete islands separated by loose stroma. Some nuclear irregularity and perinuclear clearing is present. Faint but diffuse c-KIT positivity is seen along with vimentin negativity (not shown), consistent with renal oncocytoma. However, diffuse positivity of CK7 and the nuclear cytologic irregularities raise the possibility of an alternative diagnosis such as eosinophilic chromophobe renal cell carcinoma.

and additionally found that Ep-CAM identified 100% of ChRCC with membranous or basolateral staining whereas only 29% of oncocytomas showed focal positive staining. A similar study confirmed Ep-CAM and CK7 staining in ChRCCs (80%) with no staining seen in oncocytomas.[7] Claudin 7, a distal nephron marker identified by gene expression microarray analysis, is another candidate marker recommended for use as part of a panel, identifying 76% of ChRCC and 26% of oncocytomas in immunohistochemical validation studies.[8] A further study showed the combination of Claudin 7 (membranous or mixed membranous/cytoplasmic stain positivity) and Claudin 8 (negativity) reliably differentiated ChRCC

from oncocytomas (Claudin 7-negative/Claudin 8-positive with membranous, mixed membranous/cytoplasmic or perinuclear staining).[9] Osunkoya and colleagues[10] also showed the combination of Claudin 7-positive (membranous)/Claudin 8-negative profile had an 88% positive predictive value for ChRCC whereas Claudin 7-negative/Claudin 8-cytoplasmic staining had a 100% specificity and positive predictive value for oncocytoma. S100A1, a transduction protein involved in cell-cycle progression, was reported to be expressed in 93% of oncocytomas and not expressed by ChRCC.[11] It was 1 of 4 candidate proteins subsequently reported by Carvalho and colleagues[12] to be useful in discriminating oncocytoma from its mimics—ChRCC, papillary RCC (PRCC), and CCRCC—using hierarchical and supervised cluster analyses. S100A1-positive/CK7-focal positive distinguished oncocytoma from ChRCC with 91% sensitivity and 93% specificity. The authors also found the combination of vimentin-negative/c-KIT–positive distinguished oncocytoma from CCRCC with 83% sensitivity and 86% specificity, and from PRCC with 79% sensitivity and 88% specificity (**Table 2**).

In a recent report, S100A1 combined with HNF1b showed discriminatory potential where 73% of oncocytomas and 21% of ChRCC were nuclear positive for HNF1b and 80% of oncocytomas and 8% of ChRCC were positive for S100A1. No ChRCC were positive for both markers.[13] However, these results are yet to be validated.

Clear Cell Renal Cell Carcinoma with Eosinophilic Morphology Versus Translocation-Associated Renal Cell Carcinoma

CCRCC with a predominant eosinophilic morphology is commonly seen in high-grade tumors with accompanying hemorrhage and necrosis, but is not considered a separate entity because it shares molecular characteristics with conventional CCRCC with the classic clear cell morphology.[14] The translocation-associated RCCs, characterized and defined by translocations involving MiTF/TFE family genes, may share high nuclear grade morphology and granular eosinophilic cytoplasm. When other characteristic features such as papillary architecture and psammoma bodies are absent, ancillary studies are helpful. Conventional RCC is positive for CD10, CAIX, EMA, vimentin, and negative for CK7 and high-molecular-weight cytokeratin. MiTF RCC is negative for AE1/AE3 and EMA, and negative or focally positive for vimentin. TFE3 carcinomas are positive for RCCm, CD10, AMACR, and

Table 2
Comparison of useful immunomarkers

Immunomarker	Oncocytoma	ChRCC	CCRCC	Translocation RCC		PRCC	Follicular Thyroidlike RCC	RCC, Unclass ("Low grade")	RCC, Unclass ("High grade")	eAML	HLRCC	SDH Mutation RCC
				TFE3	TFEB							
Unique marker	—	—	—	TFE3+	TFEB+	—	TTF-1 – TG –	—	—	—	FH mutation	SDHA – SDHB –
CK7	– (Focal +)	+	—	—	—	Type 1 + Type 2 –	Mostly –	+	—	—	– (Focal +)	—
Ep-CAM	Focal +	+	—	—	—	—	—	—	—	—	—	—
Claudin 7/8	–/+	+/–	+	—	—	—	—	—	—	—	—	—
S100A1	+	–	+	—	—	+	—	—	—	—	—	—
Vimentin/c-KIT	– (Mem +)/+	–/+	+/–	—	—	+/–	—	—	—	—	—	—
EMA	—	—	+	—	—	—	—	—	+	—	—	—
AE1/AE3	—	—	+	—	—	—	+	—	+	—	—	—
Vimentin	—	—	+	—	—	—		—	—	—	—	—
PAX 8	—	—	+	—	—	—	—	—	+	—	—	—
CAIX	—	—	Mem +	—	—	+	—	—	—	—	—	—
RCCm	—	+	+	+	—	+	—	—	—	—	—	—
CD10	—	—	Mem +	+	—	Lum +	—	—	—	—	—	—
AMACR	—	—	+	+	—	+	—	—	—	—	—	—
e-Cadherin	+	+	—	+	—	—	—	—	—	—	—	—
MelanA/HMB45	—	—	—	—	+	—	—	—	—	+	—	—

Abbreviations: +, positive; –, negative; CAIX, carbonic anhydrase IX; CCRCC, clear cell renal cell carcinoma; ChRCC, chromophobe renal cell carcinoma; eAML, epithelioid angiomyolipoma; FH, fumarate hydratase; HLRCC, hereditary leiomyomatosis-associated renal cell carcinoma; Lum, luminal; Mem, membranous; PRCC, papillary renal cell carcinoma; RCC, unclass, renal cell carcinoma, unclassified; SDH mutation RCC, succinate dehydrogenase mutation renal cell carcinoma.

e-cadherin. TFEB tumors are CD10 and RCCm negative or focally positive, and positive for the melanocytic markers, Melan-A and HMB-45 (rarely expressed in TFE3 tumors)[15] (see **Table 2**). Unique TFE3 and TFEB immunomarkers are highly sensitive and specific for these tumors in appropriately fixed tissue but break-apart fluorescence in situ hybridization is used for a definitive diagnosis (**Fig. 3**).

Renal Cell Carcinoma, Unclassified ("Low-Grade Oncocytic Type") Versus Oncocytoma and Chromophobe Renal Cell Carcinoma, Eosinophilic Type

An RCC is "unclassified" when morphologic features do not fit into any recognized class, or 2 or more morphologic types, or purely sarcomatoid carcinoma is present. These are usually high-grade carcinomas. However, a subset of these tumors have "low-grade" features and include an oncocytic-type characterized by solid nests or alveoli with oncocytoma-like architecture, nuclear pleomorphism and mitotic index beyond that which is acceptable for oncocytoma.[3,16] No nuclear wrinkling or perinuclear halos, as seen in the eosinophilic ChRCC are present; features that may be absent in a limited biopsy sample. "Low-grade" unclassified RCC are diffusely

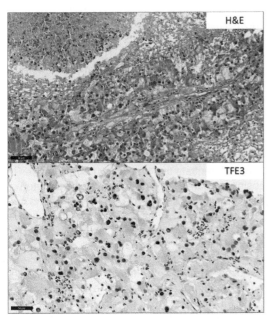

Fig. 3. High-grade clear cell cytology with marked necrosis. Voluminous clear cells are present together with pink cells with hyaline globules, suggesting a translocation-associated tumor. TFE3 immunostain is positive. Further confirmation by molecular testing should be performed.

positive for CK7, which definitively rules out oncocytoma, but does not exclude ChRCC.[3]

Follicular Thyroid-like Carcinoma Versus Papillary Renal Cell Carcinoma and Renal Cell Carcinoma, Unclassified ("Low-Grade Oncocytic Type")

A recently described and little-studied entity, follicular thyroid-like carcinoma, closely mimics well-differentiated thyroid follicular neoplasms, recapitulating the microfollicular and macrofollicular architecture, lined by amphophilic to eosinophilic cells with moderate amounts of cytoplasm and containing pink to red colloid-like secretions.[17] The uniform bland cells result in mostly low nuclear grading. This unique entity is TTF-1 and thyroglobulin negative, and immunostains should be performed to rule out a metastatic thyroid carcinoma before rendering a diagnosis. Immunohistochemically, they are mostly, but not always, CK7, CD10, Pax2, RCCm, AMACR, vimentin, ksp-cadherin, WT-1, and c-KIT/CD117 negative. Although papillary architecture is not commonly seen in this entity, it has been described in 1 report.[18] In comparison, PRCC is CK7, AMACR, and RCCm positive, and c-KIT/CD117, ksp-cadherin, parvalbumin, and WT-1 negative. Oncocytomas and RCC, unclassified ("low-grade oncocytic type", which is CK7 positive), may also show focal thyroid-like follicular features.

Epithelioid Angiomyolipoma Versus High-Grade Renal Cell Carcinoma Unclassified, Renal Cell Carcinoma with Sarcomatoid Differentiation and Translocation-Associated Carcinoma

Epithelioid angiomyolipoma, commonly seen in tuberous sclerosis patients, have sheet-like or alveolar architecture composed of 2 types of cells—clear cells with fine granular cytoplasm and small monomorphic nuclei, and eosinophilic cells with abundant cytoplasm, epithelioid morphology and large nuclei with prominent nucleoli. Focal fat and dysmorphic cells are present. The latter high-grade–type cells, in addition to the presence of mitoses, necrosis, extrarenal extension, renal vein involvement, and, rarely, distant metastases, can lead to misdiagnoses as high-grade RCC, unclassified.[19–21] Useful immunostains include Melan-A and HMB-45 positivity in epithelioid angiomyolipoma, pancytokeratin, EMA, and Pax 8 positivity in RCC unclassified and RCC with sarcomatoid differentiation. MiTF/TFE translocation-associated carcinoma shares a similar immunoprofile of positive Melan-A and HMB-45, and negative epithelial markers but is variably positive for Pax 8. As mentioned, TFE3 and TFEB immunostains and molecular studies can help to provide a definitive diagnosis.

Papillary Neoplasms with Eosinophilic Features Versus Collecting Duct Carcinoma and Urothelial Carcinoma

Diagnosing PRCC is usually not a challenge on biopsies. However, type 2 PRCC lacks the foamy macrophages and intracellular hemosiderin accumulation. High-grade cytologic atypia, eosinophilic cytoplasm, and nuclear pseudostratification are common features. Collecting duct RCC (CDRCC) and urothelial carcinoma involving the renal pelvis are differentials to consider as variable papillary growth is seen. Other morphologic features of CDRCC, such as a neutrophil-rich infiltrate and dysplastic changes in adjacent renal collecting ducts, if present, are helpful. Of note, a pseudopapillary pattern can be seen in CCRCC from cell drop-off in areas away from feeding vessels.

PRCC is positive for CK7 (type 1 more often than type 2), CD10 (luminal membranous), AMACR (cytoplasmic granular), RCC and Pax 2; either negative or focal positive for CAIX in the papillary tips or perinecrotic areas. In contrast with PRCC, CDRCC are RCC antigen and AMACR negative. Urothelial carcinoma is CK20 and ULEX-1 positive, which is not seen in PRCC or CDRCC (see **Table 1**).

Hereditary leiomyomatosis-related RCC (HLRCC) shows variable but prominent papillary architecture, admixed with cystic/tubular, solid, or cribriform patterns. Very prominent macronucleoli and perinuclear halos are key distinct morphologic features. The presence of desmoplasia and multinodularity resembles CDRCC. Cytogenetics testing for fumarate hydratase germline mutation is confirmatory. An oncocytic variant with low-grade nonoverlapping nuclei with molecular and biologic similarity to type 1 PRCC has been described.[22]

Succinate Dehydrogenase Mutant Renal Cell Carcinoma

RCC with SDHB deficiency is currently considered a provisional entity in the 2013 International Society of Urologic Pathology Vancouver Classification of renal tumors.[23] However, it begs mention because it presents as part of a syndrome that might not yet be known in the patient at the time of biopsy. Those tumors with low nuclear grade features are not associated with a true oncocytic cytoplasm, but rather have flocculent cytoplasm. However, in the largest reported series, a few of the tumors described had International Society of Urologic

Pathology nucleolar (nuclear) grade 3 cells, had high-grade areas with dense eosinophilic cytoplasm, and nested, solid sheets or focal abortive papillary architecture.[24] These tumors, aside from SDHB negativity, show SDHA, Pax 8, and limited focal EMA positivity. Rare focal CK7 staining is seen. Most cases are completely negative for cytokeratins (AE1/AE3, CK8/18, CK7, CK20) and c-KIT/CD117, the latter which mainly highlights the characteristic intratumoral mast cells.

A recent case report described the first SDHA mutant RCC, which was associated with aggressive behavior. The tumor architecture was a combination of high-grade papillary and collecting duct carcinoma with pale eosinophilic cytoplasmic inclusions.[25] Although SDHA-deficient tumors are not well-described, staining for both SDHB and SDHA should be performed when the differential is being considered.

DISCUSSION

Percutaneous renal core biopsies have been shown to play a meaningful role in the clinical management of patients, especially with the use of immunohistochemical markers, improving diagnostic accuracy of tumor subtyping and influencing the type of therapeutic intervention.[26] The oncocytic neoplasms pose the greatest challenge wherein low-grade oncocytic neoplasms include renal oncocytoma, eosinophilic ChRCC, or RCC unclassified, "low-grade oncocytic type." In the absence of characteristic cytologic features of ChRCC (crenated nuclei and perinuclear halos), the use of a single or panel of immunomarkers is favored by pathologists. CK7 has proven to be the most common single biomarker used in this scenario.[1] A review shows Ep-CAM and Claudin 7/8 have been well-studied and, although not yet commonly used in daily practice, these could prove to be effective additions.

To differentiate the 4 most common subtypes of eosinophilic renal tumors, namely, oncocytoma, ChRCC, CCRCC, and PRCC, Al-Ahmadie and colleagues recommend a panel of 5 immunomarkers (CAIX, CK7, racemase, CD117 and CD10; see **Table 2**). This panel was also used completely, or in part, in 69% of cases reported by Gellert and colleagues[26] in a larger series of 181 neoplastic lesions, including 29 low-grade oncocytic tumors (11 ChRCC, 9 oncocytomas, and 9 RCC, unclassified). Among 30 cases confirmed by nephrectomy, the reported diagnostic accuracy of tumor subtyping was 97%.

Oncocytic neoplasms with high nuclear grade features include entities with a range of clinical behavior, several of which have unique markers (translocation RCC, HLRCC, and SDH mutation RCC). Other clinical parameters, such as patient age, family history, and metachronous/synchronous tumors present at other anatomic sites, should raise one's suspicion of these entities, which could then be confirmed by specific immunomarkers or molecular testing.

Papillary architecture and high nuclear grade features can be seen in PRCC, and urothelial and collecting duct carcinoma. CK7, CK20, 34BE12, and Ulex-1 are the recommended panel for distinguishing these entities (see **Table 1**).

SUMMARY

A panel of immunostains, in conjunction with morphology, remain the holy grail of distinguishing eosinophilic renal neoplasms. We present the entities that fall into this diagnostic category and their reported immunoprofiles. With such wide-ranging neoplasms, we conclude that consideration of several sets of panels appropriate to the case being evaluated, is amenable to daily practice. On core biopsy material with limited tissue, it may not always be possible to confidently assign tumor subtype, and in such instances, excision of the tumor for full histologic assessment may be required.

REFERENCES

1. Tan PH, Cheng L, Rioux-Leclercq N, et al. Renal tumors: diagnostic and prognostic biomarkers. Am J Surg Pathol 2013;37:1518–31.

2. Al-Ahmadie HA, Alden D, Fine SW, et al. Role of immunohistochemistry in the evaluation of needle core biopsies in adult renal cortical tumors: an ex vivo study. Am J Surg Pathol 2011;35:949–61.

3. Kryvenko ON, Jorda M, Argani P, et al. Diagnostic approach to eosinophilic renal neoplasms. Arch Pathol Lab Med 2014;138:1531–41.

4. Amin MB, Paner GP, Alvarado-Cabrero I, et al. Chromophobe renal cell carcinoma: histomorphologic characteristics and evaluation of conventional pathologic prognostic parameters in 145 cases. Am J Surg Pathol 2008;32:1822–34.

5. Ng KL, Rajandram R, Morais C, et al. Differentiation of oncocytoma from chromophobe renal cell carcinoma (RCC): can novel molecular biomarkers help solve an old problem? J Clin Pathol 2014;67:97–104.

6. Liu L, Qian J, Singh H, et al. Immunohistochemical analysis of chromophobe renal cell carcinoma, renal oncocytoma, and clear cell carcinoma: an optimal and practical panel for differential diagnosis. Arch Pathol Lab Med 2007;131:1290–7.

7. Ray ER, Goodwill J, Chandra A, et al. Exploring the potential of immunohistochemistry to identify renal oncocytoma. Br J Med Surg Urol 2011;4:8–12.

8. Hornsby CD, Cohen C, Amin MB, et al. Claudin-7 immunohistochemistry in renal tumors: a candidate marker for chromophobe renal cell carcinoma identified by gene expression profiling. Arch Pathol Lab Med 2007;131:1541–6.

9. Lechpammer M, Resnick MB, Sabo E, et al. The diagnostic and prognostic utility of claudin expression in renal cell neoplasms. Mod Pathol 2008;21:1320–9.

10. Osunkoya AO, Cohen C, Lawson D, et al. Claudin-7 and claudin-8: immunohistochemical markers for the differential diagnosis of chromophobe renal cell carcinoma and renal oncocytoma. Hum Pathol 2009;40:206–10.

11. Li G, Barthelemy A, Feng G, et al. S100A1: a powerful marker to differentiate chromophobe renal cell carcinoma from renal oncocytoma. Histopathology 2007;50:642–7.

12. Carvalho JC, Wasco MJ, Kunju LP, et al. Cluster analysis of immunohistochemical profiles delineates CK7, vimentin, S100A1 and C-kit (CD117) as an optimal panel in the differential diagnosis of renal oncocytoma from its mimics. Histopathology 2011;58:169–79.

13. Conner JR, Hirsch MS, Jo VY, et al. HNF1β and S100A1 are useful biomarkers for distinguishing renal oncocytoma and chromophobe renal cell carcinoma in FNA and core needle biopsies. Cancer Cytopathol 2015;123:298–305.

14. Yang XJ, Takahashi M, Schafernak KT, et al. Does 'granular cell' renal cell carcinoma exist? Molecular and histological reclassification. Histopathology 2007;50:678–80.

15. Camparo P, Vasiliu V, Molinie V, et al. Renal translocation carcinomas: clinicopathologic, immunohistochemical, and gene expression profiling analysis of 31 cases with a review of the literature. Am J Surg Pathol 2008;32:656–70.

16. Amin MB, McKenney JK, Tickoo SK, et al. Diagnostic pathology genitourinary. Manitoba (Canada): AMIRSYS; 2010. p. 1–247.

17. Amin MB, Gupta R, Ondrej H, et al. Primary thyroid-like follicular carcinoma of the kidney: report of 6 cases of a histologically distinctive adult renal epithelial neoplasm. Am J Surg Pathol 2009;33:393–400.

18. Sterlacci W, William S, Verdorfer I, et al. Thyroid follicular carcinoma-like renal tumor: a case report with morphologic, immunophenotypic, cytogenetic, and scintigraphic studies. Virchows Arch 2008;452:91–5.

19. Nese N, Martignoni G, Fletcher CD, et al. Pure epithelioid PEComas (so-called epithelioid angiomyolipoma) of the kidney: a clinicopathologic study

of 41 cases: detailed assessment of morphology and risk stratification. Am J Surg Pathol 2011;35: 161–76.

20. Brimo F, Robinson B, Guo C, et al. Renal epithelioid angiomyolipoma with atypia: a series of 40 cases with emphasis on clinicopathologic prognostic indicators of malignancy. Am J Surg Pathol 2010;34: 715–22.

21. He W, Cheville JC, Sadow PM, et al. Epithelioid angiomyolipoma of the kidney: pathological features and clinical outcome in a series of consecutively resected tumors. Mod Pathol 2013;26: 1355–64.

22. Hes O, Brunelli M, Michal M, et al. Oncocytic papillary renal cell carcinoma: a clinicopathologic, immunohistochemical, ultrastructural, and interphase cytogenetic study of 12 cases. Ann Diagn Pathol 2006;10:133–9.

23. Srigley JR, Delahunt B, Eble JN, et al. The International Society of Urological Pathology (ISUP) Vancouver Classification of Renal Neoplasia. Am J Surg Pathol 2013;37:1469–89.

24. Gill AJ, Hes O, Papathomas T, et al. Succinate dehydrogenase (SDH)-deficient renal carcinoma: a morphologically distinct entity: a clinicopathologic series of 36 tumors from 27 patients. Am J Surg Pathol 2014;38:1588–602.

25. Yakirevich E, Ali SM, Mega A, et al. A novel SDHA-deficient renal cell carcinoma revealed by comprehensive genomic profiling. Am J Surg Pathol 2015; 39:858–63.

26. Gellert LL, Mehra R, Chen YB, et al. The diagnostic accuracy of percutaneous renal needle core biopsy and its potential impact on the clinical management of renal cortical neoplasms. Arch Pathol Lab Med 2014;138:1673–9.

Prognostic Biomarkers for Response to Vascular Endothelial Growth Factor–Targeted Therapy for Renal Cell Carcinoma

Andrew G. Winer, MD[a], Robert J. Motzer, MD[b], A. Ari Hakimi, MD[a],*

KEYWORDS

- Biomarker • Renal cell carcinoma • Tyrosine kinase inhibitor • VEGF • Targeted therapy

KEY POINTS

- Biomarker studies in advanced renal cell carcinoma attempting to predict response to VEGF-targeted therapies have largely focused on circulating proteins, tissue-based molecules, and germline polymorphisms.
- To date, such devoted studies have yielded conflicting results, therefore no definitive biomarker has emerged.
- The heterogeneity in findings may relate to interstudy inconsistencies in design, laboratory assay, and data analysis.
- Information from high-throughput molecular analyses has improved the understanding of renal cell carcinoma and is presently being used to create prediction models for response to VEGF-targeted therapies.

INTRODUCTION

Renal cell carcinoma (RCC) has an annual estimated incidence of 64,000 cases in the United States, of which the clear cell (ccRCC) histology represents the most common and aggressive subtype.[1] The incidence of this disease seems to be rising, which is largely thought to be a result of improved quality and more frequent use of cross-sectional imaging leading to a stage migration toward smaller, lower-stage tumors.[2] However, despite the observed stage migration over the past two decades, this trend has not translated into population-level improvements in survival in those diagnosed with RCC.[2,3] In fact, roughly 30% of patients with RCC present with advanced disease, which remains largely incurable.[4]

Enhanced understanding of RCC disease biology in the past several decades has led to the discovery of novel therapies targeted at specific biochemical pathways involved in renal tumorigenesis. Specifically, the identification of molecular disturbances in the von Hippel-Lindau (*VHL*) gene that, when altered, causes aberrant stabilization of the hypoxia-inducible factor (HIF)-α subunit with consequent upregulation of proangiogenic

Funding: Supported by the Sidney Kimmel Center for Prostate and Urologic Cancers.
Conflict of Interest: None.
[a] Urology Service, Department of Surgery, Memorial Sloan Kettering Cancer Center, 353 East 68th Street, New York, NY 10065, USA; [b] Genitourinary Oncology Service, Division of Solid Tumor Oncology, Department of Medicine, Memorial Sloan Kettering Cancer Center, 1275 York Ave, New York, NY 10065, USA
* Corresponding author.
E-mail address: hakimia@mskcc.org

Urol Clin N Am 43 (2016) 95–104
http://dx.doi.org/10.1016/j.ucl.2015.08.009
0094-0143/16/$ – see front matter © 2016 Elsevier Inc. All rights reserved.

urologic.theclinics.com

downstream molecules, such as vascular endothelial growth factor (VEGF). From this framework spawned the development and Food and Drug Administration approval of four inhibitor molecules directed at various targets in the tyrosine kinase signaling pathway involved in VEGF modulation, termed tyrosine kinase inhibitors (TKIs), and one monoclonal antibody directed specifically at the VEGF receptor (**Table 1**).

Although several clinical trials with such targeted agents have demonstrated improved outcomes in patients with metastatic RCC (mRCC), a clear understanding of which patients will respond remains uncertain. To address this challenge, several biomarkers have been identified to aid in patient selection for particular therapies and prediction for therapeutic response. This article provides an overview of available biomarkers that have been tested and used with respect to VEGF-targeted therapies in patients with mRCC.

CIRCULATING/BLOOD-BASED BIOMARKERS
Vascular Endothelial Growth Factor and Vascular Endothelial Growth Factor–Related Proteins

Under normal and disease conditions, VEGF is a critical regulator of angiogenesis and lymphangiogenesis.[5] On a cellular level, VEGF is persistently upregulated in ccRCC as a direct result of *VHL* gene inactivation. Given the relationship between VEGF and RCC tumorigenesis, the prognostic value of circulating VEGF levels and response to VEGF-targeted therapy has been extensively evaluated with conflicting results (**Table 2**). Biomarker analysis from two sunitinib trials demonstrated that low baseline levels of soluble VEGFR-3 and VEGF-C were found to be favorably correlated with longer progression-free survival (PFS).[6,7] Conversely, in the AVOREN phase III trial comparing interferon (IFN)-α alone with IFN-α

plus bevacizumab, the PFS benefit observed in the bevacizumab arm was not significantly different between patients with baseline VEGF levels above or below the median.[8] In a separate phase III randomized controlled trial, higher pretreatment levels of VEGF were associated with a trend toward improved PFS in sorafenib-treated patients compared with placebo (P = .096).[9,10] The same study investigated the predictive significance of changes in VEGF and soluble VEGFR-2 after 3 or 12 weeks of treatment with sorafenib; however, there was no association identified. This lack of association was similarly found between decreases in circulating VEGF-2 and response in patients treated with sunitinib.[11] On the contrary, biomarker analysis from a phase II sunitinib study revealed that patients with objective tumor responses experienced substantially larger changes in VEGF, soluble VEGFR-2, and soluble VEGFR-3 levels compared with those patients exhibiting tumor progression (P<.05).[12] The conflicting nature of the results to date may be a direct consequence of inconsistent biomarker detection methods in addition to the effect that therapy may have on the ability to accurately measure the concentrations of drug targets.

Cytokine and Angiogenic Factors

Numerous cytokines and other proteins involved in the angiogenic cascade have also been evaluated as biomarkers for response to VEGF-targeted therapies (see **Table 2**). Using data from phase II and phase III pazopanib trials, the authors identified interleukin (IL)-6, IL-8, VEGF, osteopontin (OPN), E-selectin, and hepatocyte growth factor (HGF) to be associated with tumor shrinkage and PFS. In the validation set of samples from the phase III trial, patients in the pazopanib arm with elevated concentration of IL-8 (P = .006), OPN (P = .0004), HGF (P = .010), and tissue inhibitor

Table 1
Summary of FDA-approved VEGF-directed therapies for renal cancer

Drug	Brand Name	Company	Target	Year of FDA Approval
Sorafenib	Nexavar	Bayer	Inhibits VEGFR-2, VEGFR-3, PDGFR-β, Flt-3, RAF-1, and c-KIT	2005
Sunitinib	Sutent	Pfizer	Inhibits VEGFR-2, Flt-3, c-KIT, and PDGFR-β	2006
Pazopanib	Votrient	GSK	Inhibits VEGFR-1, VEGFR-2, VEGFR-3, PDGFR-α, PDGFR-β, and c-KIT	2009
Axitinib	Inlyta	Pfizer	Inhibits VEGFR-1, VEGFR-2, and VEGFR-3	2012
Bevacizumab	Avastin	Roche	Recombinant monoclonal antibody to VEGF-A	2009

Abbreviation: FDA, Food and Drug Administration.

Table 2
Summary of circulating/blood-based biomarkers for response to VEGF-targeted therapy

Circulating Biomarker	No. of Patients	Treatment	Description of Biomarker Levels	Outcome	Ref.
VEGF and VEGF-related proteins					
VEGF	363	Sorafenib	High	Trend toward prolonged PFS (HR, 0.64; $P = .096$)	10
	63	Sunitinib	Change after treatment	Larger change in patients with PR compared with those with SD or PD (HR, NR; $P<.0001$)	12
VEGFR-2	63	Sunitinib	Change after treatment	Larger change in patients with PR compared with those with SD or PD (HR, NR; $P<.0001$)	12
VEGFR-3	33	Sunitinib	Low	Increased PFS (HR, 2.40; $P = .01$) and OS (HR, 1.68; $P = .07$)	6
	59	Sunitinib	Low	Increased PFS (HR, 0.45; $P = .006$)	7
	63	Sunitinib	Change after treatment	Larger change in patients with PR compared with those with SD or PD (HR, NR; $P<.0001$)	12
VEGF-C	59	Sunitinib	Low	Increased PFS (HR, 0.37; $P = .0006$)	7
Cytokine and angiogenic factors					
IL-6	344	Pazopanib	High	Increased PFS (HR, 0.55; $P = .009$)	13
Inflammatory markers					
CRP	41	Sunitinib	Low	Increased PFS (HR, NR; $P = .036$)	16
	52	Sunitinib, sorafenib	Low	Improved OS (HR, 1.79; $P = .01$)	17
	200	Sunitinib	High	Shorter PFS (HR, 1.14; $P = .01$) and OS (HR, 1.29; $P<.001$)	18
NLR	109	Sunitinib	NLR <3	Improved PFS (HR, 0.285; $P<.001$) and OS (HR, 0.3; $P = .043$)	19
	100	Sunitinib, sorafenib, pazopanib	NLR <3	Improved PFS (HR, NR; $P = .009$) and OS (HR, NR; 0.004)	20
Lactate dehydrogenase	375	Sunitinib	High	Shorter PFS (HR, 1.6; $P = .003$) and OS (HR, 2.0; $P<.001$)	24

Abbreviations: CRP, C-reactive protein; HR, hazard ratio; IL, interleukin; NLR, neutrophil-to-lymphocyte ratio; NR, not reported; OS, overall survival; PR, partial response; PD, progressive disease; PFS, progression-free survival; SD, stable disease.

of metalloproteinase-1 ($P = .006$) had shorter PFS than did those with low concentrations. They also found that elevated levels of IL-6 were correlated with improved PFS in the pazopanib-treated arm as compared with placebo arm ($P = .009$).[13] Additional analysis from this study generated a seven-factor angiogenic signature (IL-6, IL-8, HGF, OPN, tissue inhibitor of metalloproteinase-1, VEGF, and E-selectin) and patients were categorized into high and low groups, which were then correlated with PFS. They found that patients with higher signature scores were associated with significantly shorter PFS in the placebo ($P = .001$) and pazopanib ($P = .001$) arms.[14] In a separate investigation of cytokine and angiogenic factors as biomarkers predicting therapeutic response to sorafenib, two distinct clusters of patients emerged that were characterized either by elevated levels of proangiogenic or proinflammatory factors. A panel of six baseline mediators (OPN, VEGF, carbonic anhydrase IX [CAIX], collagen IV, VEGFR-2, and tumor necrosis factor–related apoptosis-inducing ligand) was then correlated with PFS after sorafenib. Patients negative for the six-marker signature benefitted from an improved PFS (hazard ratio [HR], 0.20 vs 2.25 in the signature negative vs positive, respectively; $P = .0002$).[15]

Inflammatory Markers

Several circulating markers of inflammation have been investigated as prognostic markers for advanced RCC treated with targeted agents (see **Table 2**). In a small series of 41 patients with mRCC treated with sunitinib, C-reactive protein (CRP) was considered as a possible biomarker for therapeutic response.[16] They found that patients with normal CRP levels had a significantly higher partial response plus stable disease rate (84.6% vs 35.7%; $P = .002$) and significantly longer PFS (median, 19.0 vs 6.0 months; $P = .036$) than patients with an elevated level of CRP. CRP was identified as an independent predictor of objective response ($P = .016$) on multivariate analysis. Nonelevated levels of CRP (<8 mg/L) was also found to be an independent predictor of improved overall survival (OS) ($P = .003$) in another small study (N = 52) that included treatment with both sunitinib and sorafenib.[17] A larger retrospective report evaluating 200 patients who received sunitinib as first-line therapy substantiated the previous findings in smaller subsets of treated patients. They found that elevated baseline CRP levels conferred a clear disadvantage with respect to PFS (8 months vs 25 months; HR, 2.48) and OS (12 months vs 50 months; HR, 3.17). Increasing baseline CRP levels was independently associated with inferior PFS in a multivariate model accounting for the variables included in the International Metastatic RCC Database Consortium model (HR, 1.14 for each doubling in CRP).[18]

Neutrophil-to-lymphocyte ratio (NLR) is an inflammatory response marker that has demonstrated prognostic value in several cancer types including RCC. This ratio has recently been examined as a tool for predicting response to VEGF-targeted agents in patients with mRCC. The first study analyzed 109 sunitinib-treated patients and compared pretreatment NLR with posttreatment outcomes.[19] They found NLR less than three to be associated with improved PFS (HR, 0.285; $P<.001$) and OS (HR, 0.38; $P = .043$). Similarly, another analysis correlated pretreatment NLR with PFS and OS in 100 patients.[20] They demonstrated an improved PFS ($P = .009$) and OS (0.004) after VEGF-directed therapy in patients with a lower baseline NLR (≤3.04). The median OS was 16 months versus 29 months in patients with NLR greater than 3.04 versus less than or equal to 3.04, respectively ($P = .004$). This association was further corroborated in a recent analysis that demonstrated high baseline NLR to be correlated with lower response rates to TKIs.[21]

Additional circulating proteins have been studied as potential biomarkers, although in a limited capacity. In a small prospective predictive marker trial of 13 patients with mRCC on TKI therapy, the authors found that the plasma granulocyte-macrophage colony–stimulating factor concentrations were significantly higher in the therapy responsive group when compared with the patients who either progressed or remained stable posttreatment ($P = .012$).[22] In a biomarker subanalysis from a phase II randomized controlled trial comparing sunitinib dose schedules, the authors correlated drug efficacy with selected serum markers. Of the 45 proteins evaluated, only two of the proteins showed statistically significant correlations with tumor response (complete and partial response vs stable and progressive disease): lower angiopoietin-2 concentrations ($P = .0215$) and higher matrix metalloproteinase-2 concentrations ($P = .0180$).[23] Lastly, in a phase III sunitinib trial, elevated lactate dehydrogenase was found to be independently associated with shorter PFS (HR, 1.575) and OS (HR, 2.01); however, the fact that lactate dehydrogenase is a robust prognostic marker in advanced RCC independent of treatment calls these findings into question.[24]

TISSUE-BASED BIOMARKERS
Vascular Endothelial Growth Factor and Vascular Endothelial Growth Factor–Related Proteins

Circulating levels of proteins often vary at any given time making them difficult to accurately evaluate. Another approach to assess the relationship between VEGF-related protein levels and treatment response has been through tumor tissue profiling. Several studies that have investigated the expression levels of VEGF and VEGF-related proteins in RCC tissue identify factors predicting susceptibility to VEGF-directed agents (**Table 3**). One such study performed immunohistochemical (IHC) staining for 10 molecular markers on 40 patients undergoing cytoreductive nephrectomy for mRCC and compared expression levels with response to sunitinib. Only strong expression of VEGFR-2 was found to be correlated with improved PFS on multivariate analysis ($P = .039$).[25] Another study evaluated tissue biomarkers using reverse transcription polymerase chain reaction (RT-PCR) on RNA extracted from 23 primary tumors in patients with mRCC treated with sunitinib to predict response. Of the 16 biomarkers analyzed, increased expression levels of soluble isoforms of VEGF (VEGF [121] and VEGF [165]) were correlated with therapeutic responses to sunitinib ($P = .04$ for both).[26]

The *VHL* downstream effector proteins in the HIF family have been demonstrated to be independent poor prognostic markers in RCC.[27] However, less is known about the predictive ability of these proteins to be used as a marker of response to VEGF-targeted therapy. In one analysis IHC of

Table 3
Summary of tissue-based biomarkers for response to VEGF-targeted therapy

Tissue Biomarker	No. of Patients	Treatment	Tissue Analysis Technique	Description of Biomarker	Outcome	Ref.
VEGF	23	Sunitinib	PCR	Increased expression	Correlated with therapeutic responses to sunitinib (HR, NR; $P = .015$)	26
VEGFR-2	40	Sunitinib	IHC	Strong staining	Improved PFS on multivariate analysis (HR, NR; $P = .039$)	25
VEGFR-3	67	Sunitinib	IHC	Strong staining	Improved PFS (HR, 0.4; $P = .012$)	28
HIF-2α	67	Sunitinib	IHC	Strong staining	Higher ORR (HR, 0.11; $P = .024$) and longer OS (HR, 0.39; $P = .048$)	28
PDGF	67	Sunitinib	IHC	Strong staining	Higher rates of ORR (HR, 0.04; $P = .026$)	28
CA-IX	94	Sunitinib, sorafenib, valatenib, bevacizumab	IHC	Strong staining	Not associated with ORR (HR, NR; $P = 1.0$) or OS (HR, NR; $P = .43$)	29
	133	Sorafenib	IHC	Strong staining	Not correlated with PFS (HR, NR; $P = .97$)	30
	42	Sunitinib	IHC	Strong staining	Independent prognostic marker for OS (HR, 0.174; $P = .011$)	31
VHL gene	43	Bevacizumab	PCR	Mutated or methylated gene	Longer TTP compared patients with wild-type *VHL* (HR, NR; $P = .06$)	32
	123	Sunitinib, sorafenib, axitinib, bevacizumab	PCR	Mutated gene	Higher ORR (HR, NR; $P = .04$)	33
	78	Pazopanib	PCR	Mutated or methylated gene	Not associated with ORR (HR, NR; $P = .17$)	34

Abbreviations: IHC, immunohistochemistry; ORR, objective response rate; PCR, polymerase chain reaction; TTP, time to progression.

eight key hypoxia-related proteins was performed in 67 primary ccRCC samples from patients with advanced RCC who received first-line sunitinib. They demonstrated that elevated expression of HIF-2α ($P = .024$) and platelet-derived growth receptor-β ($P = .026$) were correlated with higher rates of objective response according to RECIST criteria and increased VEGFR3 was associated with improved PFS ($P = .012$), whereas elevated VEGFA was associated with shorter ($P = .009$) and HIF-2α with longer ($P = .048$) OS.[28] Further studies are needed to validate the findings of this one investigation.

Carbonic Anhydrase-IX

CAIX is a transmembrane protein that is used a cellular marker for hypoxia and is frequently overexpressed in *VHL*-mutated tumors. Similar to HIF family proteins, it has been demonstrated to be independent a poor prognostic marker in RCC but its role as a predictor of response has been less well established (see **Table 3**).[27] One study evaluated tumor CAIX expression in 94 patients with mRCC treated with VEGF-directed therapy to predict response. They found that patients with high versus low tumor CAIX expression experienced similar tumor shrinkage rates ($P = .38$). Additionally, CAIX expression levels were not associated with response rate ($P = 1.0$), treatment duration ($P = .23$), and OS ($P = .43$).[29] Another study by the same authors evaluated the predictive value of CAIX in predicting response to sorafenib versus placebo in the pivotal TARGET trial. CAIX expression was evaluated in paraffin-embedded tumor samples for 133 patients. They found that the degree of CAIX expression was not correlated with PFS (5.5 months vs 5.4 months, high CAIX vs low CAIX, respectively; $P = .97$) or median tumor shrinkage (-14.9% vs -12.6%, high CAIX vs low CAIX, respectively; $P = .63$) in the sorafenib treatment arm.[30] Conflicting data from another study found that among several protein biomarkers that were associated with improved outcomes on univariate analysis, only positive immunostaining of CAIX was an independent predictor of prolonged OS in patients receiving sunitinib on multivariate analysis.[31]

von Hippel-Lindau Gene Functional Status

Given its central role in the development of ccRCC, the functional status of the VHL gene has been investigated as a possible predictive biomarker for TKI therapy response (see **Table 3**). One such study compared VHL activation status via PCR with clinical response in 43 patients receiving IFN-α plus bevacizumab. They found that patients harboring VHL loss via methylation or a mutation predicted had a longer median time to progression of 13.3 months compared with 7.4 months in patients with VHL wild-type ($P = .06$).[32] In a similar study in 123 patients with mRCC receiving VEGF-targeted therapies, the patients with loss of function VHL mutations had higher response rates (52% vs 31%; $P = .04$), which was also significant in a multivariate analysis as an independent predictor of improved response to therapy. PFS and OS were not significantly different in the VHL mutated versus wild-type cohorts.[33] Tissue from a phase II pazopanib trial of 78 patients was used to analyze biomarkers for response in the VHL/HIF pathway. Aberrations in the VHL gene were identified in 70 (90%) patients via PCR, status of HIF-1α and HIF-2α were assessed via IHC, and isolated RNA was used to evaluate gene expression in a HIF-1α transcriptional signature. They found that VHL gene status was not associated with objective response or PFS. Likewise, expression levels of HIF-1α, HIF-2α, and the HIF-1α transcriptional signature did not correlate with therapeutic response or PFS.[34] Given the virtually ubiquitous presence of VHL inactivation within ccRCC, it is unclear if the observed relationships between mutation and outcomes can reliably be used as a clinically relevant tool to predict response in this setting.

SINGLE-NUCLEOTIDE POLYMORPHISM AS BIOMARKERS FOR RESPONSE

Multiple studies have been performed to identify genomic polymorphisms that are associated with patient response to VEGF-targeted therapy (**Table 4**). Germline alterations in key genes encoding proteins related to the pharmacokinetics (CYP3A5, NR1/3, and ABCB1) and pharmacodynamics (VEGFR1, VEGFR3) of sunitinib and proangiogenic pathways (FGFR2) were associated with improved outcomes after sunitinib treatment.[35,36] In patients with mRCC receiving pazopanib, three polymorphisms in IL8 and HIF-1α and five polymorphisms in HIF-1α, NR1/2, and VEGFA showed a marginally significant association with PFS and clinical response rate.[37] Another study rigorously tested 27 single-nucleotide polymorphisms (SNPs) in 13 genes from pazopanib- or sunitinib-treated patients and found that specific polymorphisms in IL-8 are associated with poorer OS compared with those with the reference allele.[38] In the phase III AXIS trial comparing axitinib versus sorafenib in the second-line setting, germline SNPs were evaluated as predictors of response to either therapy. On univariate analysis, polymorphisms in VEGF-A in the axitinib-treated cohort and VEGFR2 in the sorafenib-treated group were associated with prolonged OS (HR, 0.39 and 0.41, respectively). However, on multivariate analysis, no single SNP predicted axitinib outcomes, whereas polymorphisms in VEGFR2 predicted improved PFS ($P = .005$) and OS ($P = .003$) for sorafenib-treated patients.[39] In a validation cohort of 333 sunitinib-treated patients, two of the previously reported SNP associations maintained significance: polymorphisms in CYP3A5, which was associated with drug dose reductions ($P = .039$), and polymorphisms in the ABCB1 haplotype, which was correlated with increased PFS ($P<.001$).[40] Another SNP biomarker effort attempted to validate findings from earlier reports by retrospectively analyzing 16 SNPs in 10 genes in 88 patients with mRCC treated with sunitinib.[41] The authors confirmed significant associations between sunitinib response and SNPs in ABCB1, NR1/2, NR1/3, and VEGFR3; however, prospective studies are required to corroborate these findings.

FUTURE DIRECTIONS

Genomic profiling has become increasingly precise and broadly applicable with the advent of next-generation sequencing. Although the current literature is relatively scarce, there have been a few recent analyses that use such technology to identify a molecular biomarker of response and resistance to VEGF-targeted therapy in patients with mRCC beyond the VHL gene alone. One such study used whole exome sequencing data on 28 tumor samples from two phenotypes of response to therapy: extreme responders versus refractory

Table 4
Summary of germline biomarkers for response to VEGF-targeted therapy compared with wild-type

Biomarker Gene	SNP ID	No. of Patients	Treatment	Gene Analysis Technique	Outcome	Ref.
VEGFR-2	rs2071559	146	Sorafenib	TaqMan assay	Predicted PFS (HR, 2.22; P = .0053) and OS (HR, 2.58; P = .0027)	39
VEGFR-3	rs307826 rs307821	89	Sunitinib	KASPar SNP genotyping system	Reduced PFS (HR, 3.57; P = .0079) Reduced PFS (HR, 3.31; P = .014)	36
	rs307826 rs307821	88	Sunitinib	Sequenom MassArray platform	Reduced OS (HR, NR; P = .013) Reduced PFS (HR, NR; P = .032) and OS (HR, NR; P = .011)	41
FGFR2	rs2981582	88	Sunitinib	Sequenom MassArray platform	Reduced PFS (HR, NR; P = .031)	41
IL8	rs1126647 rs4073	397	Pazopanib	TaqMan assay	Reduced PFS (HR, 1.8; P = .009) Reduced PFS (HR, 1.7; P = .01)	37
	rs1126647	1059	Pazopanib, sunitinib	Multiple platforms	Reduced OS (HR, 1.32; P = 8.8 × 10^{-5})	38
HIF-1α	rs11549467	397	Pazopanib	TaqMan assay	Reduced PFS (HR, 1.8; P = .03)	37
NR1/2	rs2276707	88	Sunitinib	Sequenom MassArray platform	Reduced PFS (HR, NR; P = .047)	41
NR1/3	rs2307424, rs2307418, rs4073054	136	Sunitinib	TaqMan assay	Improved PFS (HR, 1.76; P = .017)	35
	rs4073054 rs2307424	88	Sunitinib	Sequenom MassArray platform	Reduced PFS (HR, NR; P = .025) and OS (HR, NR; P = .035) Reduced OS (HR, NR; P = .048)	41
CYP3A5	rs776746	136	Sunitinib	TaqMan assay	Improved PFS (HR, 0.27; P = .032)	35
ABCB1	rs1045642, rs1128503, rs2032582	136	Sunitinib	TaqMan assay	Improved PFS (HR, 0.52; P = .033)	35
	rs1128503	88	Sunitinib	Sequenom MassArray platform	Reduced PFS (HR, NR; P = .027) and OS (HR, NR; P = .025)	41
	rs1128503, rs2032582, rs1045642	333	Sunitinib	Multiple platforms	Increased PFS (HR, 1.9; P<.001)	40

patients. Specific mutations or copy number alterations were then compared with response to therapy. In this small pilot study, the authors identified that mutations in *PBRM1* were associated with extreme response to VEGF therapy on univariate analysis ($P = .03$).[42] In a larger cohort of 260 patients that received sunitinib in the RECORD-3 trial,[43] associations between somatic mutations and treatment efficacy were investigated.[44] The authors found that mutations in the *KDM5C* gene were associated with longer PFS within the sunitinib arm (median PFS, 20.6 months in mutated vs 8.4 months in wild-type group; $P = .05$). If such findings can be reproduced in additional studies, this may suggest that epigenetic modifications within the tumor affect therapeutic response to VEGF-targeted therapy. Finally, a unique study using global transcriptomic data from patients treated with sunitinib in the first-line setting identified four ccRCC molecular subtypes that were predictive for response to therapy and could potentially be used for proper selection of patients for TKI-directed treatments.[45] This area of investigation, although promising, requires further studies to identify and validate predictive genomic biomarkers.

SUMMARY

The ability to accurately predict response to VEGF-targeted therapy in patients with mRCC is of critical import. Although an extensive amount of work has been performed on this topic, to date no definitive biomarker has been identified that would guide the proper patient selection to receive TKI therapy that would allow for maximal therapeutic efficacy. A major pitfall of the available literature lies in the heterogeneous methodology of these studies. Such variability in study design, laboratory assay, and data analysis often precludes the ability to reproduce and validate results. Thus, the first step in overcoming this challenge may lie in the standardization of the approach to biomarker evaluation. Given recent advances in genomic sequencing, development of a comprehensive molecular-level assay is warranted.

REFERENCES

1. Siegel R, Ma J, Zou Z, et al. Cancer statistics, 2014. CA Cancer J Clin 2014;64:9–29.
2. Kane CJ, Mallin K, Ritchey J, et al. Renal cell cancer stage migration: analysis of the National Cancer Data Base. Cancer 2008;113:78–83.
3. Russo P, Jang TL, Pettus JA, et al. Survival rates after resection for localized kidney cancer: 1989 to 2004. Cancer 2008;113:84–96.
4. Motzer RJ, Mazumdar M, Bacik J, et al. Survival and prognostic stratification of 670 patients with advanced renal cell carcinoma. J Clin Oncol 1999;17:2530–40.
5. Tugues S, Koch S, Gualandi L, et al. Vascular endothelial growth factors and receptors: anti-angiogenic therapy in the treatment of cancer. Mol Aspects Med 2011;32:88–111.
6. Harmon CS, DePrimo SE, Figlin RA, et al. Circulating proteins as potential biomarkers of sunitinib and interferon-alpha efficacy in treatment-naive patients with metastatic renal cell carcinoma. Cancer Chemother Pharmacol 2014;73:151–61.
7. Rini BI, Michaelson MD, Rosenberg JE, et al. Antitumor activity and biomarker analysis of sunitinib in patients with bevacizumab-refractory metastatic renal cell carcinoma. J Clin Oncol 2008;26:3743–8.
8. Escudier BJ, Ravaud A, Négrier S, et al. Update on AVOREN trial in metastatic renal cell carcinoma (mRCC): efficacy and safety in subgroups of patients (pts) and pharmacokinetic (PK) analysis. American society of clinical oncology (ASCO), 44th annual meeting. Chicago, May 30–June 3, 2008.
9. Pena C, Lathia C, Shan M, et al. Biomarkers predicting outcome in patients with advanced renal cell carcinoma: results from sorafenib phase III Treatment Approaches in Renal Cancer Global Evaluation Trial. Clin Cancer Res 2010;16:4853–63.
10. Escudier B, Eisen T, Stadler WM, et al. Sorafenib for treatment of renal cell carcinoma: final efficacy and safety results of the phase III Treatment Approaches in Renal Cancer Global Evaluation Trial. J Clin Oncol 2009;27:3312–8.
11. Gruenwald V, Beutel G, Schuch-Jantsch S, et al. Circulating endothelial cells are an early predictor in renal cell carcinoma for tumor response to sunitinib. BMC Cancer 2010;10:695.
12. Deprimo SE, Bello CL, Smeraglia J, et al. Circulating protein biomarkers of pharmacodynamic activity of sunitinib in patients with metastatic renal cell carcinoma: modulation of VEGF and VEGF-related proteins. J Transl Med 2007;5:32.
13. Tran HT, Liu Y, Zurita AJ, et al. Prognostic or predictive plasma cytokines and angiogenic factors for patients treated with pazopanib for metastatic renal-cell cancer: a retrospective analysis of phase 2 and phase 3 trials. Lancet Oncol 2012;13:827–37.
14. Liu Y, Tran HT, Lin Y, et al. Circulating baseline plasma cytokines and angiogenic factors (CAF) as markers of tumor burden and therapeutic response in a phase III study of pazopanib for metastatic renal cell carcinoma (mRCC). J Clin Oncol 29. 2011;29(15)(May 20 Supplement):4553. (Amer Soc Clinical Oncology 2318 Mill Road, Ste 800, Alexandria, VA 22314 USA, 2011).
15. Zurita AJ, Jonasch E, Wang X, et al. A cytokine and angiogenic factor (CAF) analysis in plasma for selection of sorafenib therapy in patients with metastatic renal cell carcinoma. Ann Oncol 2012;23:46–52.

16. Fujita T, Iwamura M, Ishii D, et al. C-reactive protein as a prognostic marker for advanced renal cell carcinoma treated with sunitinib. Int J Urol 2012;19:908–13.

17. Yasuda Y, Saito K, Yuasa T, et al. Prognostic impact of pretreatment C-reactive protein for patients with metastatic renal cell carcinoma treated with tyrosine kinase inhibitors. Int J Clin Oncol 2013;18:884–9.

18. Beuselinck B, Vano YA, Oudard S, et al. Prognostic impact of baseline serum C-reactive protein in patients with metastatic renal cell carcinoma (RCC) treated with sunitinib. BJU Int 2014;114:81–9.

19. Keizman D, Ish-Shalom M, Huang P, et al. The association of pre-treatment neutrophil to lymphocyte ratio with response rate, progression free survival and overall survival of patients treated with sunitinib for metastatic renal cell carcinoma. Eur J Cancer 2012;48:202–8.

20. Cetin B, Berk V, Kaplan MA, et al. Is the pretreatment neutrophil to lymphocyte ratio an important prognostic parameter in patients with metastatic renal cell carcinoma? Clin Genitourin Cancer 2013;11:141–8.

21. Templeton AJ, Heng DYC, Choueiri TK, et al. Neutrophil to lymphocyte ratio (NLR) and its effect on the prognostic value of the International Metastatic Renal Cell Carcinoma Database Consortium (IMDC) model for patients treated with targeted therapy (TT). J Clin Oncol 32. 2014;(Suppl 4):abstr470. (Amer Soc Clinical Oncology 2318 Mill Road, Ste 800, Alexandria, VA 22314 USA, 2014).

22. Yamada D, Matsushita H, Azuma T, et al. Granulocyte macrophage colony-stimulating factor as a predictor of the response of metastatic renal cell carcinoma to tyrosine kinase inhibitor therapy. Mol Clin Oncol 2014;2:1023–7.

23. Motzer RJ, Hutson TE, Hudes GR, et al. Investigation of novel circulating proteins, germ line single-nucleotide polymorphisms, and molecular tumor markers as potential efficacy biomarkers of first-line sunitinib therapy for advanced renal cell carcinoma. Cancer Chemother Pharmacol 2014;74:739–50.

24. Patil S, Figlin RA, Hutson TE, et al. Prognostic factors for progression-free and overall survival with sunitinib targeted therapy and with cytokine as first-line therapy in patients with metastatic renal cell carcinoma. Ann Oncol 2011;22:295–300.

25. Terakawa T, Miyake H, Kusuda Y, et al. Expression level of vascular endothelial growth factor receptor-2 in radical nephrectomy specimens as a prognostic predictor in patients with metastatic renal cell carcinoma treated with sunitinib. Urol Oncol 2013;31:493–8.

26. Paule B, Bastien L, Deslandes E, et al. Soluble isoforms of vascular endothelial growth factor are predictors of response to sunitinib in metastatic renal cell carcinomas. PLoS One 2010;5:e10715.

27. Klatte T, Seligson DB, Riggs SB, et al. Hypoxia-inducible factor 1 alpha in clear cell renal cell carcinoma. Clin Cancer Res 2007;13:7388–93.

28. Garcia-Donas J, Seligson DB, Riggs SB, et al. Prospective study assessing hypoxia-related proteins as markers for the outcome of treatment with sunitinib in advanced clear-cell renal cell carcinoma. Ann Oncol 2013;24:2409–14.

29. Choueiri TK, Regan MM, Rosenberg JE, et al. Carbonic anhydrase IX and pathological features as predictors of outcome in patients with metastatic clear-cell renal cell carcinoma receiving vascular endothelial growth factor-targeted therapy. BJU Int 2010;106:772–8.

30. Choueiri TK, Cheng S, Qu AQ, et al. Carbonic anhydrase IX as a potential biomarker of efficacy in metastatic clear-cell renal cell carcinoma patients receiving sorafenib or placebo: analysis from the treatment approaches in renal cancer global evaluation trial (TARGET). Urol Oncol 2013;31:1788–93.

31. Dornbusch J, Zacharis A, Meinhardt M, et al. Analyses of potential predictive markers and survival data for a response to sunitinib in patients with metastatic renal cell carcinoma. PLoS One 2013;8:e76386.

32. Rini BI, Jaeger E, Weinberg V, et al. Clinical response to therapy targeted at vascular endothelial growth factor in metastatic renal cell carcinoma: impact of patient characteristics and Von Hippel-Lindau gene status. BJU Int 2006;98:756–62.

33. Choueiri TK, Vaziri SA, Jaeger E, et al. von Hippel-Lindau gene status and response to vascular endothelial growth factor targeted therapy for metastatic clear cell renal cell carcinoma. J Urol 2008;180:860–5 [discussion: 865–6].

34. Choueiri TK, Fay AP, Gagnon R, et al. The role of aberrant VHL/HIF pathway elements in predicting clinical outcome to pazopanib therapy in patients with metastatic clear-cell renal cell carcinoma. Clin Cancer Res 2013;19:5218–26.

35. van der Veldt AA, Eechoute K, Gelderblom H, et al. Genetic polymorphisms associated with a prolonged progression-free survival in patients with metastatic renal cell cancer treated with sunitinib. Clin Cancer Res 2011;17:620–9.

36. Garcia-Donas J, Esteban E, Leandro-García LJ, et al. Single nucleotide polymorphism associations with response and toxic effects in patients with advanced renal-cell carcinoma treated with first-line sunitinib: a multicentre, observational, prospective study. Lancet Oncol 2011;12:1143–50.

37. Xu CF, Bing NX, Ball HA, et al. Pazopanib efficacy in renal cell carcinoma: evidence for predictive genetic markers in angiogenesis-related and exposure-related genes. J Clin Oncol 2011;29:2557–64.

38. Xu CF, Johnson T, Garcia-Donas J, et al. IL8 polymorphisms and overall survival in pazopanib- or

sunitinib-treated patients with renal cell carcinoma. Br J Cancer 2015;112(Suppl):1190–8.

39. Escudier B, Rini BI, Motzer RJ, et al. Genotype correlations with blood pressure and efficacy from a randomized phase III trial of second-line axitinib versus sorafenib in metastatic renal cell carcinoma. Clin Genitourin Cancer 2015;13(4):328–37.e3.

40. Diekstra MH, Swen JJ, Boven E, et al. CYP3A5 and ABCB1 polymorphisms as predictors for sunitinib outcome in metastatic renal cell carcinoma. Eur Urol 2015;68(4):621–9.

41. Beuselinck B, Karadimou A, Lambrechts D, et al. Single-nucleotide polymorphisms associated with outcome in metastatic renal cell carcinoma treated with sunitinib. Br J Cancer 2013;108:887–900.

42. Fay AP, Van Allen EP, Murray B, et al. Whole-exome sequencing (WES) predicting two extreme phenotypes of response to VEGF-targeted therapies (VEGF-TT) in patients with metastatic clear cell renal cell carcinoma (mRCC). Genitourinary Cancers Symposium (ASCO GU). Orlando, FL, February 26–28, 2015.

43. Motzer RJ, Barrios CH, Kim TM, et al. Phase II randomized trial comparing sequential first-line everolimus and second-line sunitinib versus first-line sunitinib and second-line everolimus in patients with metastatic renal cell carcinoma. J Clin Oncol 2014;32(25):2765–72.

44. Hsieh JJ, Wang P, Chen YB, et al. Identification of efficacy biomarkers in a large metastatic renal cell carcinoma (mRCC) cohort through next generation sequencing (NGS): results from RECORD-3. J Clin Oncol 2015;33(Suppl 15):4509.

45. Beuselinck B, Job S, Becht E, et al. Molecular subtypes of clear cell renal cell carcinoma are associated with sunitinib response in the metastatic setting. Clin Cancer Res 2015;21(6):1329–39.

Prognostic Role of Cell Cycle and Proliferative Markers in Clear Cell Renal Cell Carcinoma

Laura-Maria Krabbe, MD[a,b], Vitaly Margulis, MD[a],
Yair Lotan, MD[a,*]

KEYWORDS

- Renal cell carcinoma • Cell cycle markers • Markers of proliferation • Prognostic marker

KEY POINTS

- Biomarkers can provide additional information to routinely assess clinicopathologic features regarding prognosis of patients with clear cell renal cell carcinoma (ccRCC).
- Of the cell cycle and proliferative biomarkers, p53 and Ki-67 are the most studied markers and provide independent prognostic information in patients with ccRCC.
- Marker combinations of one or multiple pathways are thought to be superior to single markers due to complexity of carcinogenesis.
- Because of a lack of proper validation, no cell cycle or proliferative biomarkers are currently used in routine care to guide treatment decisions.

INTRODUCTION

Clear cell renal cell carcinoma (ccRCC) is the most common malignancy of the kidneys and comprises most of the estimated 61,560 cases of renal malignancies and 14,080 deaths in the United States in 2015.[1] With increased availability of cross-sectional imaging, more renal masses are found incidentally before the appearance of systemic symptoms.[2] The proportionate increase of small renal masses is tremendous from about 3% to 17% in the 1970s to up to 48% to 66% in current studies.[3] Although around 20% to 30% of patients with ccRCC are initially metastatic, 20% to 40% of patients will relapse after initial curatively intended surgery.[4] Unfortunately, patients who relapse often require systemic therapy and have a poor prognosis.[5]

Improved prognostic classification apart from conventional TNM staging could provide a substantial increase in information, potentially with therapeutic implications. First, a personalized surveillance protocol could be established for each patient based on their risk, such that relapses could be detected early, making salvage metastasectomy a treatment possibility to provide long-term cure. Second, improved risk stratification may be important in design of trials using adjuvant therapies for patients with advanced disease. Furthermore, tissue biomarkers can be useful to select systemic therapies in patients with advanced disease in the presurgical setting to predict response to therapy more accurately. After assessment of biomarker profiles through biopsies, treatment choices might be made in these patients with information from biomarkers in

Disclosure Statement: The authors have nothing to disclose.
a Department of Urology, UT Southwestern Medical Center at Dallas, 5323 Harry Hines Boulevard, Dallas, TX 75390-9110, USA; b Department of Urology, University of Muenster Medical Center, Albert-Schweitzer Campus 1, GB A1, Muenster D-48149, Germany
* Corresponding author.
E-mail address: Yair.Lotan@UTSouthwestern.edu

Urol Clin N Am 43 (2016) 105–118
http://dx.doi.org/10.1016/j.ucl.2015.08.010

addition to conventional histology. Last, with new targets like the recently introduced CTLA-4, PD-1, and PD-L1 inhibitors, a whole new class of drugs is available for which biomarkers are very important, and still missing, to distinguish possible responders from nonresponders as early as possible, preferably in advance. Therefore, prognostic as well as predictive biomarkers are urgently needed for patients with ccRCC.

CELL CYCLE AND CELL PROLIFERATION

The cell cycle is one of the most important regulatory mechanisms of the human body because it controls rate of cell division and proliferation. The cell cycle is subdivided into different phases (G1, S, G2, and G0), which have to be completed in a certain order before cell division is completed. Control mechanisms are found in protein complexes consisting of cyclins and cyclin-dependent kinases. These complexes control orderly progression through the cell cycle. Progression of the cell cycle is achieved by phosphorylation of key components and subsequent release of inhibition at certain checkpoints. These processes are completed thousands of times each day in a human body. Loss of cell cycle regulation is thought to be the first step in carcinogenesis and an important contributor to tumor invasion as well as development of metastases.[6]

The current article focuses on the prognostic role of cell cycle and proliferative markers in patients with ccRCC.

PROGNOSTIC VALUE OF CELL CYCLE AND PROLIFERATIVE MARKERS
p53 and TP53

p53 is one of the major regulatory proteins in cell division and is often called the guardian of the cell cycle. It acts as a tumor suppressor by inhibition of cell cycle progression and induction of apoptosis in cells that suffer DNA damage.[7] Dysfunctional p53 leads to loss of control of cell division and lack of apoptotic signals in affected cells.[8] Mutations of TP53, the gene coding for p53, leads to extended half-life of p53 and accumulation of the protein in the nucleus, making it detectable by immunohistochemistry. However, immunohistochemistry is not able to differentiate wild-type p53 versus mutant p53. TP53 mutations are among the most frequent in human cancers, found in up to 50% of cases.[9] The importance of the tumor-suppressive properties of p53 and the impact of p53 mutations becomes apparent when looking at the frequency of cancers in patients with germline mutations of p53 as in patients

with Li-Fraumeni syndrome, who develop a diverse set of malignancies, including breast carcinomas, sarcomas, and brain tumors.[10]

In ccRCC, many investigators have evaluated the role of p53 for individual tumor characteristics as well as the prognosis for oncologic outcomes. However, for the interpretation of results, it is important to consider possible pitfalls. First, the issue of cutoffs used and its implication on rate of expression must be discussed. Another issue to consider is the method of detection of p53. Most of the studies used immunohistochemistry for p53 evaluation, which harbors a large possibility for variable results. Depending on antibody (mostly DO-7) and cutoff of positivity (>1% to >20%) used in the different trials, results may differ significantly. As there are no regulations of cutoffs for p53 staining, the available studies are not always comparable. Also, validation studies are currently missing because suggested cutoffs were often developed in the datasets themselves. Nonetheless, there are still patterns that emerge regarding the significance of p53 in renal cell carcinoma.

Studies comparing primary and metastatic tumor sites found that p53 overexpression is seen more often in metastatic tissue (50%–85%) than in primary tumors (20%–35%), suggesting accumulation of mutations and dysregulation promoting aggressiveness along the course of disease.[11–13] Overall, p53 overexpression seems to be lower in ccRCC (11.9%) in comparison to other histologic subtypes (27%–70%).[12] However, it is important to emphasize that the altered expression rate is directly affected by the cutoff used to define alterations. The average range of p53 overexpression is suggested to be between 10% and 40% (**Table 1**).[12,14] Also, p53 accumulation is heterogeneous across tumor sections, further complicating interpretation.[15]

Interestingly, in multiple studies, p53 overexpression was not associated with TNM stage or grade, suggesting that as a marker it may provide information that is independent from conventionally acquired pathologic information.[12,16]

Many studies have assessed the prognostic value of p53 on oncologic outcomes.[11,12,15–48] Most recent and often better designed studies found an independent prognostic value of p53 regarding different survival outcomes (recurrence-free survival, disease-specific survival, and overall survival) (see **Table 1**).[11,12,15,16,19,21,24,27–30,32–35,37–40,42,46,47] However, some earlier and usually smaller studies did not find a correlation between p53 immunoreactivity and outcomes, which might be due to lack of statistical power to detect a

Table 1
Studies investigating the prognostic value of p53 in renal cell carcinoma

Study	No. of RCC (% ccRCC)	Cutoff for Alteration, %	Alteration Rate, %	Prognostic Value in UVA	Prognostic Value in MVA	Endpoint with Prognostic Value
Weber et al,[46] 2014	145 (100)	—[a]	—	✓	✗	↓[b] DSS
Weber et al,[45] 2013	132 (100)	>15	50.8	✗	✗	—
Noon et al,[44] 2012	97 (90)	>10	15.6	✗	✗	—
Baytekin et al,[43] 2011	104 (63.5)	>10	13.5	✗	✗	—
Dahinden et al,[48] 2010	527 (100)	NR	NR	✗	✗	—
Zubac et al,[42] 2009	160 (100)	>10	53	✓	✓	↓ DSS
Sakai et al,[41] 2009	153 (86.3)	>20	33.3	✗	✗	—
Klatte et al,[40] 2009	170 (100)	Any positive	NR	✓	✓	↓ RFS
Perret et al,[39] 2008	50 (0)	>20	48	✓	✗	↓ OS
Phuoc et al,[38] 2007	119 (100)	>10	54	✓	✓	↓ DSS
Kankuri et al,[37] 2006	117 (86)	>10	12.8	✓	✗	↓[b] DSS
Kramer et al,[36] 2005	117 (89)	>5	13.6	✗	✗	—
Cho et al,[35] 2005	92 (100)	>10	12	✓	✓	↓ DSS
Shvarts et al,[16] 2005	193 (85)	>20	7.3	✓	✓	↓ RFS
Uzunlar et al,[34] 2005	57 (77.1)	>1	35	✓	✗	↓ DSS
Zigeuner et al,[12] 2004	184 (70.7)	>1	22.8	✓	✓	↓ RFS
Kim et al,[33] 2004	318 (100)	>15	NR	✓	✓	↓ DSS
Uchida et al,[32] 2002	112 (78)	>1	13.4	✓	✓	↓ OS
Olumi et al,[31] 2001	48 (100)	>10	51	✗	✗	—
Ljungberg et al,[30] 2001	99 (74)	>5	19	✓	✗	↓[c] DFS
Girgin et al,[29] 2001	50 (62)	>20	20	✓	✗	↓ DFS
Haitel et al,[47] 2001	104 (100)	>5	NR	✓	✗	↓ DFS
Haitel et al,[28] 2000	97 (100)	>5	36	✓	✗	↓ DFS
Rioux-Leclercq et al,[27] 2000	66 (NR)	>20	17	✓	✗	↓ DFS
Sejima et al,[26] 1999	53 (NR)	NR	2	✗	✗	—
Vasavada et al,[25] 1998	39 (71)	>1	0	✗	✗	—
Sinik et al,[24] 1997	39 (100)	>10	17.9	✓	✗	↓ OS
Papadopoulos et al,[23] 1997	90 (NR)	Any positive	33	✗	✗	—
Gelb et al,[22] 1997	52 (100)	>5	2	✗	✗	—
Shiina et al,[15] 1997	72 (NR)	>10	40.3	✓	✓	↓ OS
Moch et al,[21] 1997	50 (100)	NR	16	✓	✓	↓ OS
Hofmockel et al,[20] 1996	31 (NR)	>1	16	✗	✗	—
Lipponen et al,[19] 1994	123 (NR)	Any positive	33	✓	✗	↑ RFS
Kamel et al,[18] 1994	56 (NR)	>1	11	✗	✗	—
Bot et al,[17] 1994	100 (74)	>50	32	✗	✗	—
Uhlman et al,[11] 1994	175 (NR)	>1	28	✓	✓	↓ DFS

—, not applicable; MVA, multivariate; NR, not reported; UVA, univariate; ✓, yes; ✗, no; ↑, increased survival; ↓, decreased survival.
[a] Analyzed as continuous variable.
[b] In patients with metastases/advanced disease.
[c] For non-ccRCC.

difference, due to cutoff or assay used, as well as a possible true nonsignificant effect.[17,18,20,22,23,25,26,31,36,41,43–45,48] Further explanations might be the inclusion of nonclear histology, leading to high heterogeneity and nonspecific results. For correct data interpretation, it is also important to consider publication bias in this scenario because studies without significant results are probably not published as frequently as their positive counterparts. An overview of the published results regarding p53 expression and its impact on oncologic outcomes is provided in **Table 1**.

Mutational analyses of p53 are another important avenue for evaluating p53 as a marker for ccRCC. A limitation of Immunohistochemistry is that it provides no information about wild-type or mutated protein status, and although immunohistochemical expression is often used as a surrogate for p53 mutational status, this is not entirely similar information.[49] The frequency of p53 mutations is described between 0% and 44% overall.[50–52] In most studies, single-strand conformation polymorphisms were evaluated and contained mostly the core domain between exon 4 and 8 or 5 and 8 because this is the most common site of p53 mutation.[53] Still, up to 15% of p53 mutations occur outside of the core domain and suggest underestimation of mutational status in some studies.[54] With the large differences in mutational status and protein expression, mutational analysis has not proven its utility for prognostication of outcomes yet.

It should also be noted as in later discussion that many analyses use more than one marker in combination. Many of these analyses include p53 as a key marker associated with cell cycle.

p21

p21 or cyclin-dependent kinase inhibitor 1 prevents cyclin-dependent kinases from phosphorylation of protein substrates and acts downstream of p53 regulation where it is activated by wild-type but not mutant p53.[47,55] Therefore, p21 mainly acts as a tumor suppressor by blockage of cell proliferation as well as promotion of apoptosis, and loss of p21 can lead to uncontrolled cell growth. However, it seems that p21 can act as an inhibitor of the cell cycle as well as a growth permissive and harbors proapoptotic and anti-apoptotic properties, which are p53 dependent as well as p53 independent.[56] Mutations in the gene locus of p21 are thought to be rare in renal cell carcinoma (RCC).[57]

The cutoff for normal p21 expression assessed via immunohistochemistry was suggested to be greater than 30%. In one study assessing different histologic subtypes, it was also shown that positive nuclear and cytosolic staining for p21 was lower (median expression of 20% in nuclear assays) to minimal (median 0% in cytosolic assays) in ccRCC in comparison to other tumor subtypes.[58] Interestingly, when comparing primary and metastatic tumor tissue, nuclear expression of p21 was higher and cytosolic expression was lower in the metastatic tissue.[58] p21 expression was not associated with grade or stage when evaluated for this endpoint.[59] Furthermore, high levels of p21 indicated poor prognosis in patients with metastatic disease, indicating mechanisms of therapy resistance associated with this status.[58,60] p21 protein expression with regard to prognosis was evaluated in multiple studies, and according to its function in the cell cycle, patients with high and therefore intact levels of p21 demonstrated favorable disease-specific survival in some larger studies and was an independent predictor of this endpoint in patients with organ-confined disease as well.[45,46,58] However, in previous and usually smaller studies, this association could not always be demonstrated.[40,47,48,59] An overview of the published results regarding p21 expression and its impact on oncologic outcomes is provided in **Table 2**.

p27

Another cyclin-dependent kinase inhibitor is p27. p27 inhibits cyclin-dependent kinase 2 and leads to cell cycle arrest in the G1 phase.[61] Therefore, similar to p21 to which it is structurally related, loss of p27 leads to uncontrolled cell cycle progression and cell division as well as tumor growth.[47] However, transcription of the p27 gene is not controlled by p53 as it is in p21.[47]

Depending on the cutoff used, p27 is detectable in around 60% of ccRCCs via immunohistochemistry.[62] Loss of p27 was seen in tumors with higher Fuhrman grade, larger tumor size, and higher TNM status.[62,63] Conversely, nuclear expression levels of p27 were lowest in benign tissue, higher in primary ccRCC tissue, and highest in metastatic ccRCC tissue, which seems contradictory to the known mechanism of action of p27.[62,63] However, other study groups as well found higher levels of nuclear p27 in tumor tissue than in, for example, oncocytomas, chromophobe, or benign tissue, whereas papillary RCC demonstrated slightly higher expression rates.[62,64] Most studies, however, found low nuclear expression of p27 to be associated with unfavorable oncologic outcomes.[47,48,62,65–71] Still, in some studies, no correlation of p27 expression with oncologic outcomes

Table 2
Studies investigating the prognostic value of p21 in renal cell carcinoma

Study	No. of RCC (% ccRCC)	Cutoff for Alteration, %	Alteration Rate, %	Prognostic Value in UVA	Prognostic Value in MVA	Endpoint with Prognostic Value
Weber et al,[46] 2014	145 (100)	<32.5	63	✔	✔	↓ DSS
Weber et al,[45] 2013	132 (100)	<32.5	36.6	✔	✔	↓ DSS
Dahinden et al,[48] 2010	527 (100)	NR	NR	✗	✗	—
Klatte et al,[40] 2009	170 (100)	NR	NR	✗	✗	—
Weiss et al,[58] 2007	366 (93.4)	<32.5[a]	NR	✔	✔	↓ DSS
Haitel et al,[47] 2001	104 (100)	<10	42.3	✗	✗	—
Aaltomaa et al,[59] 1999	118 (NR)	NR	NR	✗	✗	—

—, not applicable; MVA, multivariate; NR, not reported; UVA, univariate; ✔, yes; ✗, no; ↓, decreased survival.
[a] For nonmetastatic patients.

was found.[40,72] No found correlation may be partly attributed to heterogeneity in p27 expression in tumor tissue because one study found that low p27 expression at the border of invasion held prognostic significance for survival endpoints, while it did not when measured within the primary tumor.[73]

These studies, however, focused on the nuclear staining of p27. One group recently focused on the importance of cytoplasmic expression of p27.[74] The investigators found that high cytoplasmic staining for p27 was associated with unfavorable cancer-specific survival.[74] However, the importance of this finding is not clear yet because the investigators defined high cytoplasmic expression as a higher expression in tumor tissue than matched benign tissue from other parts of the kidney and low expression as similar or lower expression of cytoplasmic p27 in tumor tissue than in benign tissue. It is unclear how the relation of p27 expression in benign and tumor tissue has to be in order to have a significant impact on prognosis.

An overview of the published results regarding p27 expression and its impact on oncologic outcomes is provided in **Table 3**.

Cyclin A

The cyclins are located downstream in the p53 pathway and cell cycle and are mainly responsible for further phosphorylation of target proteins to promote progression in the cell cycle.[75] Cyclin A, among others, is responsible for phosphorylation of pRB and is mostly present in late S and G2 phase and is degraded before the M phase.[75] It can be visualized by immunohistochemistry and can be found in the cell nucleus and also the cytoplasm.[59] Intensity in tumor tissue seems to be relatively low (mean staining 1.08%).[69] High levels of cyclin A (cutoff of >1%) have been associated with higher nuclear grade and tumor volume in RCC.[59] Furthermore, it is associated with disease-free and overall survival in patients with nonmetastatic as well as metastatic RCC.[59] An overview of the published results regarding cyclin A expression and its impact on oncologic outcomes is provided in **Table 4**.

Cyclin B

Cyclin B is a cyclin of the late cell cycle and promotes progression through the G2 and M phase. So far, exploration of the prognostic importance of cyclin B has been very sparse. Cyclin B positivity in immunohistochemical staining was defined at a cutoff of greater than 10% and staining occurred almost exclusively in the cytoplasm.[76] In one study, 70% of primary tumors showed cyclin B positivity as compared with 30% in the invasion front of the primary tumor and 60% of normal kidney tissue.[76] In this study, cytoplasmic cyclin B expression was associated with adverse pathologic characteristics, whereas nuclear expression was not. Regarding survival outcomes, patients with high expression levels of cyclin B in the tumor and low expression levels in benign parenchyma seemed to be at higher risk of cancer-specific death; however, this was not confirmed by multivariate analysis.[76] An overview of the published results regarding cyclin B expression and its impact on oncologic outcomes is provided in **Table 5**.

Cyclin D

Cyclin D is responsible, when activated, to phosphorylate pRB to allow initiation of transcription,

Table 3
Studies investigating the prognostic value of p27 in renal cell carcinoma

Study	No. of RCC (% ccRCC)	Cutoff for Alteration, %	Alteration Rate, %	Prognostic Value in UVA	Prognostic Value in MVA	Endpoint with Prognostic Value
Kruck et al,[74] 2012	140 (100)	Greater than corresponding benign tissue[b]	24.3	✔	✔	↓ DSS[b]
Sgambato et al,[65] 2010	125 (80)	<20	45.5	✔	✔	↓ RFS, ↓ OS
Dahinden et al,[48] 2010	527 (100)	NR	NR	✔	✗	↓ OS
Klatte et al,[40] 2009	170 (100)	NR	NR	✗	✗	—
Liu et al,[66] 2008	482 (87.9)	<40	82.2	✔	✔	↓ RFS, ↓ DSS
Pertia et al,[67] 2009	52 (100)	No staining	30.8	✔	✔	↓ RFS, ↓ DSS
Merseburger et al,[73] 2007	251 (NR)	<5	46.2[a]	✔	✔	↓ DSS[a]
Pertia et al,[71] 2007	52 (100)	No staining	30.8	✔	✔	↓ RFS, ↓ DSS
Langner et al,[62] 2004	171 (75.4)	<50	64	✔	✔	↓ RFS
Hedberg et al,[70] 2003	218 (80.3)	<5 cells/core	24.8	✔	✔	↓ DSS
Anastasiadis et al,[72] 2003	154 (NR)	NR	NR	✗	✗	—
Hedberg et al,[68] 2002	79 (83.5)	<60	29	✔	✗	↓ DSS
Migita et al,[69] 2002	67 (100)	<50	31.3	✔	✔	↓ DSS
Haitel et al,[47] 2001	104 (100)	<70	75	✔	✔	↓ RFS

—, not applicable; MVA, multivariate; NR, not reported; UVA, univariate; ✔, yes; ✗, no; ↓, decreased survival.
[a] In the invasion front tissue.
[b] Cytoplasmic staining.

progression from G1 to S phase, and finally, DNA replication.[77] Cyclin D can be detected via immunohistochemistry. Positive immunoreactivity for cyclin D is seen in about 50% to 75% of ccRCC and oncocytomas but less often in papillary or chromophobe RCC and benign renal tissue.[78,79] However, genetic alterations of the gene locus of cyclin D are rare.[78]

Table 4
Studies investigating the prognostic value of cyclin A in renal cell carcinoma

Study	No. of RCC (% ccRCC)	Cutoff for Alteration, %	Alteration Rate, %	Prognostic Value in UVA	Prognostic Value in MVA	Endpoint with Prognostic Value
Aaltomaa et al,[59] 1999	118 (NR)	<1	NR	✔	✔	↓ RFS, ↓ OS
Migita et al,[69] 2002	67 (100)	>1	70.1	✗	✗	—

—, not applicable; MVA, multivariate; NR, not reported; UVA, univariate; ✔, yes; ✗, no; ↓, decreased survival.

Table 5
Studies investigating the prognostic value of cyclin B in renal cell carcinoma

Study	No. of RCC (% ccRCC)	Cutoff for Alteration, %	Alteration Rate, %	Prognostic Value in UVA	Prognostic Value in MVA	Endpoint with Prognostic Value
Ikuerowo et al,[76] 2006	251 (92)	>10	84	✔	✗	↓ OS

MVA, multivariate; NR, not reported; UVA, univariate; ✔. yes; ✗, no; ↓, decreased survival.

Multiple studies did not show a significant association of cyclin D with oncologic outcomes.[38,59,69] However, in further studies, low nuclear cyclin D expression (<5 positive cells per tissue core) was associated with higher tumor grade as well as larger tumor size in patients with ccRCC.[70] Kaplan-Meier survival analyses suggested lower survival of these patients as well; however, that could not be reproduced in multivariate analyses.[70] Similar results were found recently in a thorough analysis of cyclin D expression.[77] Here, a cutoff of less than 30% was used and it was found that low cyclin D expression was associated with adverse pathologic features and unfavorable survival in univariate but not in multivariate analyses.[77] In an early study, using a cutoff of less than 12%, low cyclin D expression was associated with worse disease-specific survival in univariate and multivariate analysis.[79] Therefore, the prognostic role of cyclin D is not completely resolved yet; however, to date, there are only a few established implications on survival endpoints. An overview of the published results regarding cyclin D expression and its impact on oncologic outcomes is provided in **Table 6**.

Cyclin E

Another member of the cyclin family is cyclin E. As with other cyclins, it is detectable via immunohistochemistry. More than 60% of tumor tissue show higher cyclin E expression than benign renal tissue, and positive nuclear staining is found in more than 30% of cases.[68] However, other histologic subtypes seem to express higher levels of cyclin E than ccRCC.[70] High expression of cyclin E has been linked to adverse clinicopathologic criteria; however, a demonstration of impact on prognosis has not been established yet, which might have been an issue of sample size or study goals.[68,80] An overview of the published results regarding cyclin E expression and its impact on oncologic outcomes is provided in **Table 7**.

Table 6
Studies investigating the prognostic value of cyclin D in renal cell carcinoma

Study	No. of RCC (% ccRCC)	Cutoff for Alteration, %	Alteration Rate, %	Prognostic Value in UVA	Prognostic Value in MVA	Endpoint with Prognostic Value
Lima et al,[77] 2014	109 (71.6)	<30	47.7	✔	✗	↓ DFS/OS[a]
Phuoc et al,[38] 2007	119 (100)	<10	36	✔	✗	↓ DSS
Hedberg et al,[70] 2003	218 (80.3)	<5 cells/core	54.6	✔	✗	↓ DSS
Migita et al,[69] 2002	67 (100)	<10	88.0	✗	✗	—
Aaltomaa et al,[59] 1999	118 (NR)	NR	NR	✗	✗	—
Hedberg et al,[79] 1999	80 (82.5)	<12	25	✔	✔	↓ DSS

—, not applicable; MVA, multivariate; NR, not reported; UVA, univariate; ✔, yes; ✗, no; ↓, decreased survival.
[a] Combined endpoint.

Table 7
Studies investigating the prognostic value of cyclin E in renal cell carcinoma

Study	No. of RCC (% ccRCC)	Cutoff for Alteration, %	Alteration Rate, %	Prognostic Value in UVA	Prognostic Value in MVA	Endpoint with Prognostic Value
Hedberg et al,[70] 2003	218 (80.3)	5 cells/core	65.6	✗	✗	—
Hedberg et al,[68] 2002	65 (100)	<1.16	50.7	✗	✗	—

—, not applicable; MVA, multivariate; UVA, univariate; ✗, no.

pRB and RB1

Retinoblastoma gene 1 (RB1) and its protein pRB are also involved in regulatory processes of the cell cycle and are located downstream of p53 and the cyclins. Unphosphorylated pRB acts with inhibitory properties on transcription factors, therefore pausing progression of the cell cycle.[47] After phosphorylation of pRB, cell cycle progression from G1 to S phase is promoted. Although mutations in RB1 are rare and found in less than 2% of cancer cell lines, alterations in pRB protein expression is thought to have an impact on ccRCC biology.[81]

In immunohistochemical assays, pRB is found in most RCCs (up to 95%), confirming that inactivation due to mutation of pRB is rare.[82,83] Overexpression of pRB in the phosphorylated state induces tumor growth and promotes invasion and metastases. The phosphorylated state of pRB is found in up to 50% of RCCs.[82] The cutoff suggested for pRB overexpression is 20% for immunohistochemical assays.[47] It was found to be an independent predictor of progression-free survival as well as other oncologic outcomes.[47] An overview of the published results regarding pRB expression and its impact on oncologic outcomes is provided in **Table 8**.

Overall, the data regarding pRB are sparse. This lack of data might be due to the low frequency of dysregulations in the RB gene product and the high frequency of pRB expression, suggesting that these markers are not good discriminators between different outcomes due to rarity of positive cases.

Ki-67

Ki-67 is a marker of cell proliferation and has been evaluated in almost all malignancies including RCC.[84] The nuclear antigen is present in virtually all phases of the cell cycle, G1, S, G2, and M phase, of all human cells participating in cell division.[85] Although it is detectable via immunohistochemistry as well, the adoption of the MIB1 antibody has increased the applicability of this assay as it can be performed in paraffin-embedded material.[86]

There is no consensus about the best cutoff of this marker to date. Different studies used cutoffs between greater than 10% and greater than 20%, whereas others quantified positivity as staining of greater than 50 tumor cells/mm[3].[27,40,84,86–89] With regard to the different cutoffs as well as to the different cohorts studied, Ki-67 positivity ranges between 6.5% and 73% of patients.[27,87,88] Although more advanced tumors show higher rates of Ki-67 overexpression, more recent cohorts with many low-stage tumors may report lower alteration rates than seen previously in studies that included many advanced tumor stages.[87]

Table 8
Studies investigating the prognostic value of pRB in renal cell carcinoma

Study	No. of RCC (% ccRCC)	Cutoff for Alteration, %	Alteration Rate, %	Prognostic Value in UVA	Prognostic Value in MVA	Endpoint with Prognostic Value
Haitel et al,[47] 2001	104 (100)	>20	20.1	✔	✔	↓ RFS

MVA, multivariate; UVA, univariate; ✔, yes; ↓, decreased survival.

Table 9
Studies investigating the prognostic value of Ki-67 in renal cell carcinoma

Study	No. of RCC (% ccRCC)	Cutoff for Alteration, %	Alteration Rate, %	Prognostic Value in UVA	Prognostic Value in MVA	Endpoint with Prognostic Value
Weber et al,[46] 2014	145 (100)	—[a]	—	✔	✗	↓ DSS
Teng et al,[94] 2014	378 (NR)	NR	NR	✔	✔	↓ RFS, DSS
Abel et al,[93] 2014	216 (72.2)	>1	NR	✔	✔	↓ RFS
Gayed et al,[87] 2014	452 (100)	>10	6.5	✔	✔	↓ DSS
Weber et al,[45] 2013	132 (100)	>10	6.1	✔	✔	↓ DSS
Zubac et al,[42] 2009	160 (100)	>10	66.3	✔	✔	↓ DSS
Sakai et al,[41] 2009	153 (86.3)	>5	57.5	✔	✔	↓ RFS
Klatte et al,[40] 2009	170 (100)	NR	NR	✔	✔	↓ DSS
Tollefson et al,[88] 2007	741 (100)	>50 cells/mm^2	37.9	✔	✔	↓ DSS
Phuoc et al,[38] 2007	119 (100)	>10	56	✔	✗	↓ DSS
Kankuri et al,[37] 2006	117 (86)	>10	21	✔	✗	↓[b] DSS
Kramer et al,[36] 2005	117 (89)	>10	44.4	✗	✗	—
Dudderidge et al,[86] 2005	176 (66.4)	>12	NR	✔	✔	↓ RFS
Kallio et al,[103] 2004	138 (NR)	—[a]	NR	✔	✗	↓ DSS
Lehmann et al,[102] 2004	48 (NR)	>7	NR	✔	✔	↓ RFS, DSS
Yildiz et al,[89] 2004	48 (100)	>15	NR	✔	✔	↓ DSS
Bui et al,[92] 2004	224 (100)	NR	NR	✔	✔	↓ OS
Visapää et al,[84] 2003	257 (100)	Any staining	65	✔	✔	↓ DSS
Migita et al,[69] 2002	67 (100)	>1	NR	✗	✗	—
Cheville et al,[104] 2002	80 (100)	>5	NR	✔	✗	↓ DSS
Yuba et al,[101] 2001	52 (NR)	>5.6	21.2	✔	✗	↓ DSS
Rioux-Leclercq et al,[100] 2001	73 (NR)	>20	NR	✔	✔	↓ DSS
Rioux-Leclercq et al,[27] 2000	66 (NR)	>20	34.8	✔	✔	↓ OS
Aaltomaa et al,[59] 1999	118 (NR)	NR	NR	✔	✔	↓ OS
Gelb et al,[22] 1997	52 (100)	NR	NR	✗	✗	—
Haitel et al,[99] 1997	107 (NR)	NR	NR	✔	—	↓ RFS
Aaltomaa et al,[98] 1997	111 (NR)	NR	NR	✔	✔	↓ DFS/OS
Jochum et al,[97] 1996	58 (NR)	NR	65.5	✔	✔	↓ OS
Tannapfel et al,[91] 1996	87 (NR)	NR	NR	✔	✔	↓ OS
Hofmockel et al,[20] 1995	41 (NR)	NR	NR	✔	✔	↓ RFS/DSS
Delahunt et al,[96] 1995	206 (NR)	>6	NR	✔	✔	↓ DSS
De Riese et al,[90] 1993	58 (NR)	>9	37.9	✔	✔	↓ RFS

—, not applicable; MVA, multivariate; NR, not reported; UVA, univariate; ✔, yes; ✗, no; ↓, decreased survival.
[a] Analyzed as continuous variable.
[b] In patients with metastases/advanced disease.

High tumor proliferation as indicated by increased expression of Ki-67 has been associated with adverse pathologic features like higher Fuhrman grade, high TNM stage, tumor size, presence of sarcomatoid features, lymphovascular invasion, and tumor necrosis.[20,27,37,87,88,90–92] Furthermore, it has been found to be an independent predictor of recurrence-free and cancer-specific survival in ccRCC, especially for nonmetastatic patients.[20,27,37,38,40–42,45,46,59,84,86–103] This finding is true also for the populations of low-stage (pT1) tumors in which recurrence is uncommon.[104] Furthermore, it significantly increased the accuracy of prognostic models.[20,40] Only few and generally small studies found no association of Ki-67 expression and survival outcomes.[22,36,69] An overview of the published results regarding Ki-67 expression and its impact on oncologic outcomes is provided in **Table 9**.

MARKER COMBINATIONS

One of the issues with many studies is the fact that they focus on independent prediction of outcomes but do not evaluate the improvement in prediction accuracy garnered by use of these markers. Although any one marker has minimal improvement in prediction, the use of multiple markers in combination has the potential to enhance prediction more significantly.

Multiple study groups have evaluated the prognostic significance of combined marker panels, including markers from single or multiple pathways. This approach is promising because it is highly unlikely that in a complex process as carcinogenesis and tumor invasion, a single mechanism is responsible for the whole effect. Marker panels containing cell cycle and proliferative markers in combination with other markers found increased prognostic value in prognostication of recurrence-free, disease-specific, and overall survival with a significant increase of prognostic accuracy from around 0.65 for grade, 0.73 for TNM stage, and 0.76 for University of California Los Angeles integrated staging system to up to 0.84.[33,40,45,92,95,105] One group presented a Bio-Score, incorporating clinicopathologic factors with Ki-67, surviving, as well as B7-H1 and mentioned that this score might be updated as further prognosticators are identified.[105] Another study described a nomogram combining clinical, pathologic, and molecular biomarkers that reached prognostic accuracy of 0.9 for disease-free survival.[40]

One group has focused on the thorough investigation of solely cell cycle and proliferative markers and their impact on prognosis in patients with ccRCC.[14] This investigation was done under the rationale that this might enhance the understanding of the pathway's functional status. In this study, immunohistochemical staining was done for 8 markers (cyclin D, cyclin E, p16, p21, p27, p53, p57, and Ki-67) on tissue microarray of a total of 452 patients with ccRCC. The group suggested a prognostic marker score with 0 to 4 versus greater than 4 of 8 altered markers.[14] An unfavorable marker score was found in 12.2% of patients. On univariate analysis, an unfavorable marker score was associated with significantly worse outcomes for disease-free and cancer-specific survival.[14] On multivariate analysis, the marker score was only prognostic for disease-specific, but not cancer-specific survival, which might be explained by a limited time of follow-up (median follow-up 24 months).

SUMMARY

Many studies regarding the prognostic impact of molecular markers of the cell cycle have been conducted to date. However, none of these markers are recommended for routine clinical use in the guidelines yet; this is mostly due to the high variability in design and interpretation of these marker studies and lack of prospective validation. Furthermore, no single marker has shown the ability to provide substantial independent increase in information, and the optimal marker combination has not been found yet. It would be very desirable if future marker studies would be carried out prospectively with adequately defined patient populations and appropriately powered endpoints. Molecular markers have the potential to improve risk stratification, identify patients appropriate for adjuvant trials, and provide targets for therapies.

REFERENCES

1. Siegel RL, Miller KD, Jemal A. Cancer statistics, 2015. CA Cancer J Clin 2015;65(1):5–29.
2. Gill IS, Aron M, Gervais DA, et al. Clinical practice. Small renal mass. N Engl J Med 2010;362:624–34.
3. Volpe A, Panzarella T, Rendon RA, et al. The natural history of incidentally detected small renal masses. Cancer 2004;100:738–45.
4. Lam JS, Shvarts O, Leppert JT, et al. Renal cell carcinoma 2005: new frontiers in staging, prognostication and targeted molecular therapy. J Urol 2005; 173:1853–62.
5. Gupta K, Miller JD, Li JZ, et al. Epidemiologic and socioeconomic burden of metastatic renal cell carcinoma (mRCC): a literature review. Cancer Treat Rev 2008;34:193–205.

6. Cordon-Cardo C. Mutations of cell cycle regulators. Biological and clinical implications for human neoplasia. Am J Pathol 1995;147:545–60.
7. Lane DP. Cancer. p53, guardian of the genome. Nature 1992;358:15–6.
8. Tannapfel A, Hahn HA, Katalinic A, et al. Incidence of apoptosis, cell proliferation and P53 expression in renal cell carcinomas. Anticancer Res 1997;17:1155–62.
9. Hollstein M, Rice K, Greenblatt MS, et al. Database of p53 gene somatic mutations in human tumors and cell lines. Nucleic Acids Res 1994;22:3551–5.
10. Malkin D, Li FP, Strong LC, et al. Germ line p53 mutations in a familial syndrome of breast cancer, sarcomas, and other neoplasms. Science 1990;250:1233–8.
11. Uhlman DL, Nguyen PL, Manivel JC, et al. Association of immunohistochemical staining for p53 with metastatic progression and poor survival in patients with renal cell carcinoma. J Natl Cancer Inst 1994;86:1470–5.
12. Zigeuner R, Ratschek M, Rehak P, et al. Value of p53 as a prognostic marker in histologic subtypes of renal cell carcinoma: a systematic analysis of primary and metastatic tumor tissue. Urology 2004;63:651–5.
13. Laird A, O'Mahony FC, Nanda J, et al. Differential expression of prognostic proteomic markers in primary tumour, venous tumour thrombus and metastatic renal cell cancer tissue and correlation with patient outcome. PLoS One 2013;8:e60483.
14. Gayed BA, Youssef RF, Bagrodia A, et al. Prognostic role of cell cycle and proliferative biomarkers in patients with clear cell renal cell carcinoma. J Urol 2013;190:1662–7.
15. Shiina H, Igawa M, Urakami S, et al. Clinical significance of immunohistochemically detectable p53 protein in renal cell carcinoma. Eur Urol 1997;31:73–80.
16. Shvarts O, Seligson D, Lam J, et al. p53 is an independent predictor of tumor recurrence and progression after nephrectomy in patients with localized renal cell carcinoma. J Urol 2005;173:725–8.
17. Bot FJ, Godschalk JC, Krishnadath KK, et al. Prognostic factors in renal-cell carcinoma: immunohistochemical detection of p53 protein versus clinico-pathological parameters. Int J Cancer 1994;57:634–7.
18. Kamel D, Turpeenniemi-Hujanen T, Vahakangas K, et al. Proliferating cell nuclear antigen but not p53 or human papillomavirus DNA correlates with advanced clinical stage in renal cell carcinoma. Histopathology 1994;25:339–47.
19. Lipponen P, Eskelinen M, Hietala K, et al. Expression of proliferating cell nuclear antigen (PC10), p53 protein and c-erbB-2 in renal adenocarcinoma. Int J Cancer 1994;57:275–80.
20. Hofmockel G, Tsatalpas P, Muller H, et al. Significance of conventional and new prognostic factors for locally confined renal cell carcinoma. Cancer 1995;76:296–306.
21. Moch H, Sauter G, Gasser TC, et al. p53 protein expression but not mdm-2 protein expression is associated with rapid tumor cell proliferation and prognosis in renal cell carcinoma. Urol Res 1997;25(Suppl 1):S25–30.
22. Gelb AB, Sudilovsky D, Wu CD, et al. Appraisal of intratumoral microvessel density, MIB-1 score, DNA content, and p53 protein expression as prognostic indicators in patients with locally confined renal cell carcinoma. Cancer 1997;80:1768–75.
23. Papadopoulos I, Rudolph P, Weichert-Jacobsen K. Value of p53 expression, cellular proliferation, and DNA content as prognostic indicators in renal cell carcinoma. Eur Urol 1997;32:110–7.
24. Sinik Z, Alkibay T, Ataoglu O, et al. Nuclear p53 overexpression in bladder, prostate, and renal carcinomas. Int J Urol 1997;4:546–51.
25. Vasavada SP, Novick AC, Williams BR. P53, bcl-2, and Bax expression in renal cell carcinoma. Urology 1998;51:1057–61.
26. Sejima T, Miyagawa I. Expression of bcl-2, p53 oncoprotein, and proliferating cell nuclear antigen in renal cell carcinoma. Eur Urol 1999;35:242–8.
27. Rioux-Leclercq N, Turlin B, Bansard J, et al. Value of immunohistochemical Ki-67 and p53 determinations as predictive factors of outcome in renal cell carcinoma. Urology 2000;55:501–5.
28. Haitel A, Wiener HG, Baethge U, et al. mdm2 expression as a prognostic indicator in clear cell renal cell carcinoma: comparison with p53 overexpression and clinicopathological parameters. Clin Cancer Res 2000;6:1840–4.
29. Girgin C, Tarhan H, Hekimgil M, et al. P53 mutations and other prognostic factors of renal cell carcinoma. Urol Int 2001;66:78–83.
30. Ljungberg B, Bozoky B, Kovacs G, et al. p53 expression in correlation to clinical outcome in patients with renal cell carcinoma. Scand J Urol Nephrol 2001;35:15–20.
31. Olumi AF, Weidner N, Presti JC. p53 immunoreactivity correlates with Ki-67 and bcl-2 expression in renal cell carcinoma. Urol Oncol 2001;6:63–7.
32. Uchida T, Gao JP, Wang C, et al. Clinical significance of p53, mdm2, and bcl-2 proteins in renal cell carcinoma. Urology 2002;59:615–20.
33. Kim HL, Seligson D, Liu X, et al. Using protein expressions to predict survival in clear cell renal carcinoma. Clin Cancer Res 2004;10:5464–71.
34. Uzunlar AK, Sahin H, Yilmaz F, et al. Expression of p53 oncoprotein and bcl-2 in renal cell carcinoma. Saudi Med J 2005;26:37–41.

35. Cho DS, Joo HJ, Oh DK, et al. Cyclooxygenase-2 and p53 expression as prognostic indicators in conventional renal cell carcinoma. Yonsei Med J 2005;46:133–40.

36. Kramer BA, Gao X, Davis M, et al. Prognostic significance of ploidy, MIB-1 proliferation marker, and p53 in renal cell carcinoma. J Am Coll Surg 2005;201:565–70.

37. Kankuri M, Soderstrom KO, Pelliniemi TT, et al. The association of immunoreactive p53 and Ki-67 with T-stage, grade, occurrence of metastases and survival in renal cell carcinoma. Anticancer Res 2006; 26:3825–33.

38. Phuoc NB, Ehara H, Gotoh T, et al. Immunohistochemical analysis with multiple antibodies in search of prognostic markers for clear cell renal cell carcinoma. Urology 2007;69:843–8.

39. Perret AG, Clemencon A, Li G, et al. Differential expression of prognostic markers in histological subtypes of papillary renal cell carcinoma. BJU Int 2008;102:183–7.

40. Klatte T, Seligson DB, LaRochelle J, et al. Molecular signatures of localized clear cell renal cell carcinoma to predict disease-free survival after nephrectomy. Cancer Epidemiol Biomarkers Prev 2009;18:894–900.

41. Sakai I, Miyake H, Takenaka A, et al. Expression of potential molecular markers in renal cell carcinoma: impact on clinicopathological outcomes in patients undergoing radical nephrectomy. BJU Int 2009;104:942–6.

42. Zubac DP, Bostad L, Kihl B, et al. The expression of thrombospondin-1 and p53 in clear cell renal cell carcinoma: its relationship to angiogenesis, cell proliferation and cancer specific survival. J Urol 2009;182:2144–9.

43. Baytekin F, Tuna B, Mungan U, et al. Significance of P-glycoprotein, p53, and survivin expression in renal cell carcinoma. Urol Oncol 2011;29:502–7.

44. Noon AP, Polanski R, El-Fert AY, et al. Combined p53 and MDM2 biomarker analysis shows a unique pattern of expression associated with poor prognosis in patients with renal cell carcinoma undergoing radical nephrectomy. BJU Int 2012;109:1250–7.

45. Weber T, Meinhardt M, Zastrow S, et al. Immunohistochemical analysis of prognostic protein markers for primary localized clear cell renal cell carcinoma. Cancer Invest 2013;31:51–9.

46. Weber T, Meinhardt M, Zastrow S, et al. Stage-dependent prognostic impact of molecular signatures in clear cell renal cell carcinoma. Onco Targets Ther 2014;7:645–54.

47. Haitel A, Wiener HG, Neudert B, et al. Expression of the cell cycle proteins p21, p27, and pRb in clear cell renal cell carcinoma and their prognostic significance. Urology 2001;58:477–81.

48. Dahinden C, Ingold B, Wild P, et al. Mining tissue microarray data to uncover combinations of biomarker expression patterns that improve intermediate staging and grading of clear cell renal cell cancer. Clin Cancer Res 2010;16:88–98.

49. Warburton HE, Brady M, Vlatkovic N, et al. p53 regulation and function in renal cell carcinoma. Cancer Res 2005;65:6498–503.

50. Zhang XH, Takenaka I, Sato C, et al. p53 and HER-2 alterations in renal cell carcinoma. Urology 1997; 50:636–42.

51. Chemeris G, Loktinov A, Rempel A, et al. Elevated content of p53 protein in the absence of p53 gene mutations as a possible prognostic marker for human renal cell tumors. Virchows Arch 1995;426: 563–9.

52. Reiter RE, Anglard P, Liu S, et al. Chromosome 17p deletions and p53 mutations in renal cell carcinoma. Cancer Res 1993;53:3092–7.

53. Petitjean A, Mathe E, Kato S, et al. Impact of mutant p53 functional properties on TP53 mutation patterns and tumor phenotype: lessons from recent developments in the IARC TP53 database. Hum Mutat 2007;28:622–9.

54. Soussi T, Beroud C. Assessing TP53 status in human tumours to evaluate clinical outcome. Nat Rev Cancer 2001;1:233–40.

55. Kausch I, Bohle A. Molecular aspects of bladder cancer III. Prognostic markers of bladder cancer. Eur Urol 2002;41:15–29.

56. Weiss RH. p21Waf1/Cip1 as a therapeutic target in breast and other cancers. Cancer Cell 2003; 4:425–9.

57. Papandreou CN, Bogenrieder T, Loganzo F, et al. Expression and sequence analysis of the p21(WAF1/CIP1) gene in renal cancers. Urology 1997;49:481–6.

58. Weiss RH, Borowsky AD, Seligson D, et al. p21 is a prognostic marker for renal cell carcinoma: implications for novel therapeutic approaches. J Urol 2007;177:63–8 [discussion: 8–9].

59. Aaltomaa S, Lipponen P, Ala-Opas M, et al. Expression of cyclins A and D and p21(waf1/cip1) proteins in renal cell cancer and their relation to clinicopathological variables and patient survival. Br J Cancer 1999;80:2001–7.

60. Muriel Lopez C, Esteban E, Berros JP, et al. Prognostic factors in patients with advanced renal cell carcinoma. Clin Genitourin Cancer 2012;10:262–70.

61. Sherr CJ, Roberts JM. CDK inhibitors: positive and negative regulators of G1-phase progression. Genes Dev 1999;13:1501–12.

62. Langner C, von Wasielewski R, Ratschek M, et al. Biological significance of p27 and Skp2 expression in renal cell carcinoma. A systematic analysis of primary and metastatic tumour tissues using a

tissue microarray technique. Virchows Arch 2004; 445:631–6.

63. Schultz L, Chaux A, Albadine R, et al. Immunoexpression status and prognostic value of mTOR and hypoxia-induced pathway members in primary and metastatic clear cell renal cell carcinomas. Am J Surg Pathol 2011;35:1549–56.

64. Amend B, Hennenlotter J, Scharpf M, et al. Akt signalling parameters are different in oncocytomas compared to renal cell carcinoma. World J Urol 2012;30:353–9.

65. Sgambato A, Camerini A, Genovese G, et al. Loss of nuclear p27(kip1) and α-dystroglycan is a frequent event and is a strong predictor of poor outcome in renal cell carcinoma. Cancer Sci 2010;101:2080–6.

66. Liu Z, Fu Q, Lv J, et al. Prognostic implication of p27Kip1, Skp2 and Cks1 expression in renal cell carcinoma: a tissue microarray study. J Exp Clin Cancer Res 2008;27:51.

67. Pertia A, Nikoleishvili D, Trsintsadze O, et al. Immunoreactivity of p27(Kip1), cyclin D3, and Ki67 in conventional renal cell carcinoma. Int Urol Nephrol 2009;41:243–9.

68. Hedberg Y, Davoodi E, Ljungberg B, et al. Cyclin E and p27 protein content in human renal cell carcinoma: clinical outcome and associations with cyclin D. Int J Cancer 2002;102:601–7.

69. Migita T, Oda Y, Naito S, et al. Low expression of p27(Kip1) is associated with tumor size and poor prognosis in patients with renal cell carcinoma. Cancer 2002;94:973–9.

70. Hedberg Y, Ljungberg B, Roos G, et al. Expression of cyclin D1, D3, E, and p27 in human renal cell carcinoma analysed by tissue microarray. Br J Cancer 2003;88:1417–23.

71. Pertia A, Nikoleishvili D, Trsintsadze O, et al. Loss of p27(Kip1) CDKI is a predictor of poor recurrence-free and cancer-specific survival in patients with renal cancer. Int Urol Nephrol 2007;39: 381–7.

72. Anastasiadis AG, Calvo-Sanchez D, Franke KH, et al. p27KIP1-expression in human renal cell cancers: implications for clinical outcome. Anticancer Res 2003;23:217–21.

73. Merseburger AS, Serth J, von der Heyde E, et al. Heterogeneous p27(Kip1) expression within primary renal cell cancers, their invasive margins and peritumoral renal parenchyma correlation with pathological and prognostic features. Urol Int 2007;79:164–9.

74. Kruck S, Merseburger AS, Hennenlotter J, et al. High cytoplasmic expression of p27(Kip1) is associated with a worse cancer-specific survival in clear cell renal cell carcinoma. BJU Int 2012;109:1565–70.

75. Donnellan R, Chetty R. Cyclin D1 and human neoplasia. Mol Pathol 1998;51:1–7.

76. Ikuerowo SO, Kuczyk MA, Mengel M, et al. Alteration of subcellular and cellular expression patterns of cyclin B1 in renal cell carcinoma is significantly related to clinical progression and survival of patients. Int J Cancer 2006;119:867–74.

77. Lima MS, Pereira RA, Costa RS, et al. The prognostic value of cyclin D1 in renal cell carcinoma. Int Urol Nephrol 2014;46:905–13.

78. Lin BT, Brynes RK, Gelb AB, et al. Cyclin D1 expression in renal carcinomas and oncocytomas: an immunohistochemical study. Mod Pathol 1998; 11:1075–81.

79. Hedberg Y, Davoodi E, Roos G, et al. Cyclin-D1 expression in human renal-cell carcinoma. Int J Cancer 1999;84:268–72.

80. Nauman A, Turowska O, Poplawski P, et al. Elevated cyclin E level in human clear cell renal cell carcinoma: possible causes and consequences. Acta Biochim Pol 2007;54:595–602.

81. Presti JC Jr, Reuter VE, Cordon-Cardo C, et al. Expression of the retinoblastoma gene product in renal tumors. Anticancer Res 1996;16:549–56.

82. Hedberg Y, Ljungberg B, Roos G, et al. Retinoblastoma protein in human renal cell carcinoma in relation to alterations in G1/S regulatory proteins. Int J Cancer 2004;109:189–93.

83. Maruschke M, Thur S, Kundt G, et al. Immunohistochemical expression of retinoblastoma protein and p16 in renal cell carcinoma. Urol Int 2011;86:60–7.

84. Visapää H, Bui M, Huang Y, et al. Correlation of Ki-67 and gelsolin expression to clinical outcome in renal clear cell carcinoma. Urology 2003;61: 845–50.

85. Gerdes J, Lemke H, Baisch H, et al. Cell cycle analysis of a cell proliferation-associated human nuclear antigen defined by the monoclonal antibody Ki-67. J Immunol 1984;133:1710–5.

86. Dudderidge TJ, Stoeber K, Loddo M, et al. Mcm2, Geminin, and KI67 define proliferative state and are prognostic markers in renal cell carcinoma. Clin Cancer Res 2005;11:2510–7.

87. Gayed BA, Youssef RF, Bagrodia A, et al. Ki67 is an independent predictor of oncological outcomes in patients with localized clear-cell renal cell carcinoma. BJU Int 2014;113:668–73.

88. Tollefson MK, Thompson RH, Sheinin Y, et al. Ki-67 and coagulative tumor necrosis are independent predictors of poor outcome for patients with clear cell renal cell carcinoma and not surrogates for each other. Cancer 2007;110:783–90.

89. Yildiz E, Gokce G, Kilicarslan H, et al. Prognostic value of the expression of Ki-67, CD44 and vascular endothelial growth factor, and microvessel invasion, in renal cell carcinoma. BJU Int 2004;93: 1087–93.

90. de Riese WT, Crabtree WN, Allhoff EP, et al. Prognostic significance of Ki-67 immunostaining in

nonmetastatic renal cell carcinoma. J Clin Oncol 1993;11:1804–8.

91. Tannapfel A, Hahn HA, Katalinic A, et al. Prognostic value of ploidy and proliferation markers in renal cell carcinoma. Cancer 1996;77:164–71.

92. Bui MH, Visapaa H, Seligson D, et al. Prognostic value of carbonic anhydrase IX and KI67 as predictors of survival for renal clear cell carcinoma. J Urol 2004;171:2461–6.

93. Abel EJ, Bauman TM, Weiker M, et al. Analysis and validation of tissue biomarkers for renal cell carcinoma using automated high-throughput evaluation of protein expression. Hum Pathol 2014;45:1092–9.

94. Teng J, Gao Y, Chen M, et al. Prognostic value of clinical and pathological factors for surgically treated localized clear cell renal cell carcinoma. Chin Med J (Engl) 2014;127:1640–4.

95. Zheng K, Zhu W, Tan J, et al. Retrospective analysis of a large patient sample to determine p53 and Ki67 expressions in renal cell carcinoma. J BUON 2014;19:512–6.

96. Delahunt B, Bethwaite PB, Thornton A, et al. Proliferation of renal cell carcinoma assessed by fixation-resistant polyclonal Ki-67 antibody labeling. Correlation with clinical outcome. Cancer 1995;75:2714–9.

97. Jochum W, Schroder S, al-Taha R, et al. Prognostic significance of nuclear DNA content and proliferative activity in renal cell carcinomas. A clinicopathologic study of 58 patients using mitotic count, MIB-1 staining, and DNA cytophotometry. Cancer 1996;77:514–21.

98. Aaltomaa S, Lipponen P, Ala-Opas M, et al. Prognostic value of Ki-67 expression in renal cell carcinomas. Eur Urol 1997;31:350–5.

99. Haitel A, Wiener HG, Migschitz B, et al. Proliferating cell nuclear antigen and MIB-1. An alternative to classic prognostic indicators in renal cell carcinomas? Am J Clin Pathol 1997;107:229–35.

100. Rioux-Leclercq N, Epstein JI, Bansard JY, et al. Clinical significance of cell proliferation, microvessel density, and CD44 adhesion molecule expression in renal cell carcinoma. Hum Pathol 2001;32: 1209–15.

101. Yuba H, Okamura K, Ono Y, et al. Growth fractions of human renal cell carcinoma defined by monoclonal antibody Ki-67. Predictive values for prognosis. Int J Urol 2001;8:609–14.

102. Lehmann J, Retz M, Nurnberg N, et al. The superior prognostic value of humoral factors compared with molecular proliferation markers in renal cell carcinoma. Cancer 2004;101:1552–62.

103. Kallio JP, Hirvikoski P, Helin H, et al. Renal cell carcinoma MIB-1, Bax and Bcl-2 expression and prognosis. J Urol 2004;172:2158–61.

104. Cheville JC, Zincke H, Lohse CM, et al. pT1 clear cell renal cell carcinoma: a study of the association between MIB-1 proliferative activity and pathologic features and cancer specific survival. Cancer 2002;94:2180–4.

105. Parker AS, Leibovich BC, Lohse CM, et al. Development and evaluation of BioScore: a biomarker panel to enhance prognostic algorithms for clear cell renal cell carcinoma. Cancer 2009;115:2092–103.

Current Clinical Applications of Testicular Cancer Biomarkers

Maria C. Mir, MD, PhD[a], Nicola Pavan, MD[a,b],
Mark L. Gonzalgo, MD, PhD[a,*]

KEYWORDS

- Testicular germ cell tumors • Tumor markers • microRNAs • Serum • Markers • Mitochondrial DNA

KEY POINTS

- Aside from classic serum tumor markers for testicular cancer (human chorionic gonadotropin, alpha fetoprotein, lactate dehydrogenase), limited data on additional molecular biomarkers have been published or validated.
- Larger series with consistent results from independent groups are required to validate new testicular cancer biomarkers.
- microRNA-371-3 has potential utility as a molecular biomarker for germ cell tumor detection and prognosis.

INTRODUCTION

Most germ cell tumors (GCTs) originate in the testes and account for approximately 95% of testicular cancers. Occasionally, GCTs originate in extragonadal sites, such as the mediastinum or retroperitoneum. Clinical and pathologic heterogeneity is an important feature of GCTs. Benign forms demonstrate extensive somatic differentiation (teratoma), whereas malignant GCTs are divided into seminoma and nonseminomatous GCTs (NSGCT).

Serum tumor markers (STMs) are prognostic factors and are important for diagnosis and staging. STM should be determined before and following orchiectomy. The 3 classic STMs for testicular cancer diagnosis and staging are alpha fetoprotein (AFP), which is produced by yolk sac cells; human chorionic gonadotropin (HCG), which is expressed by trophoblasts; and lactate dehydrogenase (LDH).

STMs are increased in approximately 60% of testicular cancer cases. AFP and HCG are increased in 50% to 70% and in 40% to 60% of patients with NSGCTs, respectively. Approximately 90% of NSGCTs present with an increase in one or 2 of these markers. Up to 30% of seminomas can present with or develop an elevated HCG level during the course of the disease.

LDH is a less specific marker with its concentration being proportional to tumor volume. Its level may be elevated in up to 80% of patients with advanced testicular cancer. Negative marker levels do not exclude the diagnosis of a GCT. Placental alkaline phosphatase (PLAP) is an optional marker for monitoring patients with pure seminoma but may have limited value in smokers.

Disclosure statement: The authors have identified no professional or financial affiliations related to this work for themselves or their spouses/partners.
[a] Department of Urology, Sylvester Comprehensive Cancer Center, University of Miami Miller School of Medicine, Miami, FL 33136, USA; [b] Department of Medical, Surgical and Health Science, Urology Clinic, University of Trieste, Trieste, Italy
* Corresponding author. University of Miami Miller School of Medicine, 1120 Northwest 14th Street, Suite 1560, Miami, FL 33136.
E-mail address: m.gonzalgo@miami.edu

Traditional STMs are not only specific for testicular cancer. Elevations in HCG are commonly seen in a wide variety of carcinomas (gastric, pancreatic, neuroendocrine, lung, head and neck, lymphoma, leukemia). Similarly, elevations of AFP can be observed in hepatocellular carcinoma and benign liver disease.

A biomarker has been defined as "any substance, structure, or process that can be measured in the body or its products and influence or predict the incidence of outcome or disease" by the World Health Organization. An ideal biomarker for testicular cancer would be an easily detectable molecule that would be unique for GCTs.

Limited contemporary data have been published regarding the use of biomarkers for testicular cancer diagnosis and prognosis in addition to traditional STMs (AFP, HCG, LDH). Cytogenetic and molecular markers based on microRNA (miRNA), cell-circulating mitochondrial DNA, or DNA methylation are available at limited centers but at present are not commonly used in clinical practice (**Table 1**).

CLINICAL UTILITY OF TRADITIONAL SERUM TUMOR MARKERS
Screening Utility of Serum Tumor Markers

In the context of screening for GCTs, no role of STM has been demonstrated because of the low incidence and mortality of testicular cancer.[1] It is very unlikely that STM as a screening tool would decrease mortality because of the natural history of the disease.

Diagnostic Utility of Serum Tumor Markers

STMs have been shown to assist in determining the origin of GCTs and in some clinical scenarios will dictate treatment. For example, if only seminoma is observed in an orchiectomy specimen, but increased AFP is detected, patients will be treated according to NSGCT protocols. Few conditions other than GCTs cause extreme elevation of STM, but moderate elevations are not as uncommon. See **Table 2** for conditions that may cause elevation of STMs.

Ataxia-telangiectasia is a hereditary from of ataxia associated with various skin conditions. More than 95% of affected patients have elevated AFP.[2] Hereditary tyrosinemia is caused by various enzyme deficiencies in the tyrosine degradation pathway. This condition progresses to liver and kidney failure. Because of liver dysfunction, extreme elevations of AFP are present in affected individuals.[3] Similarly, in patients with cirrhotic liver disease and hepatocellular carcinoma, AFP can be elevated but is not always diagnostic of disease (40% of cirrhotic patients have elevation of AFP due to hepatomas).

In primary hypogonadism, a decline in testosterone may cause increased levels of LH.[4] LH is known to have cross reactivity with HCG in some immunoassays. Marijuana use may also result in elevation of HCG.

Table 1
Current clinical testicular cancer biomarkers

Molecular Marker	Target	Characteristics	Able to Differentiate GCT from Healthy Controls	Correlation with GCT Stage
miRNA	miRNA367-3p, 371a-3p, 372-3p, 373-3p	Noncoding RNA; very stable; interfere in the translation of mRNA to protein	Y	Y
mtDNA	mtDNA-79; mtDNA-220	Short length, simple structure	Y	N
CircDNA	—	Same methylation pattern as tumor cells	Y	N
CpG island hypermethylation	Gene silencing (APC, GSTP1, p14, p16, PTGS2, RASSF1A)	Easy to detect methylation; techniques already established	Y	N
CTC	—	Easy to detect; molecular techniques	Y	Y

Abbreviations: CircDNA, cell-free circulating plasma DNA; CTC, circulating tumor cell; mRNA, messenger RNA; mtDNA, mitochondrial DNA; N, no; Y, yes.

Table 2
Summary of key information for traditional STMs of GCTs

	AFP	HCG	LDH
Normal limits	1 mg/L to 10–15 mg/L of serum or plasma	1 U/L to 5–10 U/L	Depends on assay method used
Half-life (d)	5–7	1.5–3.0	Not reported
Seminoma GCT	Never elevated in pure seminoma	Yes (15%–20%)	Yes (40%–60%)
Nonseminoma GCT	Yes (10%–20% localized disease; 40%–60% advanced disease)	Yes (10%–20% localized disease; 40%–60% advanced disease)	Yes (40%–60%)
Other malignancies	Hepatocellular carcinoma, gastric, lung, colon, pancreatic	Neuroendocrine, bladder, kidney, lung, head and neck, gastrointestinal, cervix, uterus, vulva, lymphoma, leukemia	Lymphoma, small-cell lung, Ewing sarcoma, osteogenic sarcoma
Nonmalignant conditions	Alcohol abuse, hepatitis, cirrhosis, biliary tract obstruction, hereditary persistence	Marijuana, hypogonadism	Several

Staging Utility of Serum Tumor Markers

STMs cannot only help to establish a diagnosis, but the degree of elevation at diagnosis has prognostic significance.

According to NCCN guidelines, the role of STM in preorchiectomy and postorchiectomy is for staging purposes.[5] Before initiation of any treatment (surgical, chemotherapy, or radiotherapy), STMs should be measured. The magnitude of STM variability (International Germ Cell Cancer Collaborative Group [IGCCCG] classification) is used to determine chemotherapy regimens as well as for evaluation of response to chemotherapy.[6]

Measurement of Response to Treatment by Serum Tumor Markers

The use of STMs to monitor the response to chemotherapy is encouraged as increasing concentrations of markers in seminoma may imply disease progression and the need for salvage therapy.

For patients that undergo radical orchiectomy, the rate of decline of STM should coincide with the half-lives of the STMs. If the STMs remain elevated or decline slower than the expected half-life, this may indicate slowly growing metastatic disease. If STMs are elevated and there is no evidence of retroperitoneal disease on imaging, this is considered clinical stage IS disease. Use of STMs may also allow patients with residual disease to be differentiated from cancer-free patients.[5]

Decline after Treatment of Metastatic Disease

The standard chemotherapy regimen for testicular cancer includes bleomycin, etoposide, and cisplatin (BEP) or etoposide and cisplatin (EP). The number of cycles administered depends on the disease risk classification. Salvage chemotherapy is indicated for men who relapse or progress through primary chemotherapy. Finally, high-dose chemotherapy with autologous bone marrow transplant is indicated in poor-prognosis patients in whom standard chemotherapy regimens and/or salvage therapies have failed.

STMs should be measured the day before starting chemotherapy in order to accurately stratify patients according to IGCCCG classification.[6] Thereafter, STMs should be obtained at the beginning of each cycle. Serial measurements are encouraged as it correlates with the amount of viable tumor tissue remaining. Some studies have demonstrated a correlation between STM decline in the first 2 cycles of chemotherapy and oncologic outcomes (complete response, overall survival).[7] The results of a prospective randomized trial in patients with poor-prognosis according to IGCCCG criteria were recently published.[8] Patients were classified according to their response to the first cycle of BEP chemotherapy. Classification was established by the decline in STMs (normalized after first cycle). The group of patients with unfavorable decline received dose-dense chemotherapy that was associated with an improvement in progression-free and overall survival.

Despite these findings, a return to normal STMs does not always indicate a complete response. Up to 20% of patients who receive systemic chemotherapy for retroperitoneal disease demonstrate viable tumor at pathologic examination of lymph nodes.[9]

AVAILABLE BIOMARKERS FOR TESTICULAR CANCER

The introduction of more sensitive and specific biomarkers for diagnosis, staging, and surveillance of testicular cancer would allow clinicians to better select patients for further treatment. Surgery, chemotherapy, or radiotherapy may be associated with a variety of side effects that have the potential to impact the quality of life in a young patient population. Few studies have examined the clinical applicability of molecular biomarkers (miRNA, circulating mitochondrial DNA, circulating tumor cells) for early detection, staging, and surveillance of testicular cancer.

Increased expression of embryonic miRNA clusters (miR-371–3 and miR-302–367) can be detected in the serum of patients with GCT at higher rates compared with controls.[10–12] These findings hold promise for the clinical management of GCT, especially for seminoma because traditional STMs have limited utility for diagnosis or surveillance.

miRNAs are a new class of noncoding RNA. They are not only involved in physiologic processes (cell differentiation) but they are also involved in pathologic responses (carcinogenesis). miRNAs interfere with the translation of a given messenger RNA to protein; thus, they can act as a tumor-suppressor gene or oncogene. miRNAs are characterized by strong stability in body fluids once released from tumor cells.[13,14] In testicular cancer, miRNAs have shown to mimic the effects of mutated p53. miRNA expression has also been studied in other genitourinary malignancies.[15]

Testicular GCTs arise from carcinoma in situ cells that resemble malignant (pluripotent) primordial germ cells. They persist in the testis during puberty and early adulthood and then progress to seminoma or NSGCT. The miRNA profile of a cell may change during the course of malignant transformation.

Elevated levels of miR-371-3 have been observed in patients with GCTs compared with controls with a significant decrease in the level of miR-371-3 following orchiectomy. The rapid decline following surgery and the correlation of miRNA levels with tumor aggressiveness hold promise for the clinical utility of this biomarker.[10] This miRNA has also been shown to be elevated

in thyroid cancer, and it is not exclusively specific for GCT.[16] The level of miR-371a-3p in blood and other body fluids has also been investigated.[17] The study included 25 patients with GCT, 6 with testicular intraepithelial neoplasia, 20 healthy men, and 24 patients with nontesticular malignancies. Moreover, 5 patients with GCT and 5 healthy controls had testicular vein blood examined for miR-371a-3p in an effort to demonstrate local release of miRNA. Increased levels of miR-371a-3p were observed in GCTs with rapid decay after orchiectomy. No correlation was found between the miRNA levels in testicular intraepithelial neoplasia (TIN) cases and controls. Although these results are promising, larger series with standardized results (miRNA technique for measurement seems to be controversial among investigators at normalization) need to be reported in order to become the standard of care.

Serum miR-367-3p, miR-371a-3p, miR-372-3p, and miR-373-3p have also been found to be significantly increased in patients with GCT compared with healthy controls.[18] The sensitivity and specificity of miR-371a-3p for the detection of GCT was 84.7% and 99.0%, respectively. These results were consistent with what has been reported in other previously published series.[19]

The unique characteristics of the mitochondrial genome, such as short length, simple molecular structure, and high copy number, have made monitoring aberrant changes of mitochondrial DNA (mtDNA) quantity a promising molecular marker for early tumor detection with advantages over nuclear genome-based methods. Recently, circulating cell-free (ccf) mtDNA in blood has emerged as a noninvasive diagnostic and prognostic biomarker for solid tumors.[20] Accumulating evidence suggests that plasma or serum ccf mtDNA levels are significantly different between patients with cancer and healthy individuals. Furthermore, quantification of ccf mtDNA levels in blood may assist in differentiating affected individuals from cancer-free patients.

A significant increase in short (79 bp) and large (220 bp) mtDNA fragments in patients with seminoma and NSGCT were detected compared with healthy controls.[21] No correlation with clinicopathological variables (clinical stage, pathologic stage, or lymph node invasion) was observed. mtDNA-79 showed an improved capacity (against traditional STMs) to distinguish between patients and healthy controls (mtDNA sensitivity 60%, specificity 94%).

Cell-free circulating plasma DNA (circDNA) is DNA found in blood plasma that is not associated with any cell fraction. circDNA is generally shed from normal cells, including. Among individuals with cancer, a proportion of circDNA is derived from tumor cells and contains the same mutations and methylation patterns as the primary tumor.[22] Furthermore, studies have demonstrated that circDNA can be detected in most patients harboring solid tumors with advanced disease as well as in a lower fraction of patients with localized disease.[23] Thus, tumor-specific methylation in circDNA is a potential target for the development of noninvasive, blood-based assays for cancer diagnosis. A 9-fold increase in the level of circDNA among patients with testicular cancer compared with healthy controls has been described. No correlation between circDNA and STM, age, or histologic subtype was observed.[24]

One of the surprising aspects of cancer biology that has emerged from The Cancer Genome Atlas (TCGA) sequencing projects was the wide diversity of mutations associated with cancer.[25] Even within a single tumor type, mutational profiles may be very different between patients. It is not unusual for even the most commonly altered genes to be mutated in less than half of cases. The TCGA ovarian cancer sequencing project identified 7 significantly mutated genes, but these were only present in 2% to 6% of samples.[26] Limited data are available regarding GCT. This mutational heterogeneity provides a challenge for the development of cancer diagnostic tests based on DNA sequence changes, because large proportions of the genome would need to be interrogated to provide a test of adequate sensitivity.

The variability of cancer mutational profiles contrasts with the stability of DNA methylation changes that are a hallmark of oncogenic transformation. Given the greater consistency of DNA methylation changes in cancer compared with mutations, methylation is a promising target for biomarker development. CpG island hypermethylation of promoter regions is associated with gene silencing and has been reported for several genes in testicular cancer tissues (APC, GSTP1, p14 [ARF], p16 [INK], PTGS2, RASSF1A).[27] Detection of methylation changes is feasible in blood samples and has potential utility as a specific biomarker for testicular cancer.

Various levels of aberrant DNA methylation have been detected in up to 50% of patients with testicular cancer (APC, p14 [ARF], p16 [INK], PTGS2, RASSF1A).[28] Although the potential feasibility of hypermethylation as a testicular cancer biomarker has been investigated, limited data exist that examines the correlation between methylation, stage of disease, or tumor aggressiveness.

Finally, circulating tumor cells (CTCs) have been investigated as a potential biomarker for detection of testicular cancer. CTCs are cells that have shed into the vasculature from a primary tumor and circulate in the bloodstream. Several studies suggest that very small tumors shed cells at less than 1.0% per day.[29] CTCs are derived from clones in the primary tumor. A correlation between the incidence of CTCs in the peripheral blood of patients with testicular cancer and stage of disease/recurrence after chemotherapy has been reported.[30] A higher concentration of CTCs was described when testicular vein blood was analyzed. Other investigators have previously reported detection of CTCs in patients with GCTs.[31]

FUTURE BIOMARKERS FOR TESTICULAR CANCER UNDER INVESTIGATION

Recently, newly discovered biomarkers have been reported to differentiate between histologic subtypes of testicular cancer. These biomarkers include High Mobility Group A (HMGA), POZ-AT hook-zinc finger protein (PATZ), Aurora-B, Nek-2, Octamer Binding Transcription Factor 3/4 (OCT3/4), c-kit, PLAP, NANOG, SOX2, and CDK10.

HMGA1 and HMGA2 are proteins that are expressed depending on the state of differentiation of GCT. HMGA1 is overexpressed in seminoma. HMGA1 and HGMA2 are overexpressed in pluripotential embryonal carcinoma cells. HMGA1 expression is lost in yolk sac tumors, and expression of both proteins is lost in adult teratoma tissue.[32]

PATZ functions as a nuclear transcriptional repressor. PATZ and HMGA1 cytoplasmic delocalization associates with estrogen receptor downregulation in seminomas. Moreover, the PATZ interacting protein RNF4 is overexpressed in spermatocytes. RNF4 is not expressed in dedifferentiated tumors (embryonal carcinoma, yolk sac), suggesting a role in progression of GCT. Aurora-B is expressed in carcinoma in situ (CIS), seminoma, and embryonal carcinomas but not in teratoma and yolk sac carcinomas.[33,34]

OCT3/4 is another marker that has been reported in testicular cancer. OCT is a transcription factor of the family of octamer-binding proteins known as the key regulators of pluripotency.[35] Its expression has been reported in carcinoma in situ, seminoma, and embryonal carcinoma. Although OCT is a potential biomarker for testicular cancer, OCT has also been expressed in normal testicular tissue in some studies. However, there may be technical challenges related to the consistency of the antibody used for OCT detection.[36,37]

SOX2 is a transcription factor that has been reported in embryonal carcinomas, the undifferentiated part of nonseminomas, but absent in seminomas, yolk sac tumors, and normal spermatogenesis. SOX17 has also been shown to discriminate carcinoma in situ and seminoma from embryonal carcinoma.[38] No clinical applicability of the use of the aforementioned biomarkers has been reported to date. CDK10 is a nuclear structural protein that has been expressed in seminoma.[39]

In summary, new testicular cancer biomarkers for diagnosis, staging, or follow-up remain promising but still lack evidence from large clinical studies to determine if traditional STMs can be replaced. A better understanding of the molecular mechanisms underlying the development of GCT may provide new insight into more effective diagnosis and treatment of GCT.

REFERENCES

1. Siegel RL, Miller KD, Jemal A. Cancer statistics, 2015. CA Cancer J Clin 2015;65:5–29.
2. Chun HH, Gatti RA. Ataxia-telangiectasia, an evolving phenotype. DNA Repair (Amst) 2004;3: 1187–96.
3. Scott CR. The genetic tyrosinemias. Am J Med Genet C Semin Med Genet 2006;142C:121–6.
4. Fowler JE Jr, Platoff GE, Kubrock CA, et al. Commercial radioimmunoassay for beta subunit of human chorionic gonadotropin: falsely positive determinations due to elevated serum luteinizing hormone. Cancer 1982;49:136–9.
5. Motzer RJ, Agarwal N, Beard C, et al. NCCN clinical practice guidelines in oncology: testicular cancer. J Natl Compr Canc Netw 2009;7:672–93.
6. Mead GM, Stenning SP. The International Germ Cell Consensus Classification: a new prognostic factor-based staging classification for metastatic germ cell tumours. Clin Oncol 1997;9:207–9.
7. Mazumdar M, Bajorin DF, Bacik J, et al. Predicting outcome to chemotherapy in patients with germ cell tumors: the value of the rate of decline of human chorionic gonadotrophin and alpha-fetoprotein during therapy. J Clin Oncol 2001;19:2534–41.
8. Fizazi K, Pagliaro L, Laplanche A, et al. Personalised chemotherapy based on tumour marker decline in poor prognosis germ-cell tumours (GETUG 13): a phase 3, multicentre, randomised trial. The Lancet. Oncology 2014;15:1442–50.
9. Eggener SE, Carver BS, Loeb S, et al. Pathologic findings and clinical outcome of patients undergoing retroperitoneal lymph node dissection after multiple chemotherapy regimens for metastatic testicular germ cell tumors. Cancer 2007;109:528–35.
10. Belge G, Dieckmann KP, Spiekermann M, et al. Serum levels of microRNAs miR-371-3: a novel class of serum biomarkers for testicular germ cell tumors? Eur Urol 2012;61:1068–9.
11. Murray MJ, Halsall DJ, Hook CE, et al. Identification of microRNAs from the miR-371~373 and miR-302 clusters as potential serum biomarkers of malignant germ cell tumors. Am J Clin Pathol 2011;135:119–25.
12. Murray MJ, Coleman N. Testicular cancer: a new generation of biomarkers for malignant germ cell tumours. Nature reviews. Urology 2012;9:298–300.
13. Reis LO, Pereira TC, Lopes-Cendes I, et al. MicroRNAs: a new paradigm on molecular urological oncology. Urology 2010;76:521–7.
14. Weber JA, Baxter DH, Zhang S, et al. The microRNA spectrum in 12 body fluids. Clin Chem 2010;56: 1733–41.
15. Du M, Shi D, Yuan L, et al. Circulating miR-497 and miR-663b in plasma are potential novel biomarkers for bladder cancer. Sci Rep 2015;5:10437.
16. Rippe V, Dittberner L, Lorenz VN, et al. The two stem cell microRNA gene clusters C19MC and miR-371-3 are activated by specific chromosomal rearrangements in a subgroup of thyroid adenomas. PLoS One 2010;5:e9485.
17. Spiekermann M, Belge G, Winter N, et al. MicroRNA miR-371a-3p in serum of patients with germ cell tumours: evaluations for establishing a serum biomarker. Andrology 2015;3:78–84.
18. Syring I, Bartels J, Holdenrieder S, et al. Circulating serum miRNA (miR-367-3p, miR-371a-3p, miR-372-3p and miR-373-3p) as biomarkers in patients with testicular germ cell cancer. J Urol 2015;193:331–7.
19. Gillis AJ, Rijlaarsdam MA, Eini R, et al. Targeted serum miRNA (TSmiR) test for diagnosis and follow-up of (testicular) germ cell cancer patients: a proof of principle. Mol Oncol 2013;7:1083–92.
20. Fernandes J, Michel V, Camorlinga-Ponce M, et al. Circulating mitochondrial DNA level, a noninvasive biomarker for the early detection of gastric cancer. Cancer Epidemiol Biomarkers Prev 2014;23:2430–8.
21. Ellinger J, Albers P, Muller SC, et al. Circulating mitochondrial DNA in the serum of patients with testicular germ cell cancer as a novel noninvasive diagnostic biomarker. BJU Int 2009;104:48–52.
22. Schwarzenbach H, Hoon DS, Pantel K. Cell-free nucleic acids as biomarkers in cancer patients. Nat Rev Cancer 2011;11:426–37.
23. Bettegowda C, Sausen M, Leary RJ, et al. Detection of circulating tumor DNA in early- and late-stage human malignancies. Sci Transl Med 2014;6:224ra24.
24. Ellinger J, Wittkamp V, Albers P, et al. Cell-free circulating DNA: diagnostic value in patients with testicular germ cell cancer. J Urol 2009;181:363–71.
25. Vogelstein B, Papadopoulos N, Velculescu VE, et al. Cancer genome landscapes. Science 2013;339: 1546–58.
26. Integrated genomic analyses of ovarian carcinoma. Nature 2011;474:609–15.
27. Koul S, McKiernan JM, Narayan G, et al. Role of promoter hypermethylation in cisplatin treatment response of male germ cell tumors. Mol Cancer 2004;3:16.
28. Ellinger J, Albers P, Perabo FG, et al. CpG island hypermethylation of cell-free circulating serum

DNA in patients with testicular cancer. J Urol 2009; 182:324–9.

29. Pantel K, Brakenhoff RH, Brandt B. Detection, clinical relevance and specific biological properties of disseminating tumour cells. Nat Rev Cancer 2008; 8:329–40.

30. Nastaly P, Ruf C, Becker P, et al. Circulating tumor cells in patients with testicular germ cell tumors. Clin Cancer Res 2014;20:3830–41.

31. Hautkappe AL, Lu M, Mueller H, et al. Detection of germ-cell tumor cells in the peripheral blood by nested reverse transcription-polymerase chain reaction for alpha-fetoprotein-messenger RNA and beta human chorionic gonadotropin-messenger RNA. Cancer Res 2000;60:3170–4.

32. Franco R, Esposito F, Fedele M, et al. Detection of high-mobility group proteins A1 and A2 represents a valid diagnostic marker in post-pubertal testicular germ cell tumours. J Pathol 2008;214: 58–64.

33. Pero R, Lembo F, Chieffi P, et al. Translational regulation of a novel testis-specific RNF4 transcript. Mol Reprod Dev 2003;66:1–7.

34. Pero R, Lembo F, Di Vizio D, et al. RNF4 is a growth inhibitor expressed in germ cells but not in human testicular tumors. Am J Pathol 2001;159:1225–30.

35. Looijenga LH, Stoop H, de Leeuw HP, et al. POU5F1 (OCT3/4) identifies cells with pluripotent potential in human germ cell tumors. Cancer Res 2003;63: 2244–50.

36. de Jong J, Looijenga LH. Stem cell marker OCT3/ 4 in tumor biology and germ cell tumor diagnostics: history and future. Crit Rev Oncog 2006;12: 171–203.

37. de Jong J, Stoop H, Dohle GR, et al. Diagnostic value of OCT3/4 for pre-invasive and invasive testicular germ cell tumours. J Pathol 2005;206: 242–9.

38. de Jong J, Stoop H, Gillis AJ, et al. Differential expression of SOX17 and SOX2 in germ cells and stem cells has biological and clinical implications. J Pathol 2008;215:21–30.

39. Leman ES, Magheli A, Yong KM, et al. Identification of nuclear structural protein alterations associated with seminomas. J Cell Biochem 2009;108: 1274–9.

MicroRNAs in Testicular Cancer Diagnosis and Prognosis

Hui Ling, MD, PhD[a], Lisa Krassnig, BSc[b],
Marc D. Bullock, MD, PhD[a], Martin Pichler, MD[a,b,*]

KEYWORDS

- MicroRNA • Testicular cancer • Biomarkers • Detection • Prognosis

KEY POINTS

- MicroRNAs are important regulators of testicular cancer initiation, progression, and metastatic spread.
- Potential serum-based biomarkers miR-371, miR-372, miR-373, and miR-367 demonstrate diagnostic sensitivity of 98% in patients with testicular cancer.
- MicroRNAs may affect sensitivity of testicular cancer to cisplatin treatment.

INTRODUCTION

Testicular cancer represents the most common form of cancer in men of Caucasian ancestry aged 15 to 40 years.[1] In addition to the different histologic growth patterns (isolated vs mixed histology), testicular cancer can be divided into seminomatous or nonseminomatous tumors, which are clinically distinct in terms of therapy, surveillance requirements, and prognosis. Nonseminomatous germ cell tumors (GCTs) contain 1, 2, or several proportions of the following major histologic subtypes: embryonal carcinoma, yolk sac tumor, choriocarcinoma, or teratoma.[2]

These microscopic differences are mirrored by differences in biological phenotype, in terms of metastatic potential, uptake of radioisotopes in medical imaging, drug sensitivity, and radioresistance. The cellular and molecular mechanisms that underpin each histologic subtype are also distinct.[2] In general, patients with testicular cancer are present with symptoms of local disease or less commonly with signs of metastatic spread (eg, respiratory symptoms in case of lung metastases or localized pain in case of bone metastases).[2]

Serum-based tumor markers (including alpha-fetoprotein [AFP], human chorionic gonadotropin [HCG], and lactate dehydrogenase [LDH]) have an established role in diagnosis and prognostic risk stratification of patients with testicular cancer.[3] However, these biomarkers are limited by relatively high false-negativity rates (only 60% through all testicular cancer subtypes can be detected) at the time of presentation coupled by the potential for false-positive detection associated with nonspecific alterations related to other diseases (eg, AFP increase associated with liver diseases).[4] In particular, the proportion of patients with seminomas and embryonal carcinomas presenting with elevated tumor markers is low, as AFP is predominantly associated with yolk sac tumors and HCG with choriocarcinoma histology.[2]

The authors have nothing to disclose.
[a] Department of Experimental Therapeutics, The University of Texas M.D. Anderson Cancer Center, Houston, TX 77054, USA; [b] Division of Oncology, Department of Internal Medicine, Medical University of Graz (MUG), Graz, Austria
* Corresponding author. Department of Experimental Therapeutics, The University of Texas M.D. Anderson Cancer Center, Unit 1950, PO Box 301429, Houston, TX 77230-1429.
E-mail address: mart.pichler@gmx.net

It is therefore clear that improved detection and risk stratification in early-stage disease, and the use of biomarkers to guide decision making around the use of adjuvant therapy and local surgical resection would have considerable clinical utility.

The biological importance of microRNAs (miRNAs) was identified in the early 1990s, when several groups reported the regulation of developmental processes in worms by small non–protein-coding RNA molecules.[5] MiRNAs are small (approximately 20 nucleotides in length) RNA molecules that do not translate into peptides or proteins,[6] but regulate the expression of larger messenger RNAs (mRNAs) by sequence complementarity, and block protein translation or accelerate mRNA degradation.[7]

In the past 20 years, this class of small regulatory RNAs has been associated with the pathogenesis of cancer and the mechanisms that govern metastatic spread.[6,8,9] They have been implicated in all of the hallmark processes of cancer, including but not restricted to genome instability,[10] cancer stem cells,[11] and response to anticancer therapies.[12] In the context of cancer initiation and progression, miRNAs can either act as tumor suppressors or oncogenic drivers, depending on the regulated genes, the cellular context, and the cancer type.[13] In this review, we provide an overview of the molecular role of miRNAs specifically in the context of testicular cancer and we discuss their potential utility as diagnostic and prognostic biomarkers in the clinical setting.

MOLECULAR ASPECTS OF MICRORNA BIOGENESIS

Human miRNAs originated from the cell nucleus, and are encoded by genes commonly assembled in clusters.[14] On activation by various transcription factors, RNA polymerase II transcribes the gene information to a primary miRNA ("pri-miRNA") molecule, which in turn is processed into a precursor form ("pre-miRNA") by the ribonuclease (RNase) III enzyme Drosha in association with the binding protein Pasha (DGCR8).[14] The hairpin structure of pre-miRNA allows the nuclear export into the cytoplasm by the transporter exportin-5 and its associated protein GTPase Ran.[5] In the cytoplasm, the RNase III endonuclease Dicer cleaves the hairpin loop and produces small, 19 to 22 nucleotides long miRNAs. Mature miRNAs in the cytoplasm then interact with complementary target mRNAs within the RNA-induced silencing complex, and regulate mRNA stability or protein translation. **Fig. 1** summarizes the process of miRNA biogenesis. It has been estimated that more than one-third of human protein-coding genes are controlled by miRNAs.[14]

MICRORNAS IN TESTICULAR CANCER

Current hypotheses assume that GCTs develop from noninvasive intratubular germ cell neoplasia unclassified (IGCNU), also known as carcinoma in situ (CIS), cells that are for whatever reasons prevented from maturation.[15] Under normal conditions, germ cells migrate after embryogenesis into the genital ridge to become gonocytes and later on spermatogonia. Particular underlying and yet unknown triggers lead to the development of CIS cells.[16] They often persist until puberty and then start to proliferate, presumably as a consequence of endocrine signals, which might result in the progression to seminomatous or nonseminomatous tumors.[17] CIS cells mimic embryonic stem cells in their pluripotent properties, which enable the conversion to multiple lineages, including germ cell lineage, embryonal carcinoma, somatic lineage teratoma, and yolk sac tumors or choriocarcinoma (**Fig. 2**).[2]

By controlling protein-coding genes involved in cancer development, miRNAs may affect every aspect of testicular cancer pathogenesis from initiation to progression to metastatic spread. Early in 2006, Voorhoeve and colleagues[18] identified miRNA-372 and miRNA-373 as oncogenic drivers in testicular cancer by using high-throughput screening with a library of miRNA expression vectors. They found that expression levels of miR-372 and miR-373 determine the fate of proliferation and apoptosis under the stress induced by rat sarcoma viral oncogene homolog (RAS) in the wild-type p53 background. Further analysis showed that these 2 miRNAs directly target large tumor suppressor kinase 2 (LATS2) to abrogate the cell cycle arrest initiated by p53-p21-CDK signaling, and consequently increase proliferation of testicular germ cells.[18] Similarly, Gillis and colleagues[19] reported in 2007 that the miRNA-371 to 373 cluster, including miR-371a, miR-371b, miR-372, and miR373, are significantly upregulated in type II and III (ie, testicular germ cell tumors of adolescents and adults can be subdivided into seminomas and nonseminomas, all referred to as type II GCTs, whereas the other type [type III germ cell tumor] is the so-called spermatocytic seminoma) human GCTs. They also noted that the expression of the hsa-miR-302 to 367 cluster, including miR-302a, miR-302b, miR-302c, miR-302d, miR-302a, and hsa-miR-367, are downregulated on differentiation, suggesting functional involvement of these miRNAs in controlling stem cell differentiation in GCTs.[19] Echoing these findings,

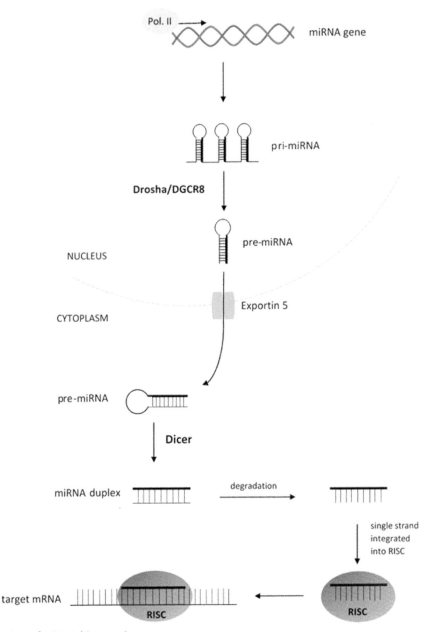

Fig. 1. Illustration of miRNA biogenesis.

Barroso-del Jesus and colleagues[20] surmised that the miR-302 to 367 cluster is transcriptionally activated by Oct3/4, Sox2, and Nanog, and potentially regulates stemness in embryonic stem cells. Furthermore, Palmer and colleagues[21] showed that the miR-371 to 373 and miR-302 clusters are overexpressed in all types of malignant GCTs, regardless of histology, tumor site, or patient age. The same group subsequently performed a global analysis of mRNAs that are downregulated in testicular cancers, and discovered an enrichment of mRNAs containing 3′UTR sequence of GCACTT, which is complementary to the seed sequence (AAGUGC) contained within the previously discussed miRNAs.[22] This enrichment of miRNA-targeted mRNAs provides strong evidence on the functional relevance of aberrant miRNA expression in testicular cancer.

Crucially, testicular cancers appear to express a unique and consistent miRNA signature, that is, the enhanced expression of the miR-371 to 373 cluster located at chromosome 19q13. This indicates an intrinsic link between the expressions of this miRNA cluster and an essential characteristic

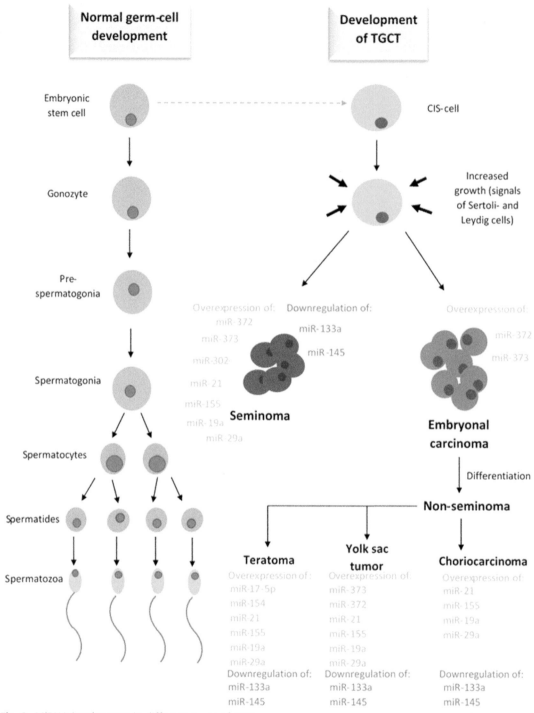

Fig. 2. MiRNA involvement in different types of GCTs.

of testicular cancers. Zhou and colleagues[23] examined the mechanisms underlying this unique upregulation pattern of miRNAs in germ cell cancers. They identified a feedback loop between the miR-371 to 373 cluster and the Wnt/β-catenin signaling pathway, whereby miR-372 and miR-

373, transcriptionally activated by Wnt signaling, inhibit DKK1, a key antagonist of Wnt/β-catenin signaling. Wnt signaling plays critical roles in regulating cell stemness, and thus it appears that the miR-371 to 373 cluster contributes to the maintenance of stem cell status. In support of this hypothesis, one study showed that the miR-371 to 373 cluster functions as a self-renewal miRNA to induce and maintain the pluripotent state of stem cells. A further study showed higher expression of miR-371 to 373 cluster miRNAs in stem cells than differentiated cells, which again supports an association between miR-371 to 373 miRNAs and stem cell status in testicular cancer.[24]

Other miRNAs also have been reported to associate with testicular cancer. Several reports from the Chan group showed that miR-199a is downregulated in testicular cancer,[25] largely due to hypermethylation at the miR-199a promoter region,[25,26] and overexpression of miR-199a inhibits testicular cancer growth and metastasis by targeting the embryonal carcinoma antigen, podocalyxin-like protein 1 (PODXL).[25] Male infertility has been associated with increased risk of developing testicular cancer. Lian and colleagues[27] proposed miR-383 as a link between male infertility and testicular cancer, based on the findings of reduced miR-383 expression in testicular tissues of infertile patients, and in vitro effect of miR-383 on germ cell proliferation, probably via regulating the tumor suppressor gene, interferon regulator factor1 (IRF1). However, unlike the miR-371 to 373 cluster and the miR-302 to 367 cluster that are consistently linked with testicular cancer by multiple groups, the significance of miR-199a and miR-383 in this type of cancer remains to be verified by further studies.

MICRORNAS AS DIAGNOSTIC BIOMARKERS IN TESTICULAR CANCER

Traditional serum-based testicular tumor markers (AFP, HCG, LDH) have an established role in managing patients with testicular GCTs.[2] However, because only 60% of all patients with testicular GCT display elevated expression of at least one of these markers, there is clearly an unmet need for novel biomarkers with greater sensitivity and specificity. As previously discussed, patterns of miRNA deregulation in testicular cancer are highly characteristic and may therefore be used to provide enhanced prognostic and diagnostic accuracy in this context.

One of the first efforts to subdivide testicular cancers in terms of unique miRNA expression profiles came in a study by Gillis and colleagues.[19] In this study, the investigators report a high-throughput screen of 156 miRNAs in a series of type II and III GCTs using a quantitative polymerase chain reaction–based approach. Patient samples, both normal and malignant, clustered predominantly according to their maturation status. The investigators stated that this finding parallels normal embryogenesis, rather than chromosomal anomalies in the tumors. Interestingly, normal non-neoplastic testicular tissue expressed many of the discriminating miRNAs at a higher level than seminomas and spermatocytic seminomas.[19] More specifically, the miR-302 cluster was expressed in embryonic stem cells as well as in seminomas, but not in other subtypes.[19] Similar results were shown for miR-17-5p and miR-154, which were both suppressed in teratomas.[19] In addition, miR-21 and miR-155 show high expression in seminomas and type III GCTs; tumor-specific miR-19a was upregulated in seminomas and type III GCTs, and miR-29a was overexpressed in type III tumors alone. Furthermore, both miR-133a and miR-145 were downregulated in seminomas and type III GCTs compared with normal testicular tissue.[16,19] MiR-301 upregulation occurs in more differentiated tissues, such as spermatocytic seminomas, yolk sac tumors, or teratomas, and was not detectable in embryonic stem cells and embryonal carcinoma.[19] Moreover, differentiated nonseminomas showed upregulation of particular discriminating miRNAs.[19] Remarkably, this study demonstrated for the first time the potential of using miRNAs as diagnostic biomarkers to differentiate between different types of testicular cancer.

Another interesting study came from Ruf and colleagues[28] who examined blood-based rather than tissue-based miRNA signatures to differentiate between metastatic and nonmetastatic seminomas. The simplicity of blood as a specimen for biomarker analysis in patients with cancer is a great advantage and is frequently referred to by the term "liquid biopsy."[29] Ruf and colleagues[28] isolated miRNAs from a relatively small cohort of patients (n = 5) that included patients with lymph node metastases, occult and patients who were free of metastasis. They submitted these samples for miRNA next-generation sequencing. Using the patients without metastasis as the reference group, the investigators selected at least 50 reads and a difference of at least a twofold change of expression levels in the blood as their criteria for a candidate screen. Overall, 137 small RNAs fulfilled this criteria and univariate logistic regression analyses detected 35 different small RNAs that significantly discriminated patients with lymphogen/occult/combined metastasis from patients without metastasized seminoma. Interestingly, when combining 2 of these small RNAs, the investigators could completely discriminate metastasized from nonmetastasized seminoma irrespective of the metastasis subtype. Although this study provides a proof-of-principle, the true value of these diagnostic miRNAs has yet to be validated in larger prospective cohorts.

In another larger study of Gillis and colleagues,[30] conducted in 80 subjects with testicular GCTs, among 47 controls, serum levels were screened for the most promising miRNAs miR-371 to miR-373 and miR-367, which demonstrated a significant increase in their levels in patients with tumors compared with healthy subjects. The serum levels of these miRNAs were even higher in patients with metastasis than in patients with their tumors restricted only to the testis. Interestingly, patients monitored after orchiectomy had baseline tumor marker serum levels similar to healthy subjects. MiR-371 to miR-373 and miR-367 showed a sensitivity of 98%, in comparison with traditional tumor markers AFP and HCG, which had a significantly lower rate of approximately 36% and 57%.

In line with these data, Dieckmann and colleagues[31] carried out a study in 20 patients with stage I seminoma, as well as 4 with metastatic tumors before and after treatment and 17 healthy patients for controls. As in previous studies, upregulation of miR-371/-373 cluster as well as miR-302 was observed. Preoperative serum levels of each miRNA were significantly higher than those in the controls, and, following orchiectomy, serum levels of the corresponding miRNAs decreased again. Among the measured miRNAs, miR-371a-3p showed the most significant changes between preoperative increase and postoperative decrease.[31] The investigators furthermore reported a significant decrease in serum levels after the first cycle of chemotherapy in metastatic tumors.[31] This study showed impressively that circulating miRNAs are not only released from the primary tumor, but also from metastatic lesions. Again when compared with established serum markers, among the 20 patients with seminomas, only 1 of 4 responded to AFP and HCG, but 85% showed decreased expression of miR-371a-3p.[31]

Recently, Rijlaarsdam and colleagues[32] conducted a serum-based high-throughput profiling study of more than 700 miRNAs in 14 patients with seminoma, 10 without seminoma, and 11 control patients. Besides affirming the importance of miR-371/-372, several other miRNAs, including miR-511, miR-26b, miR-769, miR-23a, miR-106b, miR-365, miR-598, and miR-340, were shown to discriminate patients with testicular GCTs from healthy controls with high sensitivity/specificity.

In another study, Syring and colleagues[33] followed an interesting strategy: they used a selected panel of 7 serum miRNAs for assessing the diagnostic accuracy in a small screening cohort and then validated the most promising candidates in a larger cohort. More specifically, they used miR-302a-3p, 302b-3p, 302c-3p, 367-3p, 371a-3p, 372-3p, and 373-3p in a subcohort of 30 patients

with testicular GCT and 18 healthy subjects. Importantly, they validated their results in 76 patients treated with inguinal exploration due to suspicion of testicular GCT, of whom 59 had cancer and 17 had benign disease, and in 84 healthy male subjects. They proposed the serum levels of miR-367-3p, -371a-3p, 372-3p, and 373-3p as significantly increased in patients with testicular GCT compared with healthy individuals and patients with nonmalignant testicular disease. In particular, miR-371a-3p diagnosed testicular GCTs with a sensitivity of 84.7% and specificity of 99%, thus outperforming established markers, such as human chorionic gonadotropin or α1-fetoprotein serum. In addition, miR-367-3p was increased in nonseminoma compared with seminoma cases. Serum miRNA levels were increased in patients with advanced local stage and metastasis. In 9 patients with localized (clinical stage 1A) testicular GCT, serum miR-371a-3p levels decreased postoperatively, indicating tumor-specific release.[33] **Table 1** summarizes important miRNAs previously involved in testicular GCT.

MICRORNAS, PROGNOSIS, AND CISPLATIN-BASED TREATMENT

Testicular GCTs are chemosensitive and radiosensitive tumors and a platinum-based chemotherapy has been the mainstay of therapy for more than 2 decades.[34] In addition to cisplatin/carboplatin, testicular cancers are also sensitive to other agents, such as etoposide, ifosfamide, bleomycin, and vinblastine.[34] Depending on clinical and biological factors, approximately 80% of metastatic testicular cancers are potentially curable by administration of a combination of these agents.[34]

Several molecular factors have been proposed to explain the highly chemosensitive biological behavior of testicular cancer. These include high intratumoral levels of the proapoptotic BCL2-associated X protein, low levels of the antiapoptotic BCL2 protein, and a low frequency of mutations in the gatekeeper p53 tumor suppressor gene.

As miRNAs have been implicated in drug response and resistance mechanisms in many types of cancer,[35] it is logical to evaluate their potential as prognostic biomarkers in patients with testicular cancer in terms of predicting the response to cisplatin and other chemotherapy agents.

A study of Liu and colleagues[36] identified an association between high miR-302a expression and increased sensitivity of testicular cancer cells to cisplatin in vitro (in 2 independent cell lines, NT2

Table 1
Deregulated microRNAs in testicular cancer

Differentially Expressed microRNAs	Regulation	Reference
miR-372, miR-373	Overexpressed in seminomas, embryonal carcinomas, yolk sac tumors	Voorhoeve et al,[18] 2006 McIver et al,[16] 2012
miR-302	Overexpression in seminomas	Gillis et al,[19] 2007
miR-17-5p and miR-154	Overexpressed in teratomas	Gillis et al,[19] 2007
miR-21 and miR-155	Overexpressed in seminomas and type III tumors	Gillis et al,[19] 2007 McIver et al,[16] 2012
miR-19a	Overexpressed in seminomas and type III tumors	Gillis et al,[19] 2007 McIver et al,[16] 2012
miR-29a	Overexpressed in type III tumors	Gillis et al,[19] 2007 McIver et al,[16] 2012
miR-133a and miR-145	Downregulated in seminomas and type III tumors	Gillis et al,[19] 2007 McIver et al,[16] 2012
miR-301	Spermatocytic seminomas, yolk sac tumors, or teratomas	Gillis et al,[19] 2007

and NCCIT). MiR-302a reinforces the cisplatin-induced G2/M phase arrest, which leads to increased apoptosis rate. Moreover, miR-302a increases apoptotic susceptibility in cells after cisplatin treatment by reducing the apoptotic threshold of the cells. This effect can be partly explained by the downregulation of p21. In this context, another group demonstrated that high cytoplasmic p21 levels in testicular embryonic carcinoma cells mediate cisplatin resistance and that p21 itself seems to be regulated by miR-106b seed family members.[37]

Huang and colleagues[38] found that miR-383 inhibits the phosphorylation of H2A histone family member X (gamma-H2AX), a DNA damage marker, by targeting phosphatase 1, regulatory subunit 10 (PNUTS), which leads to cell-cycle arrest. Furthermore, forced expression of miR-383 increased the in vitro sensitivity of testicular cancer cells toward cisplatin exposure.

Summarizing the current evidence, miRNAs have the capacity to influence the sensitivity of testicular cancer to anticancer drugs. However, the clinical significance of miRNAs in testicular cancer as predictive biomarkers for drug response remains to be verified by more clinical studies.

REFERENCES

1. Siegel R, Ma J, Zou Z, et al. Cancer statistics, 2014. CA Cancer J Clin 2014;64(1):9–29.
2. Albers P, Albrecht W, Algaba F, et al. EAU guidelines on testicular cancer: 2011 update. Eur Urol 2011; 60(2):304–19.
3. Oldenburg J, Fossa SD, Nuver J, et al. Testicular seminoma and non-seminoma: ESMO Clinical Practice Guidelines for diagnosis, treatment and follow-up. Ann Oncol 2013;24(Suppl 6):vi125–32.
4. Vaughn DJ. Primum non nocere: active surveillance for clinical stage I testicular cancer. J Clin Oncol 2015;33(1):9–12.
5. Lee RC, Feinbaum RL, Ambros V. The C. elegans heterochronic gene lin-4 encodes small RNAs with antisense complementarity to lin-14. Cell 1993; 75(5):843–54.
6. Bezan A, Gerger A, Pichler M. MicroRNAs in testicular cancer: implications for pathogenesis, diagnosis, prognosis and therapy. Anticancer Res 2014;34(6):2709–13.
7. Croce CM, Calin GA. miRNAs, cancer, and stem cell division. Cell 2005;122(1):6–7.
8. Stiegelbauer V, Perakis S, Deutsch A, et al. MicroRNAs as novel predictive biomarkers and therapeutic targets in colorectal cancer. World J Gastroenterol 2014;20(33):11727–35.
9. Troppan K, Wenzl K, Deutsch A, et al. MicroRNAs in diffuse large B-cell lymphoma: implications for pathogenesis, diagnosis, prognosis and therapy. Anticancer Res 2014;34(2):557–64.
10. Vincent K, Pichler M, Lee GW, et al. MicroRNAs, genomic instability and cancer. Int J Mol Sci 2014; 15(8):14475–91.
11. Schwarzenbacher D, Balic M, Pichler M. The role of microRNAs in breast cancer stem cells. Int J Mol Sci 2013;14(7):14712–23.
12. Wagner A, Mayr C, Bach D, et al. MicroRNAs associated with the efficacy of photodynamic therapy in biliary tract cancer cell lines. Int J Mol Sci 2014; 15(11):20134–57.

13. Di Leva G, Calin GA, Croce CM. MicroRNAs: fundamental facts and involvement in human diseases. Birth Defects Res C Embryo Today 2006;78(2):180–9.

14. Ling H, Fabbri M, Calin GA. MicroRNAs and other non-coding RNAs as targets for anticancer drug development. Nat Rev Drug Discov 2013;12(11):847–65.

15. Horwich A, Shipley J, Huddart R. Testicular germ-cell cancer. Lancet 2006;367(9512):754–65.

16. McIver SC, Stanger SJ, Santarelli DM, et al. A unique combination of male germ cell miRNAs coordinates gonocyte differentiation. PLoS One 2012;7(4):e35553.

17. Novotny GW, Belling KC, Bramsen JB, et al. MicroRNA expression profiling of carcinoma in situ cells of the testis. Endocr Relat Cancer 2012;19(3):365–79.

18. Voorhoeve PM, le Sage C, Schrier M, et al. A genetic screen implicates miRNA-372 and miRNA-373 as oncogenes in testicular germ cell tumors. Cell 2006;124(6):1169–81.

19. Gillis AJ, Stoop HJ, Hersmus R, et al. High-throughput microRNAome analysis in human germ cell tumours. J Pathol 2007;213(3):319–28.

20. Barroso-del Jesus A, Lucena-Aguilar G, Menendez P. The miR-302-367 cluster as a potential stemness regulator in ESCs. Cell Cycle 2009;8(3):394–8.

21. Palmer RD, Murray MJ, Saini HK, et al. Malignant germ cell tumors display common microRNA profiles resulting in global changes in expression of messenger RNA targets. Cancer Res 2010;70(7):2911–23.

22. Murray MJ, Saini HK, van Dongen S, et al. The two most common histological subtypes of malignant germ cell tumour are distinguished by global micro-RNA profiles, associated with differential transcription factor expression. Mol Cancer 2010;9:290.

23. Zhou AD, Diao LT, Xu H, et al. beta-Catenin/LEF1 transactivates the microRNA-371-373 cluster that modulates the Wnt/beta-catenin-signaling pathway. Oncogene 2012;31(24):2968–78.

24. Stadler B, Ivanovska I, Mehta K, et al. Characterization of microRNAs involved in embryonic stem cell states. Stem Cells Dev 2010;19(7):935–50.

25. Cheung HH, Davis AJ, Lee TL, et al. Methylation of an intronic region regulates miR-199a in testicular tumor malignancy. Oncogene 2011;30(31):3404–15.

26. Gu S, Cheung HH, Lee TL, et al. Molecular mechanisms of regulation and action of microRNA-199a in testicular germ cell tumor and glioblastomas. PLoS One 2013;8(12):e83980.

27. Lian J, Tian H, Liu L, et al. Downregulation of microRNA-383 is associated with male infertility and promotes testicular embryonal carcinoma cell proliferation by targeting IRF1. Cell Death Dis 2010;1:e94.

28. Ruf CG, Dinger D, Port M, et al. Small RNAs in the peripheral blood discriminate metastasized from non-metastasized seminoma. Mol Cancer 2014;13:47.

29. Heitzer E, Auer M, Gasch C, et al. Complex tumor genomes inferred from single circulating tumor cells by array-CGH and next-generation sequencing. Cancer Res 2013;73(10):2965–75.

30. Gillis AJ, Rijlaarsdam MA, Eini R, et al. Targeted serum miRNA (TSmiR) test for diagnosis and follow-up of (testicular) germ cell cancer patients: a proof of principle. Mol Oncol 2013;7(6):1083–92.

31. Dieckmann KP, Spiekermann M, Balks T, et al. MicroRNAs miR-371-3 in serum as diagnostic tools in the management of testicular germ cell tumours. Br J Cancer 2012;107(10):1754–60.

32. Rijlaarsdam MA, van Agthoven T, Gillis AJ, et al. Identification of known and novel germ cell cancer-specific (embryonic) miRs in serum by high-throughput profiling. Andrology 2015;3(1):85–91.

33. Syring I, Bartels J, Holdenrieder S, et al. Circulating serum miRNA (miR-367-3p, miR-371a-3p, miR-372-3p and miR-373-3p) as biomarkers in patients with testicular germ cell cancer. J Urol 2015;193(1):331–7.

34. Killock D. Chemotherapy. After 25 years, therapy for poor-prognosis GCTs advances. Nat Rev Clin Oncol 2015;12(1):3.

35. Pichler M, Winter E, Stotz M, et al. Down-regulation of KRAS-interacting miRNA-143 predicts poor prognosis but not response to EGFR-targeted agents in colorectal cancer. Br J Cancer 2012;106(11):1826–32.

36. Liu L, Lian J, Zhang H, et al. MicroRNA-302a sensitizes testicular embryonal carcinoma cells to cisplatin-induced cell death. J Cell Physiol 2013;228(12):2294–304.

37. Koster R, di Pietro A, Timmer-Bosscha H, et al. Cytoplasmic p21 expression levels determine cisplatin resistance in human testicular cancer. J Clin Invest 2010;120(10):3594–605.

38. Huang H, Tian H, Duan Z, et al. microRNA-383 impairs phosphorylation of H2AX by targeting PNUTS and inducing cell cycle arrest in testicular embryonal carcinoma cells. Cell Signal 2014;26(5):903–11.

The Emerging Role and Promise of Biomarkers in Penile Cancer

Camille Vuichoud, MD, Julia Klap, MD,
Kevin R. Loughlin, MD, MBA*

KEYWORDS

- Penile • Biomarkers • Prognostic • Molecular • Squamous cell carcinoma

KEY POINTS

- Penile cancer is a rare malignancy, making it difficult to extrapolate the results of many investigations in this domain.
- There is no reliable biomarker routinely available to help clinicians predict outcomes and select patients for further treatment after excision of the primary lesion.
- Knowledge of the link between human papillomavirus (HPV) and carcinogenesis of penile cancer is improving, allowing better identification of the prognostic significance of HPV.
- Other promising markers are under investigation, including plasmatic SCC and cytogenetic markers.

INTRODUCTION
Epidemiology

Penile carcinoma is a rare disease, accounting for only 1640 new cases diagnosed in the United States in 2014.[1] The incidence is higher among men in developing countries of Asia, South America, and Africa. Risk factors for penile carcinoma include chronic inflammation, lichen sclerosis, phimosis, and tobacco use[2]; one-third of cases can be attributed to human papillomavirus (HPV) infection.[3] Because of its localization, this malignancy can be a source of potentially devastating psychosexual distress, in addition to the other factors associated with malignancies.

Pathology

Penile squamous cell carcinoma (pSCC) is the most common malignant disease of the penis, accounting for more than 95% of cases of penile carcinomas. The American Joint Committee of Cancer recognizes 4 subtypes of SCC:

- Verrucous
- Papillary squamous
- Warty
- Basaloid

The verrucous subtype is known to be of low malignant potential, whereas the other types have a worse prognosis.

Management

The current guidelines of the American Urologic Association recommend a surgical amputation of the primary tumor. Prognostic factors after treating the primary lesions mainly depend on the presence of regional lymph nodes metastases (LNM), which are found in 25% of men at presentation.[4,5] Hence, establishing the lymph node status for

The authors have nothing to disclose.
Division of Urology, Brigham and Women's Hospital, Harvard Medical School, 45 Francis Street, Boston, MA 02115, USA
* Corresponding author.
E-mail address: KLOUGHLIN@PARTNERS.ORG

urologic.theclinics.com

each patient is relevant at baseline to determine the prognosis and, thus, the need for further treatment and following.

The biology of pSCC is such that it exhibits a prolonged locoregional phase before distant dissemination, also providing a rationale for the therapeutic value of lymphadenectomy, what has demonstrated survival benefits.[6] Yet, it has been suggested that 20% of men with pSCC have nodal metastases that are not clinically evident at the time of initial presentation.[7]

Clinical examination to determine the lymph node status is unreliable in inguinal lymph nodes; the incidence of occulted metastases varies between 2% and 66%.[8] The sensitivity and specificity of computed tomography or MRI are not sufficient as 50% of enlarged nodes show no malignancy.[9] Other methods like the PET with fludeoxyglucose 18 scanner have been suggested for nodal staging, but the results have been inconclusive. Minimally invasive techniques, such as fine-needle biopsy or sentinel node biopsy, have been used for nodal staging.[7,10] Based on recent results, dynamic sentinel lymph node biopsy (DSNB), which relies on the injection of the primary lesion with blue dye and a radioactive tracer, was shown to have a false-negative rate of 7.0% and a complication rate of 4.7%.[11] Association with fine-needle aspiration of suspicious lymph nodes can help to improve DSNB sensitivity. But these techniques require a multidisciplinary team consisting of urologists, nuclear medicine physicians, and pathologists in addition to specialized equipment and training.[12] So far, the gold standard to determine the inguinal lymph node status is inguinal lymph node resection, which is an invasive procedure associated with significant morbidity.[13] Even if the therapeutic benefits outweigh these complications for patients who have lymph node involvement, only 20% of those with clinically nonpalpable lymph nodes will harbor occult metastasis.

To select candidates for inguinal lymphadenectomy for patients with clinically negative inguinal nodes, guidelines[3] are mainly based on primary penile histology, including stage, lymphovascular invasion, and grade of primary tumor[14]; but a recent prospective study stipulates that these criteria alone are still insufficient, with many patients (82%) being subjected to unnecessary lymphadenectomy with this method of selection.[15]

These limitations to penile cancer stage provide the underpinning for the identification of more reliable penile cancer biomarkers.

Currently, there are no existing biomarkers for pSCC routinely available; but ongoing research has identified biomarkers, which can be classified into several types:

- Plasmatic biomarkers
- Proliferation associated markers
- HPV-related markers
- P53
- Cytogenetic markers

PLASMATIC BIOMARKERS
Squamous Cell Carcinoma Antigen

Squamous cell carcinoma antigen (SCCAg) is a tumor-associated glycoprotein and a member of the serine protease inhibitor family. It can be measured using a microparticle enzyme immunoassay. In cervical and anal carcinoma, SCCAg has been successfully used in both staging and following the course of the disease.[16,17]

There are few clinical studies examining the reliability of SCCAg in penile cancer.

Laniado and colleagues[18] found that SCCAg was elevated in patients with LNM and demonstrated that an elevated SCCAg level had a sensitivity of 57% and a specificity of 100% for predicting nodal metastases at the 1.50 μg/L cutoff. This same study demonstrated that SCCAg was a useful tool in following patients after excision of the primary lesion. In this study, levels of SCCAg increased exponentially in patients who subsequently developed nodal metastases and before any clinical or radiological evidence of nodal involvement.

More recently, a prospective study evaluated the clinical use of SCCAg in 16 patients with penile cancer and suggested that the sequential measurement of plasma SCCAg might indicate the presence of LNMs and/or distant metastases before they are detected clinically or by imaging, allowing early and potentially curative inguinal nodes dissections. It also demonstrated that SCCAg was useful for monitoring patients' response to treatment.[19]

In a larger series including 54 patients, Hungerhuber and colleagues[20] reported a correlation between tumor burden and SCCAg, which increased significantly with extensive lymph node involvement and metastatic disease. They also reported that SCCAg was powerful for monitoring treatment control and early detection of recurrence after treatment.

The prospective series of Zhu and colleagues,[21] based on the data of 63 patients with penile cancer, showed that despite the confirmation that SCCAg is significantly associated with nodal status, it could not accurately predict the presence of occult inguinal metastasis. These investigators further demonstrated that SCCAg was an independent prognostic factor in node positive cases and was an important predictor of progression-free survival in patients with penile cancer.

However, despite these promising results, these data are not yet sufficient to include the use of SCCAg in the guidelines for the management of patients with penile cancer, primarily because of the low number of patients involved in theses studies. It seems that SCCAg correlates with tumor burden and is useful for following the disease course and detecting early recurrence. Regarding the ability of this biomarker to predict the presence of occult LNM, data are controversial. There is a need for a larger prospective study to ascertain the clinical utility of this biomarker.

C-Reactive Protein

C-reactive protein (CRP) is a protein produced by the liver in response to microbial infection, trauma, infarction, autoimmune diseases, or malignancies. Its production occurs in response to an inflammatory stimulus involving increased cytokine expression[22]; it is already a cheap, simple, and routinely performed marker for infection. Various mechanisms can explain the elevation of CRP during malignancies: inflammation caused by tumor growth, immune response to tumor antigen, or the chronic inflammation itself, which can be an etiologic factor for carcinogenesis.[23]

High levels of plasma CRP have been linked to a poor prognosis in various cancers, including urologic cancers, such as renal cell carcinoma and urothelial carcinoma.[24,25]

Recently, Saito and Kihara[26] suggested that CRP could be a useful biomarker for many urologic cancers and that the analysis of dynamic changes in CRP concentrations over time could predict tumor aggressiveness and potential treatment efficacy.

Two studies evaluated CRP blood levels as a prognostic marker in penile cancer. Steffens and colleagues,[27] in a retrospective study counting 79 patients with penile cancer, found that an elevated preoperative serum CRP level is significantly associated with reduced cancer-specific survival but failed to define CRP as an independent prognostic factor.

Another retrospective study based on data from 51 patients found that CRP serum level correlated significantly with LNM.[28]

These preliminary data based on retrospective studies suggest that CRP could be an interesting noninvasive prognostic marker and that it could help identify patients with pSCC who may benefit from an inguinal lymph nodes dissection. This finding needs to be confirmed by further studies.

PROLIFERATION ASSOCIATED BIOMARKERS
Ki-67

Ki-67 is a nonhistone nuclear matrix protein expressed in all cell-cycle phases except G0. An assessment of Ki-67 protein expression is a reliable mean of the evaluation of tumor cell proliferation.[29] It has already been found as a prognostic factor in various cancers,[30] but the data remain controversial in the case of penile carcinoma.

In a retrospective study of 44 samples of pSCC, there was a significant association only between Ki-67 and tumor grade and a tendency toward higher Ki labeling index with tumor stage, nodal metastasis, and clinical disease progression.[31] In a larger retrospective study on 148 patients, Stankiewicz and colleagues[32] found a similar significant association between Ki-67 and tumor grade but failed to find an association with LNM or survival. Similarly, in the larger multicentric study with 153 patients with pSCC,[33] it has been found that Ki-67, even if it reflects a more aggressive behavior with a positive correlation with histologic tumor grade, is not an independent prognostic factor for the cancer-specific survival.

For instance, only one small study found a positive association between Ki-67 and LNM.[34] Conversely, Guimarães and colleagues[35] found an inverse association between LNM and the Ki-67 expression level in both univariate and multivariate analysis.

According to these results, Ki-67 seems to have a positive correlation with tumor grade; but its prognostic value for LNM or survival remains elusive.

Proliferating Cell Nuclear Antigen

Proliferating cell nuclear antigen (PCNA) is a protein found in the nucleus and is essential for replication. Thus, it is as Ki-67, a marker of cell proliferation, which has also been studied in penile cancer. In a quantitative analysis, Martins and colleagues[36] found that PCNA expression was significantly associated with LNM but did not find a correlation between PCNA immune expression and prognosis.

More recently, in a study of 125 patients with penile carcinoma, Guimarães and colleagues[35] found that PCNA was an independent prognostic factor for LNM but not survival.

There are few data on the prognostic significance of this biomarker; it is important to mention that there are no standardizations in the execution and interpretation of PCNA, making comparison of results challenging.

HUMAN PAPILLOMAVIRUS

Human Papillomavirus: a Risk Factor for Penile Cancer

HPV is a family of double-stranded DNA viruses, which is generally sexually transmitted. It is associated with several malignancies, including cancer of the penis, cervix, anus, and oropharynx; it seems to be an important factor in the development of in situ and invasive epithelial tumors.[37]

It is estimated that one-third of pSCCs can be attributed to HPV-related carcinogenesis.[3] The reported prevalence of HPV DNA in penile cancer ranges between 20% and 80%, this variation is likely due to the method used for the detection and the geographic variance.[38]

It has been established that prevalence varies with histologic subtype: high HPV prevalence is found in basaloid subtypes and warty pSCCs, whereas verrucous and papillary pSCCs are associated with HPV in one-third of cases.[39]

Thus, it has been suggested that penile carcinogenesis can follow 2 distinct pathways: one associated by HPV infection and the other related to nonviral factors, such as phimosis, chronic inflammation, or lichen sclerosus.[39,40]

Studies have demonstrated that HPV 16 and 18 are the most common types of HPV found in penile cancer.[41]

The studies on cervical SCC have provided the most convincing model for understanding the molecular mechanism by which HPV promotes carcinogenesis. It seems to rely on the integration of the viral genome into the host cell's chromosomal DNA. It results in an overexpression of 2 viral oncogenes, E6 and E7, which disturb cellular differentiation, proliferation, and apoptosis through their involvement with p53 tumor suppressor and the retinoblastoma RbE2F, which in turn leads to accumulation of P16^{INK4a}.[42] This is thought to be the most likely mechanism of HPV-related penile cancer.

Human Papillomavirus: Prognostic Marker for Penile Cancer

Prognostic marker for survival

HPV status has proven to be a significant prognostic factor for survival and therapeutic response in some head and neck SCCs,[43,44] and a similar trend can be reasonably expected in penile carcinomas. However, although HPV has been associated with high-grade tumors,[45] the impact on outcomes is unclear.

Several studies did not find any correlation between HPV infection and survival.[46–48] Hernandez and colleagues[48] did not find any relation between HPV status and survival in a cohort of 79 cases, neither did Bezerra colleagues[47] after analyzing the data on a group of 82 patients.

Lont and colleagues[49] reported a controversial study in a large cohort of 176 patients with pSCC. In this series, HPV positivity was linked to favorable outcomes with improved disease-specific survival. These results were recently confirmed in a Dutch cohort of 212 penile cancer cases.[50]

Interpretation of these studies should be made with caution. Further evaluation and confirmation studies must be performed before any reliable conclusion can be made about the presence of HPV as a prognostic marker for survival in pSCC.[38]

Prognostic factors for lymph node metastasis

Although an association has been found between HPV status and lymphatic embolization, Bezerra and colleagues[47] did not find any association between HPV status and LNM. Similarly, 2 other studies[49,51] found that the isolated presence of HPV DNA cannot be considered as a predictive variable for LNM.

Thus, available data suggest no association between HPV detection and the presence of LNM.

The Prognostic Significance of a Human Papillomavirus Marker: P16^{INK4a}

P16^{INK4a} is a tumor suppressor gene that induces cell cycle arrest and prevents cell division by G1 cyclin-dependent kinase 4 and 6 inhibition. It is known to accumulate in HPV-related tumors, in response to inactivation due to viral E7 protein, and seems to be a reliable marker for high-risk HPV infection in pSCC cases.[40,52,53] However, recent studies have stipulated that this diagnosis must be confirmed by P16^{INK4a} immunostaining that is diffuse, continuous, and strongly nuclear and cytoplasmic.[54,55]

As a marker of the presence of HPV, and because of the promising prognostic value of HPV in penile cancer, P16^{INK4A} has been thought to have a prognostic significance in this disease. In a small series, Ferrándiz-Pulido and colleagues[56] found a tendency toward a positive association between P16^{INK4a} overexpression and a better prognosis. This finding is supported by a multi-institutional study including 92 cases of pSCC that found that P16^{INK4a} independently predicted improved cancer-specific survival.[57] Similarly, a Canadian study of 43 cases found that the lack of p16 immunostaining was an independent factor for decreased survival.[58] Recently, Steinestel and colleagues[55] confirmed that P16^{INK4a} and high-risk HPV status indicated a less aggressive behavior but failed to provide prognostic contribution of P16[INK4a] status for node involvement or survival.

This prognostic role might be explained by its implication in cell cycle control, notably by mediating G1 arrest; this could explain the positive significance in terms of prognosis of HPV positivity found in some of the studies mentioned earlier.

Regarding the association between P16[INK4a] and lymph node status, Poetsch and colleagues[59] found an inverse relation, with a lack of P16[INK4a] predicting an increased risk of LNM.

In a retrospective cohort including 119 patients, Tang and colleagues[60] found that a lack of P16[INK4a] expression was significantly associated with recurrences only when there were positive lymph nodes found at diagnosis. Despite the large number of cases, they failed to find an association with survival. This finding suggests that P16[INK4a] could have an important role in the subgroup of patients with positive lymph nodes at baseline to predict the prognosis and help determine the choice of further treatment.

These results support the fact that this protein marker could be an important prognostic marker regarding the natural history of the disease, with the limitation that all these studies used a variable definition of P16[INK4a] positivity.[60]

P53
Is There a Link Between p53 and Human Papillomavirus Infection?

Inactivation of the tumor suppressor gene is a crucial step in cell transformation leading to oncogenesis. The tumor suppressor gene TP53, located in the short arm of chromosome 17, is known to be mutated in approximately 70% of adult solid tumors[61]; the protein p53 has been implicated in the pathogenesis of numerous tumors.[62]

Mutation in the TP53 gene results in an anomalous protein in 90% of cases or an absence of protein in 10% of cases. In cases of the mutated protein, it accumulates in the nucleus of tumor cells and can be identified by an immunohistochemical reaction.[63] However, in cases of HPV infection, the HPV oncogenic product E6 inactivates p53 expression and induces its degradation; thus, it is thought that p53 immuno-expression is regulated in HPV-induced penile cancer.[64] Several studies have investigated the relationship between p53 expression and HPV infection.

p53 overexpression or mutation have been reported to vary between 26% and 91% in penile carcinoma[51,65–67] with a suggested positive correlation with HPV infection.[65,66] However, several reports have shown an inverse or a negative relationship between p53 expression and HPV status.[68,69] Others have found that p53 overexpression can be found in HPV-positive and HPV-negative tumors, suggesting that the 2 pathways mentioned earlier are not mutually exclusive.[58]

The Prognostic Role of p53 in Penile Cancer

Lopes and colleagues[51] reported data on 82 patients who were primarily treated for pSCC with penile amputation and bilateral lymphadenectomy and found that p53 positivity was an independent prognostic factor for LNM. Similarly, Martins and colleagues[36] found that there was a positive association between p53 immunostaining and LNM and cancer-specific survival. This finding was confirmed by Gunia and colleagues[70] who found that p53 expression represented an adverse prognostic sign in terms of cancer-specific survival.

More interestingly, Zhu and colleagues[21] found that p53 positivity was an independent prognostic factor for LNM and survival, even in patients with positive nodal disease; moreover, in a subgroup analysis, they found that it had a predictive role for T1 patients, helping to distinguish those at risk for LNM.

On the other hand, Bethune and colleagues[58] did not find a significant association between p53 and survival or LNM.

Despite these promising results, the variability in the sampling method and lack of standardization of the p53 positives threshold in theses studies make it difficult to conclude a direct correlation between p53 status and the prognosis of pSCC.

CYTOGENETIC MARKERS
Genetic Imbalances

Genetic imbalance in penile carcinoma was first described by Alves and colleagues[71] based on an analysis of 23 samples of penile carcinoma by comparative genomic hybridization. Recently, Busso-Lopes and colleagues[72] evaluated DNA copy-number alteration by comparative genomic hybridization with the aim to define some novel prognostic molecular markers. They reported findings where copy-number alterations of 3p, 3q, and 8p were related to a worse prognosis as well as reduced cancer-specific survival and disease-free survival. This association between genomic alteration and poor prognosis may help to select patients who might require adjuvant treatment.

Among these copy-number alterations, amplification of the MYC gene was identified, which has been investigated by several teams. The MYC gene is a proto-oncogene, located in the 8q24 chromosome, encoding a transcription factor that seems to regulate cellular proliferation, differentiation, and apoptosis.[73] MYC gene gain and amplification have been described in several tumors, and frequent integration of HPV DNA at the 8q24 locus in cancer of the cervix has been reported.[74] Similarly, MYC gene gains have been described in pSCC,[71] with a likely direct activation of MYC by HPV.[74] More interesting, Masferrer and colleagues[75] found an increase in MYC numerical aberration, in parallel to the progression of pSCC from in situ carcinoma to metastasis, a fact that seems to be independent from HPV status. They also noted that a high copy number of MYC was significantly associated with poor cancer-specific outcomes. Busso-Lopes and colleagues[72] confirmed an increased MYC gene amplification in pSCC without any correlation with HPV infection but did not find any prognostic significance for this genomic alteration.

According to one study, another type of genetic imbalance, loss of heterozygosity (LOH) on chromosome 6, 9, and 12, has been found to be associated with metastasis and stage.[76] Moreover, in this study, the allelic loss in the chromosomal loci 6p22 to 23 was significantly associated with a poor prognosis among patients with penile cancer.[76] These results suggest the presence of an important tumor suppressor gene in this region and the potential prognostic value of detecting LOH in penile cancer.

According to these observations, the role of cytogenetic change in clinical management of patients with pSCC seems promising as potential prognostic markers but requires further investigation.

Epigenetic Modifications

Epigenetic modifications are potentially reversible alterations, such as DNA methylation, histone modifications, and regulation by noncoding RNA-regulated gene expression, which can play a key role in malignant transformation. Thus far, the data on epigenetic alterations and their significance in penile cancer outcomes are limited.[77]

In penile cancer, one of the most studied epigenetic alterations is the hypermethylation of the CDKN2A gene promoter, which is present in 0% to 42% of samples.[77] The CDKN2A locus encodes 2 tumor suppressor proteins, including P16^{INK4A}.

The epigenetic inactivation of the thrombospondin-1 gene by hypermethylation seems to confer prognostic significance in only one study (n = 24).[78]

Promising results were presented by Feber and colleagues,[79] who evaluated the methylation profile of 38 pSCC samples. They identified epi-signatures related to HPV status and found an epigenetic signature associated with LNM, with a predicative accuracy of 93%. The predicative accuracy of this 4-gene epi-signature has been successfully confirmed in an independent cohort with results that seem at least comparable with the sensitivity of sentinel lymph node biopsy.

Kuasne and colleagues[80] found a different methylation profile according to histologic grade. They found that low BDNF gene methylation was associated with LNM and a shorter disease-specific survival, but this was not confirmed on multivariate analysis. This association would require additional study to evaluate BDNF as a potential prognostic molecular marker for pSCC.

SUMMARY/DISCUSSION

We are in a period of change in the management of malignancies. The discovery of new biomarkers offers the possibility of a personalized medicine, based on the molecular and genetics of each tumor. These innovations would allow more appropriate treatment tailored to the individual tumors and patients.

Current methods available to predict outcomes are suboptimal, and there is a need to develop new noninvasive markers for penile cancer. Several promising biomarkers for penile cancer have been investigated; but none can be included in the current nomogram,[81] mainly because of a lack of power of these studies due to the relative low incidence of this tumor.

The development of the International Penile Cancer Trial,[82] a collaborative multinational clinical study under the initiative of the International Rare Cancer Initiative, is the first step toward a collaborative initiative. This project involves investigators from Europe, Canada, the United States, and South America and has the aim to study a different multimodal therapeutic approach in the treatment of pSCC. In the future, it will be important to create molecular and translational research collaborations, notably with the formation of a centralized tumor bank.[82] Such multi-institutional collaborations offer the best opportunity for improved penile cancer biomarkers in the future.

REFERENCES

1. American Cancer Society: cancer facts and figures 2014. Available at: http://www.cancer.org/research/cancerfactsstatistics/cancerfactsfigures2014/. Accessed May 25, 2015.
2. Daling JR, Madeleine MM, Johnson LG, et al. Penile cancer: importance of circumcision, human papillomavirus and smoking in in situ and invasive disease. Int J Cancer 2005;116:606–16.

3. Hakenberg OW, Compérat EM, Minhas S, et al. EAU guidelines on penile cancer: 2014 update. Eur Urol 2015;67:142–50.

4. Solsona E, Iborra I, Rubio J, et al. Prospective validation of the association of local tumor stage and grade as a predictive factor for occult lymph node micrometastasis in patients with penile carcinoma and clinically negative inguinal lymph nodes. J Urol 2001;165:1506–9.

5. Horenblas S. Lymphadenectomy for squamous cell carcinoma of the penis. Part 1: diagnosis of lymph node metastasis. BJU Int 2001;88:467–72.

6. Kroon BK, Horenblas S, Lont AP, et al. Patients with penile carcinoma benefit from immediate resection of clinically occult lymph node metastases. J Urol 2005;173:816–9.

7. Graafland NM, Lam W, Leijte JA, et al. Prognostic factors for occult inguinal lymph node involvement in penile carcinoma and assessment of the high-risk EAU subgroup: a two-institution analysis of 342 clinically node-negative patients. Eur Urol 2010;58:742–7.

8. Horenblas S, Van Tinteren H, Delemarre JF, et al. Squamous cell carcinoma of the penis: accuracy of tumor, nodes and metastasis classification system, and role of lymphangiography, computerized tomography scan and fine needle aspiration cytology. J Urol 1991;146:1279–83.

9. Persky L, deKernion J. Carcinoma of the penis. CA Cancer J Clin 1986;36:258–73.

10. Hughes B, Leijte J, Shabbir M, et al. Non-invasive and minimally invasive staging of regional lymph nodes in penile cancer. World J Urol 2009;27:197–203.

11. Yeung LL, Brandes SB. Dynamic sentinel lymph node biopsy as the new paradigm for the management of penile cancer. Urol Oncol 2013;31:693–6.

12. Pettaway CA, Crook J, Hegarty PK, et al. Penile cancer update 2011: a case-based approach. Urol Oncol 2012;30:956–8.

13. Bevan-Thomas R, Slaton JW, Pettaway CA. Contemporary morbidity from lymphadenectomy for penile squamous cell carcinoma: the M.D. Anderson Cancer Center Experience. J Urol 2002;167:1638–42.

14. McDougal WS. Advances in the treatment of carcinoma of the penis. Urology 2005;66:114–7.

15. Hegarty PK, Kayes O, Freeman A, et al. A prospective study of 100 cases of penile cancer managed according to European Association of Urology guidelines. BJU Int 2006;98:526–31.

16. Petrelli NJ, Palmer M, Herrera L, et al. The utility of squamous cell carcinoma antigen for the follow-up of patients with squamous cell carcinoma of the anal canal. Cancer 1992;70:35–9.

17. Maruo T, Yoshida S, Samoto T, et al. Factors regulating SCC antigen expression in squamous cell carcinoma of the uterine cervix. Tumour Biol 1998;19:494–504.

18. Laniado ME, Lowdell C, Mitchell H, et al. Squamous cell carcinoma antigen: a role in the early identification of nodal metastases in men with squamous cell carcinoma of the penis. BJU Int 2003;92:248–50.

19. Touloupidis S, Zisimopoulos A, Giannakopoulos S, et al. Clinical usage of the squamous cell carcinoma antigen in patients with penile cancer. Int J Urol 2007;14:174–6.

20. Hungerhuber E, Schlenker B, Schneede P, et al. Squamous cell carcinoma antigen correlates with tumor burden but lacks prognostic potential for occult lymph node metastases in penile cancer. Urology 2007;70:975–9.

21. Zhu Y, Ye DW, Yao XD, et al. The value of squamous cell carcinoma antigen in the prognostic evaluation, treatment monitoring and follow-up of patients with penile cancer. J Urol 2008;180:2019–23.

22. Pepys MB, Hirschfield GM. C-reactive protein: a critical update. J Clin Invest 2003;111:1805–12.

23. Heikkilä K, Ebrahim S, Lawlor DA. A systematic review of the association between circulating concentrations of C reactive protein and cancer. J Epidemiol Community Health 2007;61:824–33.

24. Yoshida S, Saito K, Koga F, et al. C-reactive protein level predicts prognosis in patients with muscle-invasive bladder cancer treated with chemoradiotherapy. BJU Int 2008;101:978–81.

25. Hu Q, Gou Y, Sun C, et al. The prognostic value of C-reactive protein in renal cell carcinoma: a systematic review and meta-analysis. Urol Oncol 2014;32:50.e1–8.

26. Saito K, Kihara K. C-reactive protein as a biomarker for urological cancers. Nat Rev Urol 2011;8:659–66.

27. Steffens S, Al Ghazal A, Steinestel J, et al. High CRP values predict poor survival in patients with penile cancer. BMC Cancer 2013;13:223.

28. Al Ghazal A, Steffens S, Steinestel J, et al. Elevated C-reactive protein values predict nodal metastasis in patients with penile cancer. BMC Urol 2013;13:53.

29. Scholzen T, Gerdes J. The Ki-67 protein: from the known and the unknown. J Cell Physiol 2000;182:311–22.

30. Scholzen T, Endl E, Wohlenberg C, et al. The Ki-67 protein interacts with members of the heterochromatin protein 1 (HP1) family: a potential role in the regulation of higher-order chromatin structure. J Pathol 2002;196:135–44.

31. Berdjis N, Meye A, Nippgen J, et al. Expression of Ki-67 in squamous cell carcinoma of the penis. BJU Int 2005;96:146–8.

32. Stankiewicz E, Ng M, Cuzick J, et al. The prognostic value of Ki-67 expression in penile squamous cell carcinoma. J Clin Pathol 2012;65:534–7.

33. May M, Burger M, Otto W, et al. Ki-67, mini-chromosome maintenance 2 protein (MCM2) and geminin have no independent prognostic relevance for cancer-specific survival in surgically treated

squamous cell carcinoma of the penis. BJU Int 2013; 112:E383–90.

34. Protzel C, Knoedel J, Zimmermann U, et al. Expression of proliferation marker Ki67 correlates to occurrence of metastasis and prognosis, histological subtypes and HPV DNA detection in penile carcinomas. Histol Histopathol 2007;22:1197–204.

35. Guimarães GC, Leal ML, Campos RS, et al. Do proliferating cell nuclear antigen and MIB-1/Ki-67 have prognostic value in penile squamous cell carcinoma? Urology 2007;70:137–42.

36. Martins ACP, Faria SM, Cologna AJ, et al. Immunoexpression of p53 protein and proliferating cell nuclear antigen in penile carcinoma. J Urol 2002; 167:89–92 [discussion: 92–3].

37. Walboomers JM, Jacobs MV, Manos MM, et al. Human papillomavirus is a necessary cause of invasive cervical cancer worldwide. J Pathol 1999; 189:12–9.

38. Muneer A, Kayes O, Ahmed HU, et al. Molecular prognostic factors in penile cancer. World J Urol 2009;27:161–7.

39. Rubin MA, Kleter B, Zhou M, et al. Detection and typing of human papillomavirus DNA in penile carcinoma: evidence for multiple independent pathways of penile carcinogenesis. Am J Pathol 2001;159: 1211–8.

40. Mannweiler S, Sygulla S, Winter E, et al. Two major pathways of penile carcinogenesis: HPV-induced penile cancers overexpress p16ink4a, HPV-negative cancers associated with dermatoses express p53, but lack p16ink4a overexpression. J Am Acad Dermatol 2013;69:73–81.

41. Heideman DA, Waterboer T, Pawlita M, et al. Human papillomavirus-16 is the predominant type etiologically involved in penile squamous cell carcinoma. J Clin Oncol 2007;25:4550–6.

42. Ferreux E, Lont AP, Horenblas S, et al. Evidence for at least three alternative mechanisms targeting the p16INK4A/cyclin D/Rb pathway in penile carcinoma, one of which is mediated by high-risk human papillomavirus. J Pathol 2003;201:109–18.

43. Ang KK, Harris J, Wheeler R, et al. Human papillomavirus and survival of patients with oropharyngeal cancer. N Engl J Med 2010;363:24–35.

44. Lassen P. The role of human papillomavirus in head and neck cancer and the impact on radiotherapy outcome. Radiother Oncol 2010;95:371–80.

45. Gregoire L, Cubilla AL, Reuter VE, et al. Preferential association of human papillomavirus with high-grade histologic variants of penile-invasive squamous cell carcinoma. J Natl Cancer Inst 1995;87: 1705–9.

46. Wiener JS, Effert PJ, Humphrey PA, et al. Prevalence of human papillomavirus types 16 and 18 in squamous-cell carcinoma of the penis: a retrospective analysis of primary and metastatic lesions by differential polymerase chain reaction. Int J Cancer 1992;50:694–701.

47. Bezerra AL, Lopes A, Santiago GH, et al. Human papillomavirus as a prognostic factor in carcinoma of the penis: analysis of 82 patients treated with amputation and bilateral lymphadenectomy. Cancer 2001;91:2315–21.

48. Hernandez BY, Goodman MT, Unger ER, et al. Human papillomavirus genotype prevalence in invasive penile cancers from a registry-based United States population. Front Oncol 2014;4:9.

49. Lont AP, Kroon BK, Horenblas S, et al. Presence of high-risk human papillomavirus DNA in penile carcinoma predicts favorable outcome in survival. Int J Cancer 2006;119:1078–81.

50. Djajadiningrat RS, Jordanova ES, Kroon BK, et al. Human papillomavirus prevalence in invasive penile cancer and association with clinical outcome. J Urol 2015;193:526–31.

51. Lopes A, Bezerra AL, Pinto CA, et al. p53 as a new prognostic factor for lymph node metastasis in penile carcinoma: analysis of 82 patients treated with amputation and bilateral lymphadenectomy. J Urol 2002;168:81–6.

52. Cubilla AL, Lloveras B, Alejo M, et al. Value of p16(INK)4(a) in the pathology of invasive penile squamous cell carcinomas: a report of 202 cases. Am J Surg Pathol 2011;35:253–61.

53. Chaux A, Cubilla AL, Haffner MC, et al. Combining routine morphology, p16(INK4a) immunohistochemistry, and in situ hybridization for the detection of human papillomavirus infection in penile carcinomas: a tissue microarray study using classifier performance analyses. Urol Oncol 2014;32: 171–7.

54. Darragh TM, Colgan TJ, Thomas Cox J, et al. The lower anogenital squamous terminology standardization project for HPV-associated lesions: background and consensus recommendations from the College of American Pathologists and the American Society for Colposcopy and Cervical Pathology. Int J Gynecol Pathol 2013;32:76–115.

55. Steinestel J, Al Ghazal A, Arndt A, et al. The role of histologic subtype, p16(INK4a) expression, and presence of human papillomavirus DNA in penile squamous cell carcinoma. BMC Cancer 2015;15:220.

56. Ferrándiz-Pulido C, Masferrer E, de Torres I, et al. Identification and genotyping of human papillomavirus in a Spanish cohort of penile squamous cell carcinomas: correlation with pathologic subtypes, p16(INK4a) expression, and prognosis. J Am Acad Dermatol 2013;68:73–82.

57. Gunia S, Erbersdobler A, Hakenberg OW, et al. p16(INK4a) is a marker of good prognosis for primary invasive penile squamous cell carcinoma: a multi-institutional study. J Urol 2012;187:899–907.

58. Bethune G, Campbell J, Rocker A, et al. Clinical and pathologic factors of prognostic significance in penile squamous cell carcinoma in a North American population. Urology 2012;79:1092–7.

59. Poetsch M, Hemmerich M, Kakies C, et al. Alterations in the tumor suppressor gene p16(INK4A) are associated with aggressive behavior of penile carcinomas. Virchows Arch 2011;458:221–9.

60. Tang DH, Clark PE, Giannico G, et al. Lack of P16ink4a over expression in penile squamous cell carcinoma is associated with recurrence after lymph node dissection. J Urol 2015;193:519–25.

61. Hollstein M, Sidransky D, Vogelstein B, et al. p53 mutations in human cancers. Science 1991;253:49–53.

62. Vogelstein B, Kinzler KW. p53 function and dysfunction. Cell 1992;70:523–6.

63. Rogel A, Popliker M, Webb CG, et al. p53 cellular tumor antigen: analysis of mRNA levels in normal adult tissues, embryos, and tumors. Mol Cell Biol 1985;5:2851–5.

64. Hafkamp HC, Speel EJ, Haesevoets A, et al. A subset of head and neck squamous cell carcinomas exhibits integration of HPV 16/18 DNA and overexpression of p16INK4A and p53 in the absence of mutations in p53 exons 5-8. Int J Cancer 2003;107:394–400.

65. Levi JE, Rahal P, Sarkis AS, et al. Human papillomavirus DNA and p53 status in penile carcinomas. Int J Cancer 1998;76:779–83.

66. Lam KY, Chan AC, Chan KW, et al. Expression of p53 and its relationship with human papillomavirus in penile carcinomas. Eur J Surg Oncol 1995;21:613–6.

67. Gentile V, Vicini P, Giacomelli L, et al. Detection of human papillomavirus DNA, p53 and ki67 expression in penile carcinomas. Int J Immunopathol Pharmacol 2006;19:209–15.

68. Pilotti S, Donghi R, D'Amato L, et al. HPV detection and p53 alteration in squamous cell verrucous malignancies of the lower genital tract. Diagn Mol Pathol 1993;2:248–56.

69. Ranki A, Lassus J, Niemi KM. Relation of p53 tumor suppressor protein expression to human papillomavirus (HPV) DNA and to cellular atypia in male genital warts and in premalignant lesions. Acta Derm Venereol 1995;75:180–6.

70. Gunia S, Kakies C, Erbersdobler A, et al. Expression of p53, p21 and cyclin D1 in penile cancer: p53 predicts poor prognosis. J Clin Pathol 2012;65:232–6.

71. Alves G, Heller A, Fiedler W, et al. Genetic imbalances in 26 cases of penile squamous cell carcinoma. Genes Chromosomes Cancer 2001;31:48–53.

72. Busso-Lopes AF, Marchi FA, Kuasne H, et al. Genomic profiling of human penile carcinoma predicts worse prognosis and survival. Cancer Prev Res (Phila) 2015;8:149–56.

73. Dang CV. MYC on the path to cancer. Cell 2012;149:22–35.

74. Peter M, Rosty C, Couturier J, et al. MYC activation associated with the integration of HPV DNA at the MYC locus in genital tumors. Oncogene 2006;25:5985–93.

75. Masferrer E, Ferrándiz-Pulido C, Lloveras B, et al. MYC copy number gains are associated with poor outcome in penile squamous cell carcinoma. J Urol 2012;188:1965–71.

76. Poetsch M, Schuart B-J, Schwesinger G, et al. Screening of microsatellite markers in penile cancer reveals differences between metastatic and nonmetastatic carcinomas. Mod Pathol 2007;20:1069–77.

77. Kuasne H, Marchi FA, Rogatto SR, et al. Epigenetic mechanisms in penile carcinoma. Int J Mol Sci 2013;14:10791–808.

78. Guerrero D, Guarch R, Ojer A, et al. Hypermethylation of the thrombospondin-1 gene is associated with poor prognosis in penile squamous cell carcinoma. BJU Int 2008;102:747–55.

79. Feber A, Arya M, de Winter P, et al. Epigenetics markers of metastasis and HPV-induced tumorigenesis in penile cancer. Clin Cancer Res 2015;21:1196–206.

80. Kuasne H, Cólus IM, Busso AF, et al. Genome-wide methylation and transcriptome analysis in penile carcinoma: uncovering new molecular markers. Clin Epigenetics 2015;7:46.

81. Kattan MW, Ficarra V, Artibani W, et al. Nomogram predictive of cancer specific survival in patients undergoing partial or total amputation for squamous cell carcinoma of the penis. J Urol 2006;175:2103–8 [discussion: 2108].

82. Nicholson S, Kayes O, Minhas S. Clinical trial strategy for penis cancer. BJU Int 2014;113:852–3.

Index

Printed and bound by CPI Group (UK) Ltd, Croydon, CR0 4YY

03/10/2024

01040382-0012